Social Integration in the
Second Half of Life

Social Integration in the Second Half of Life

EDITED BY

Karl Pillemer

Phyllis Moen

Elaine Wethington

Nina Glasgow

THE JOHNS HOPKINS UNIVERSITY PRESS
Baltimore & London

© 2000 The Johns Hopkins University Press
All rights reserved. Published 2000
Printed in the United States of America on acid-free paper
9 8 7 6 5 4 3 2 1

The Johns Hopkins University Press
2715 North Charles Street
Baltimore, Maryland 21218-4363
www.press.jhu.edu

Library of Congress Cataloging-in-Publication Data will be found at the
end of this book.
A catalog record for this book is available from the British Library.

ISBN 0-8018-6453-4
ISBN 0-8018-6454-2 (pbk.)

To those people who keep us socially integrated:

To my wife, Clare, and to my daughters, Hannah and Sarah (KP)

To my husband, Dick Shore, and to our daughters Melanie, Deborah, Linda, and Roberta (PM)

To Dave, and to my parents, Olga and Jerome Wethington (EW)

To my mother, Ethel Glasgow, whose successful aging inspires me, and to my husband, David Brown, whose love and support sustain me (NG)

Contents

Acknowledgments   ix
Contributors   xi

Introduction   1

PART ONE
OVERVIEW OF MAJOR ISSUES AND APPROACHES

1   Social Integration and Aging: Background and Trends   19

Karl Pillemer and Nina Glasgow

2   Multiple Roles, Social Integration, and Health   48

Elaine Wethington, Phyllis Moen, Nina Glasgow,
and Karl Pillemer

PART TWO
SOCIAL INTEGRATION IN MAJOR DOMAINS OF LATER LIFE

3   A Life-Course Approach to Retirement and Social
Integration   75

Phyllis Moen, Vivian Fields, Heather E. Quick,
and Heather Hofmeister

4   Transportation Transitions and Social Integration of
Nonmetropolitan Older Persons   108

Nina Glasgow

5   Social Integration and Family Support: Caregivers to
Persons with Alzheimer's Disease   132

Karl Pillemer and J. Jill Suitor

6   Future Housing Expectations in Late Midlife: The Role of
     Retirement, Gender, and Social Integration 158

     Julie T. Robison and Phyllis Moen

7   Neighboring as a Form of Social Integration
     and Support 190

     Elaine Wethington and Allison Kavey

8   Social Integration and the Move to a Continuing Care
     Retirement Community 211

     *Mary Ann Erickson, Donna Dempster-McClain,
     Carol Whitlow, and Phyllis Moen*

PART THREE

INTERVENTIONS TO PROMOTE SOCIAL INTEGRATION
IN LATER LIFE

9   An Intervention to Improve Transportation
     Arrangements 231

     Nina Glasgow

10 Fostering Integration: A Case Study of the Cornell Retirees
     Volunteering in Service (CRVIS) Program 247

     *Phyllis Moen, Vivian Fields, Rhoda Meador,
     and Helene Rosenblatt*

11 Peer Support for Alzheimer's Caregivers: Lessons from an
     Intervention Study 265

     *Karl Pillemer, J. Jill Suitor, L. Todd Landreneau,
     Charles R. Henderson, Jr., and Sharon Brangman*

12 Closing Thoughts and Future Directions 287

     *Phyllis Moen, Karl Pillemer, Elaine Wethington,
     Nina Glasgow, and Galyn Vesey*

     Author Index 305
     Subject Index 313

Acknowledgments

This volume is the product of many years of research by the editors and the chapter co-authors on issues relating to social support, multiple roles, community participation, and family relationships. The book is more directly influenced, however, by the fact that all contributors to this volume have worked together within an organizational framework, the Cornell Gerontology Research Institute (CGRI). It is fair to say that without the resources and organizational framework provided by the institute, this book would not have come into being.

The Cornell Gerontology Research Institute is one of five Edward R. Roybal Centers on Applied Gerontology, which are funded by the National Institute on Aging (NIA). The goal of the Roybal Centers program is to translate basic behavioral and social science research into practical outcomes to improve the quality of life of older people and promote productive aging. We are grateful to the NIA for this generous support, which we have received since 1993 (1 P50 AG11711–01). A number of NIA staff members involved with the Roybal Centers program have helped guide the development of our institute, including Jared Jobe, Marcia Ory, and Sidney Stahl, as well as former staff member Katrina Johnson.

Several other sources of funding have supported portions of the work presented in this volume. These include the John D. and Catherine T. MacArthur Foundation Research Network on Successful Midlife Development, the Van Ameringen Foundation, support from donors for the Pathways to Life Quality Project, and grants to the Cornell Employment and Family Careers Institute from the Alfred P. Sloan Foundation.

We have also benefited immensely from several academic advisers to CGRI: David Morgan (Portland State University), Benjamin Gottlieb (University of Guelph, Canada), and Martha Bruce (Cornell University Medical College). Urie Bronfenbrenner has provided us with inspiration and ideas throughout the existence of the center. Several practitioners have served as CGRI advisers or collaborators, including Irene Stein (Tompkins County Office for the Aged), William Smith (Aging in America/Morningside House Nursing Home), Betsy Harris and Deb Koen (Career Development Services), Marc Freedman (Civic Ventures), Donna Anderson (National Retiree Volunteer Coalition), Carol Hegeman (Foundation for Long Term Care), and Terry Eisenman (Rides Unlimited of Niagara, Inc.). We are also indebted to Robert H. Binstock, Consulting Editor for this series, for his encouragement in the early stages of this book.

The interrelated CGRI research projects conducted by this volume's editors have relied on many dedicated staff persons and colleagues. In particular, we would like to acknowledge the contributions of Leslie Schultz, Bonnie Pelenur, Vivian Fields, Madhurima Agarwal, Sarah Jaenike Demo, Laurie Todd, Shin-Kap Han, Donna Dempster-McClain, Bill Erickson, Clare Holmes, Nina Deligatti, Ilene West, Sandy Rightmyer, Lisa Guido, Pierre Gingrich, Roger Brunson, Catherine Ayres, Lilly Maisel, Mark Reardon, Musarrat Islam, Liane O'Brien, Joanne Jordan, and Alexis Krulish. We are also grateful to Deborah Smith, Emma Dentinger, and the many other graduate and undergraduate students who assisted in data collection, coding, and analysis.

Contributors

Sharon Brangman, M.D., is division chief, Geriatrics, State University of New York Health Sciences Center, Syracuse, New York. Her research interests include care of patients with Alzheimer's disease, and aging in minority communities.

Donna Dempster-McClain, Ph.D., is associate director, Bronfenbrenner Center for Life Course Studies, Cornell University, Ithaca, New York. Her research focuses on life-course transitions, multiple roles and well-being, and longitudinal research methods.

Mary Ann Erickson, Ph.D., is director of research for the Pathways to Life Quality study at Cornell University, Ithaca, New York. Her research focuses on residential mobility, social roles, and perceived health in later life.

Vivian Fields, Ph.D., formerly research associate, Cornell Gerontology Research Institute, is now an independent consultant on research methodology.

Nina Glasgow, Ph.D., is senior research associate in the Department of Rural Sociology, Cornell University, Ithaca, New York. Dr. Glasgow's research focuses primarily on aging in rural environments. Her publications include studies of the demographic aspects of aging in rural environments, poverty status, services utilization, retirement migration, and transportation arrangements of rural older people.

Charles R. Henderson, Jr., M.S., is senior research associate, Department of Human Development. He directs the Methodology Core of the Cornell Gerontology Research Institute.

Heather Hofmeister, Ph.D. candidate in sociology, Cornell University, Ithaca, New York, is a predoctoral fellow at the Cornell Employment and Family Careers Institute. Her research focuses on couples' work and family experiences and their community context.

Allison Kavey, former research assistant in the Cornell Gerontology Research Institute, is a Ph.D. student in the history of medicine at the Johns Hopkins University, Baltimore, Maryland.

L. Todd Landreneau, Ph.D., former research associate in the Cornell Gerontology Research Institute, is a senior analyst for Blue Cross of California.

Rhoda Meador, M.S., is senior extension associate in the Department of Human Development at Cornell University and dissemination coordinator for the Cornell Gerontology Research Institute, Ithaca, New York. Her interests include aging policy and the workforce, intergenerational relations, and social networks.

Phyllis Moen, Ph.D., is the Ferris Family Professor of Life Course Studies as well as professor of sociology and human development at Cornell University, Ithaca, New York. Her research focuses on work/ family and life-course transitions. She directs the Cornell Employment and Family Careers Institute, funded by the Alfred P. Sloan Foundation, and co-directs the Cornell Gerontology Research Institute.

Karl Pillemer, Ph.D., is professor of human development at Cornell University and co-director of the Cornell Gerontology Research Institute. His major research interests focus on family relationships in later life, social networks, and aging and long-term-care policy.

Heather E. Quick, Ph.D., is research scientist in education and human development at the American Institutes for Research. Her research interests include psychological and structural influences on life decisions, and the relationships between work, family, and community involvement over the life course.

Julie T. Robison, Ph.D., is senior scientist at the Braceland Center for Mental Health and Aging at the Institute of Living, Hartford (Connecticut) Hospital. Her research focuses on long-term care, social integration, and mental health.

Helene Rosenblatt is a research assistant in the Cornell Gerontology Research Institute, Ithaca, New York. Her projects have included intergenerational relationships, caregiving for Alzheimer's patients, and retirement and well-being studies.

J. Jill Suitor, Ph.D., is professor of sociology at Louisiana State University, Baton Rouge, Louisiana. Her recent research focuses on the impact of life-course transitions on social networks and social support.

Galyn Vesey, Ph.D., formerly a postdoctoral research fellow in the Cornell Gerontology Research Institute, is associate professor of social work at Alabama A&M University. His research focuses on aspects of aging in minority populations, with a particular emphasis on African Americans.

Elaine Wethington, Ph.D., is associate professor in the Departments of Human Development and of Sociology at Cornell University, Ithaca, New York. Her research focuses on life events, illness, and social support.

Carol Whitlow, M.A., is research support specialist in the Bronfenbrenner Center for Life Course Studies, Cornell University, Ithaca, New York. Her work focuses on examining the quality of life of older persons across residential settings.

Social Integration in the
Second Half of Life

Introduction

*Karl Pillemer, Phyllis Moen, Elaine Wethington,
and Nina Glasgow*

*Human beings are not meant to live solitary lives. Computer buffs would
say that we are "hard-wired," genetically programmed, to develop and
function by interacting with others. Talking, touching, and relating to
others is essential to our well-being. These facts are not unique to children or to older men and women; they apply to all of us, from birth to
death.*

—J. W. Rowe and R. L. Kahn, Successful Aging

The theme of this book, as the title indicates, is the integration of
persons in midlife and beyond into the web of roles and relationships
we refer to as "society." This theme is often blurred by contradictory
images of the social embeddedness of people in later life. On the one
hand, older persons are seen as an integral component of family and
community life, frequently providing continuity, care, and service
where other people are not available to do so. On the other hand, there
is also a pervasive popular impression that older persons (and especially those in their seventies, eighties, and beyond) are increasingly
isolated as they move out of major economic and family roles and
witness the mortality of friends, kin, and neighbors.

Both of these themes—integration and isolation—have long been
features of aging. To illustrate these differing perceptions of integration and isolation, we begin by drawing from two works of fiction.
Each is a well-known short story, and both have found their way into
anthologies of fiction about growing older.

Bertolt Brecht, best known as a poet and playwright, wrote the story
"The Unseemly Old Lady" (Brecht, 1991). Told from the perspective

of the title character's grandson, the story describes an elderly woman in the early part of this century, who spent most of her life quietly raising five children in impoverished circumstances. After the children moved away, she was expected to live sensibly, modestly, and alone. However, at the age of 72, she radically changed her life. To the dismay of her children, she began to go to the movies (an unseemly pursuit at that time) and to attend lively social gatherings at a cobbler's shop in the town. She started taking her meals at an inn and befriended a young, slightly "feeble-minded" girl with whom she played cards and went to the cinema. Brecht tells us that she was "not at all lonely."

When she died at age 74, her sympathetic grandson reported: "I have seen a photograph of her which was taken for the children and shows her laid out. What you see is a tiny little face, very wrinkled, and a thin-lipped, wide mouth. Much that is small, but no smallness. She had savoured to the full the long years of servitude and the short years of freedom and consumed the bread of life to the last crumb" (Brecht, 1991: 272).

The other story, perhaps better known, is Tillie Olsen's "Tell Me a Riddle" (1992). In it, an elderly woman is trapped in an unhappy marriage. A Jewish immigrant from Russia, she was unwilling or unable to forge social connections beyond her family. When a devastating illness strikes her, she feels keenly the loss of the traditional community she knew as a child. She takes little pleasure in her children, whom she visits in turn. Bereft of meaningful ties, with the exception of support from a dutiful granddaughter, she dies a lonely death far from her home.

The truth likely lies somewhere between these two classic portrayals. Informal observation of friends and relatives is enough to confirm the immense variability of social relationships in later life. Some individuals remain embedded in a stable convoy of social support until the end of their lives. Others manage to replace significant relationships they have lost with new social ties. And still others are unable to recover from loss, and suffer loneliness and isolation.

This book aims to shed light on several questions: What leads to social integration (or, conversely, social isolation) in the second half of life? What are the consequences of social integration, in terms of psychological well-being, life satisfaction, and physical health? This volume, and the interrelated research projects on which it is based, respond to what we see as a key component of successful aging: remaining socially integrated until the end of life.

SUMMARY OF THE PROBLEM

Social integration and its consequences have been of central interest to social scientists for at least a century. Over the past several decades, gerontologists also have shown a sustained interest in this topic. Early research suggested that for many elderly persons, continued activity and engagement in social roles is related to high morale (Havighurst, 1964). Conversely, classic studies by Rosow (1967) and Lowenthal and Haven (1968) identified some older persons as vulnerable to the problems of loss of roles and significant attachments.

Since that time, a large body of research has documented that an optimal quantity of social roles, a stable role trajectory, and the availability of social support are positively related to psychological and physical health. Studies in sociology, psychology, and anthropology have supported this central insight: greater social integration leads to positive outcomes in the second half of life. Findings from this research are detailed in Chapters 1 and 2.

As the literary examples presented above illustrate, however, the path to a stable and satisfying set of social relationships is not always smooth. Indeed, as middle-aged and older adults move through the life course, they experience critical transitions that can make them vulnerable to threats to social integration. Although such transitions can under certain circumstances also enhance integration, social relationships may be negatively affected in a number of ways.

First, owing to changes in occupational and educational status, some children and other relatives may be widely dispersed. This geographic mobility can be problematic, because the major factor in determining the frequency of contact with kin is physical proximity. Numerous studies have found that intergenerational contact is greatly affected by geographical distance between households, with more distant children interacting less often with parents. A similar pattern has been found in relationships with grandchildren. To be sure, research has established that few older people are totally isolated from kin. However, some older persons—particularly those in areas with heavy out-migration of the young—lack networks of emotionally and instrumentally supportive family relationships.

Second, compounding the problem of geographical distance from potential supporters is the loss of network members through death. The transition to widowhood is particularly stressful, both immediately following the spouse's death and in the long term. Research indicates that low morale and loneliness are common in the years following a spouse's death (Lichenstein et al., 1996; Kalish, 1985; Umberson, et al., 1992). Other long-term intimate relationships—with friends, siblings, and other kin—are also likely to be lost in later life. If no replacement is found for these important ties, isolation and psychological distress can result (Arbuckle & de Vries, 1995; Dykstra, 1995).

Geographical dispersion and widowhood have contributed to a striking demographic shift over the past several decades: the growth in the number of elderly persons living alone (U.S. Bureau of the Census, 1993; Wolf, 1995). Population projections suggest that this proportion is likely to increase even further for the baby-boom generation, given their lower rates of marriage and high rates of marital disruption (Easterlin, 1996; Macunovich et al., 1993). Although living alone does not necessarily imply social isolation, we know that marriage is linked to well-being and happiness (Easterlin, 1996; George, 1996).

Third, declining health is another transition that can reduce social integration. The risk of chronic disease increases dramatically with age (Jette, 1996; Manton, 1990). Although many Americans are living longer and healthier than ever before, it is estimated that approximately 86 percent of persons over the age of 64 have at least one chronic illness, and that one in five requires some assistance with activities of daily living (Stephens, 1990). The greater likelihood of chronic impairment, with its accompanying limitations on mobility, increases the risk of social isolation.

Fourth, the loss of the work role is a critical life-course transition that can reduce social integration. Although retirement is a positive experience for some individuals (Gall, Evans, & Howard, 1997), it nevertheless represents an exit from a highly valued role—that of paid employee—and, in many cases, to the loss of most work relationships. If new, meaningful roles are not found, retirement can represent a serious break in social integration. Researchers are increasingly viewing retirement as a complex process, with shifts in work, family, and community roles and expectations (for a review, see Chapter 3, this volume). Riley, Kahn, and Foner (1994), along with Bronfenbrenner et al. (1996) and Moen (1996), point to the need for increasing the options for integrative, productive activity as lives—and the period of retirement—lengthen.

Fifth, life-course transitions can place *family members* of older people at risk of social isolation. A consistent finding across a range of studies has been the benefits of social support for family caregivers. The literature (reviewed in Chapter 5 of this volume) indicates that social support reduces caregiver burden and psychological stress and promotes physical health. However, some caregivers experience a decrease in such support as a result of becoming a caregiver. Research suggests that transitions related to caregiving, such as placement in a nursing home, are highly stressful for family members (Pillemer et al., 1998).

In sum, the evidence from diverse bodies of research underscores the value of social integration as a research topic and a mechanism for enhancing the quality of life. Existing knowledge indicates that (1) greater social integration, particularly in the form of social support and the availability of meaningful roles, promotes well-being among middle-aged and older persons and their families; (2) individuals may be at particular risk of social isolation during transitions and turning points; and (3) transitions that have a negative impact on social integration can multiply in later life. We need to address in more detail the life-course pathways to social integration, as well as the institutional arrangements facilitating integration. Generating such knowledge has both practical and theoretical relevance, requiring an understanding of trajectories, transitions, and context.

APPROACH OF THIS BOOK

The present volume brings a temporal and institutional focus to the topic of social integration, examining transitions and trajectories in the context of existing and emerging institutional arrangements that can facilitate or hamper life transitions, ongoing integrative ties, and subsequent quality of life. Key life transitions shift the focus from *state* to *process;* individuals and families come into contact with and require institutional support as they undergo or anticipate transition. Therefore, this book is both theoretically and practically relevant. Its focus is on institutional transitions (such as retirement and residential mobility), as well as more private, less institutional status passages (such as ceasing to drive a car or becoming a family caregiver). Some key features of the volume are as follows.

Life-Course Analysis

Our life-course perspective highlights the importance of *linked lives* (e.g., between spouses, across generations) and *institutional context*, as well as *processes of development and change* over the life span (Elder et al., 1996; Moen, 1995). We examine how different developmental paths and transitions throughout adulthood—work, family, and other role choices and constraints—are linked to changes in social integration and, in turn, may have an impact on physical, psychological, and economic well-being.

A Focus on the Second Half of Life

Much research on older people focuses exclusively on the later years, ignoring the ways in which individuals come to be old—their life histories of role involvements and relationships throughout adulthood. In contrast, we recognize that individuals in late midlife are embedded in changing social, cultural, and economic environments, as well as being products of lifetime biographies of events, relationships, and behavior. The contributions to this volume therefore deal with actual and anticipated life-course transitions, as well as practical ways to promote social integration and life quality in the face of these transitions.

Contexts

A key theme in the chapters concerns *gender*. Gender has a pervasive influence both on the structure and function of social networks and on the role options of men and women. To some extent, both men and women face threats to social integration in later life. However, the life-course challenges they confront may affect men and women in different ways (Moen, 1995). That women have been allocated the primary responsibility for the care of family members has limited their participation in roles outside the home. Further, women's social integration can also become circumscribed by loss of family roles that comes with advancing age. As noted earlier, women are more likely to spend both midlife and later adulthood alone, without the presence (and potential support) of a spouse, owing to divorce, widowhood, and low remarriage rates.

Women's growing participation in and attachment to the labor force has enormous implications for their midlife transitions and aging (Moen, 1992, 1995). Yet we have little knowledge about the implications of these changes for the lives of older women and their families. In this volume, the chapters on retirement and well-being in particular attend to the various life patterns of women and men, as well as which of these patterns are the most psychologically and physiologically adaptive.

We also recognize the importance of *geographical context* in understanding social integration, considering in particular the special population of rural older persons. It is widely acknowledged that formal services are less likely to be available in rural than in urban environments (Coward, 1987; Coward & Cutler, 1989; Krout, 1994). The way in which nonmetropolitan older persons and their families cope with this deficit in formal services has not been explored in detail. Researchers have refuted the notion that rural older persons have more intimate and more extensive informal support resources (Coward & Cutler, 1989; Coward et al., 1993; Lee & Cassidy, 1985; Lee & Whitbeck, 1987). In fact, in declining rural communities, helping networks may shrink as potential supporters relocate.

Moreover, older rural residents have had persistently lower incomes and higher poverty rates than older urban residents (Glasgow & Brown, 1997; Glasgow et al., 1993). These factors affect the ability to give and the need to receive assistance from kin. Older rural residents receive more financial assistance from kin than similarly placed older urbanites, but they are less likely to receive assistance requiring an expenditure of time (Hofferth & Iceland, 1998). Krout and Coward (1998) argue against the persistent myth that rural older people live in well-integrated communities, which take special care to ensure that older people's needs are met. Therefore, several contributors to this volume focus on older persons living in rural areas (see Chapters 4 and 9), in particular the relationship between driving and transportation transitions and social integration.

A NOTE ON TERMINOLOGY

Two concepts—both reflected in this volume's title—require clarification: *social integration* and *the second half of life.*

Social Integration

Our review of the literature found no consensus on a precise definition of social integration. Here, we provide our definition of the concept, so that readers will at least know what we mean by the term. In addition, each chapter includes more precise definitions of the particular aspects of social integration under study, as well as specific measures of social integration variables.

The research literature suggests two basic uses of the expression "social integration." One is commonly employed in the study of social networks, where social integration is a technical term indicating the number of interpersonal ties an individual has (for example, the number of members of his or her social network). Persons with more social ties (and, in some definitions, organizational memberships) are considered to be more "socially integrated" (cf. Lee & Whitbeck, 1987). Although we have no objection to this usage, we view the concept as having a substantially broader meaning, such as that provided in the work of Emile Durkheim and of Irving Rosow (discussed in Chapter 1).

As we employ the term in this volume, "social integration" means *the entire set of an individual's connections to others in his or her environment.* In contrast to the narrow definition just described, we employ social integration in a more general sociological sense to refer to both participation in meaningful roles and the network of social contacts. At the other end of the continuum is social isolation, or the lack of significant relationships with kin, neighbors, coworkers, and friends, and of fulfilling roles.

Our definition is consistent with two well-articulated analyses of the concept of integration, both of which focus on the term *embeddedness.* (Indeed, given the confusion and lack of clear definition of social integration, *social embeddedness* may ultimately be the more useful term.) In Booth, Edwards, and Johnson's (1991) framework, a key component of social integration involves "the degree to which an individual is embedded in a broader network of social relations." As such, integration "involves the formation and maintenance of a set of relations in which a person gives and receives affective support and social approval. To say an individual is highly integrated in this sense requires the existence of a social network of ties. Most proximate among these are friendships and affiliations with community organizations, particularly those in which there is face-to-face interaction and a process of identification has taken place" (209).

Our definition is also consistent with Barrera's (1986) formulation of social embeddedness, which he defines as "the connections that individuals have to significant others in their social environments" (415). Such social connectedness is key to a psychological sense of community. Components of social embeddedness in Barrera's conceptualization include key social ties like marriage, participation in organizations, and contact with friends and family. Our broad view of social integration includes these aspects of social embeddedness, as well as the social support functions that are supplied by network members.

Second Half of Life

More straightforward is the age group this volume is concerned with. The chapters focus on individuals in midlife and older; hence, the "second half" of life. However, it is more precise to say that much of the research reported here is based on samples of persons in later midlife (age 50) and beyond. Given our own ages, we are not eager to characterize the age of 50 as "later midlife." But it is demographically clear that the vast majority of people who reach that age have already lived three fifths or more of their likely life span.

There are obvious difficulties in selecting a term to refer to this entire group, because it is so heterogeneous. In general, when referring to this period of the life course, we term it "later life." Individuals in this age group we have usually referred to as "persons in late midlife and beyond," and "older persons." The chapters that specifically deal with persons aged 65 and over often use the word "elderly," which, although an imperfect and controversial term, is widely used and understood today.

PLAN OF THE BOOK

Part One: Overview of Major Issues and Approaches contains two chapters devoted to conceptual and theoretical background.

Chapter 1 ("Social Integration and Aging: Background and Trends") is an overview of social integration in later life within the context of contemporary gerontology. The authors review data in several domains to explore the question, Is social integration particularly problematic in later life? Areas addressed include marital status and living arrangements, intergenerational relationships, geographic mobility, social network participation, work and retirement, and volunteering.

Chapter 2 ("Multiple Roles, Social Integration, and Health") includes a review of theoretical approaches to social integration and social support in later life, with a special focus on the life-course perspective on human development that underlies the chapters in this volume. Elaine Wethington and colleagues examine mechanisms by which social integration, social participation, and social support improve health and well-being. They treat the issue of social selection in models relating social factors to health; that is, the possibility that healthy people are more apt to be engaged in multiple roles and multifaceted social networks precisely because they are healthier. The authors also discuss several measurement issues and, in particular, current attempts to develop contextual measures of social integration, participation, and support.

Part Two: Social Integration in Major Domains of Later Life builds on the perspectives laid out in Part One, examining in detail six key issues. Each chapter combines a review of the literature with original data collected in association with the Cornell Gerontology Research Institute.

In Chapter 3 ("A Life-Course Approach to Retirement and Social Integration"), Phyllis Moen and colleagues argue for the utility of applying a life-course approach to the analysis of social integration following the retirement transition. The authors shed light on the social participation of both older (not-yet-retired) workers and retirees, and the influences of social context, timing, and the process of change for social integration and well-being in the retirement years. In addition to examining the work role, the chapter also takes into account participation in clubs and volunteer work that may replace paid employment as a key means of social integration in retirement. This chapter introduces important life-course themes and discusses the need to conceptualize *pathways* to social integration following retirement. It then draws on data from the *Cornell Retirement and Well-Being Study* to shed light on the effects of the retirement transition on social integration for 1990s retirees.

Chapter 4 ("Transportation Transitions and Social Integration of Nonmetropolitan Older Persons") focuses on effective transportation arrangements as a means of facilitating social integration among older people, especially rural residents. Nina Glasgow adopts a life-course perspective to address issues related to the timing, context, and process of transitions and trajectories in the use of different modes of transportation. The chapter highlights the relinquishment of driving as a key life-course transition in old age, one with profound consequences for personal mobility and social integration of all older people, especially those in rural communities. Glasgow analyzes these and related issues using findings from the *Cornell Transportation and Social Integration of Nonmetropolitan Older Persons Study.*

In Chapter 5 ("Social Integration and Family Support: Caregivers to Persons with Alzheimer's Disease"), Karl Pillemer and Jill Suitor explore several issues related to the role of social networks and support in the lives of Alzheimer's caregivers. The authors begin by addressing the question of whether caregivers are at risk of social isolation. They then propose a theoretical model for understanding family caregiving, based on conceptualizing caregiving as a life-course transition. The major implication of this theoretical model is the critically important role of similar others in promoting social integration. The authors provide several illustrative findings from longitudinal research involving family caregivers.

In Chapter 6 ("Future Housing Expectations in Late Midlife: The Role of Retirement, Gender, and Social Integration"), Julie Robison and Phyllis Moen address housing experiences and expectations in the later years of adulthood, reviewing research on housing for older people and later-life residential patterns in relation to issues of social integration. Their model of expectations about later adulthood residential arrangements draws on a life-course perspective, retirement migration theory, and economic theories of expectations and intentions. Robison and Moen employ data from the *Cornell Retirement and Well-Being Study* to explore links between older workers' and recent retirees' later-life housing expectations and dispositions and various measures of their social integration.

In Chapter 7 ("Neighboring as a Form of Social Integration and Support"), Elaine Wethington and Allison Kavey propose that a key informal source of social integration in later life is neighboring—regular social interaction with those living in close proximity. The authors develop a theoretical model of neighboring as an aspect of social support and examine the dependence of neighboring on other social-support resources. They present illustrative data from two pilot studies on the relationship between neighboring and health, examining such factors as the availability of family support, personality characteristics believed to promote sociability, physical characteristics of different neighborhoods, and pre-existing levels of health.

Chapter 8 ("Social Integration and the Move to a Continuing Care Retirement Community") contains an exploration of the ways in which social contact, social roles, and social integration are affected by a move to a continuing care retirement community (CCRC). Erickson and colleagues develop hypotheses about the effects of relocation to a CCRC on social contact, social role participation, and perceived social integration and test them on a sample of older adults before and after their move to a CCRC. They ground their hypotheses in the social-ecological perspective and in continuity theory, coupled with the overarching life-course theme. Their research on a sample of persons who moved into a CCRC indicates that changes in social-structural opportunities and constraints associated with a residential move produce corresponding shifts in social contacts, social role participation, and the subjective assessment of social integration. However, they found that individuals strive to maintain previous levels of these factors.

Part Three: Interventions to Promote Social Integration in Later Life moves the book to a more practical level. In this section the chapter authors describe model intervention programs designed to increase social support and assistance or to provide meaningful social roles.

In Chapter 9 ("An Intervention to Improve Transportation Arrangements") Nina Glasgow describes an effort to improve the well-being of rural older persons with respect to their transportation arrangements. An educational intervention was implemented with older persons who reported the inability to go places as often as they wanted to. The educational intervention was designed to encourage these "transportation disadvantaged" individuals to modify the organization of their transportation arrangements in ways that were durable over time and that enhanced their social integration. Glasgow discusses the content and methods employed in conducting the educational intervention and the evaluation of its effectiveness, and she makes recommendations for future programs of this kind.

In Chapter 10 ("Fostering Integration: A Case Study of the Cornell Retirees Volunteering in Service Program") Phyllis Moen and colleagues present qualitative data describing an innovative program to foster the volunteer participation of retirees. The authors begin with the challenge of growing numbers of retirees spending more years in retirement. They then offer a case study of one potential solution for organized volunteer involvement of retirees, supplementing this case example with survey data from the *Cornell Retirement and Well-Being Study* to document factors that shape the circumstances, motivation, and volunteer participation of retirees. The authors suggest implications for policy, research, and practice. Their conclusion examines the potential that this untapped portion of the population—retirees—offers for themselves, their communities, and society.

In Chapter 11 ("Peer Support for Alzheimer's Caregivers: Lessons from an Intervention Study"), Karl Pillemer and colleagues describe a social network intervention program for family caregivers that is grounded in theory and research relating to life-course transitions and their impact on interpersonal relationships. The theoretical framework was used to design a peer support intervention in which trained volunteers (who themselves had been caregivers) visited persons caring for relatives with Alzheimer's disease. In this chapter the authors discuss the results of this randomized, controlled study and the implications for caregiver support programs.

Chapter 12 ("Closing Thoughts and Future Directions") brings together major themes of the volume and provides suggestions for future work on social integration in later life. Here, the focus is on the implications of our life-course approach to social integration for intervention, research, and policy.

REFERENCES

Arbuckle, N. W., & de Vries, B. (1995). The long-term effects of later life spousal and parental bereavement on personal functioning. *The Gerontologist, 35,* 637–647.

Barrera, M., Jr. (1986). Distinctions between social support concepts, measures, and models. *American Journal of Community Psychology, 14,* 413–445.

Booth, A., Edwards, J. N., & Johnson, D. R. (1991). Social integration and divorce. *Social Forces, 70,* 207–224.

Brecht, B. (1991). The unseemly old lady. In M. Fowler & P. McCutcheon (Eds.), *Songs of experience: An anthology of literature on growing old* (268–272). New York: Ballantine.

Bronfenbrenner, U., McClelland, P., Wethington, E., Moen, P., & Ceci, S. J. (1996). *The changing state of Americans.* New York: Free Press.

Coward, R. T. (1987). Factors associated with the configuration of the helping networks of noninstitutionalized elders. *Journal of Gerontological Social Work, 10,* 113–132.

Coward, R. T., & Cutler, S. (1989). Informal and formal health care systems for the rural elderly. *Health Services Research, 23,* 785–806.

Coward, R. T., Lee, G. R., & Dwyer, J. W. (1993). The family relations of rural elders. In C. N. Bull (Ed.), *Aging in rural America* (216–231). Newbury Park, CA: Sage.

Dykstra, P. A. (1995). Loneliness among the never and formerly married: The importance of supportive friendships and a desire for independence. *Journals of Gerontology: Social Sciences, 50B,* S321–S329.

Easterlin, R. A. (1996). Economic and social implications of demographic patterns. In R. H. Binstock & L. K. George (Eds.), *Handbook of aging and the social sciences,* 4th ed. (73–93). San Diego: Academic Press.

Elder, G. H., Jr., George, L. K., & Shanahan, M. J. (1996). Psychosocial stress over the life course. In H. B. Kaplan (Ed.), *Psychosocial stress: Perspectives on structure, theory, life course, and methods* (247–292). San Diego: Academic Press.

Gall, T. L., Evans, D. R., & Howard, J. (1997). The retirement adjustment process: Changes in the well-being of male retirees across time. *Journals of Gerontology: Psychological Sciences, 51B,* 43–52.

George, L. K. (1996). Social factors and illness. In R. H. Binstock & L. K. George (Eds.), *Handbook of aging and the social sciences,* 4th ed. (229–252). San Diego: Academic Press.

Glasgow, N., & Brown, D. (1997). *Gender differences in driving behavior among nonmetropolitan older residents: Problems and prospects.* Paper presented to Gerontological Society of America Annual Meeting, Cincinnati.

Glasgow, N., Holden, K., McLaughlin, D., & Rowles, G. (1993). The rural elderly and poverty. In Rural Sociological Task Force on Persistent Rural Poverty (Eds.), *Persistent poverty in rural America.* Boulder, CO: Westview Press.

Havighurst, R. (1964). Changing status and roles during the adult life cycle: Significance for adult education. In H.W. Burns (Ed.), *Social backgrounds of adult education* (17–38). Boston: Center for the Study of Liberal Education for Adults.

Hofferth, S. L., & Iceland, J. (1998). Social capital in rural and urban communities. *Rural Sociology, 63,* 574–598.

Jette, A. M. (1996). Disability trends and transitions. In R. H. Binstock & L. K. George (Eds.), *Handbook of aging and the social sciences,* 4th ed. (94–116). San Diego: Academic Press.

Kalish, R. A. (1985). The social context of death and dying. In R. H. Binstock & E. Shanas (Eds.), *Handbook of aging and the social sciences*, 2d ed. (149–170). New York: Van Nostrand Reinhold.

Krout, J. A. (Ed.) (1994). *Providing community-based services to the rural elderly.* Thousand Oaks, CA: Sage.

Krout, J. A., & Coward, R. T. (1998). Aging in rural environments. In R. T. Coward & J. A. Krout (Eds.), *Aging in rural settings: Life circumstances and distinctive features* (3–14). New York: Springer.

Lee, G. R., & Cassidy, M. L. (1985). Family and kin relationships of the rural elderly. In R. T. Coward & G. R. Lee (Eds.), *The elderly in rural society* (151–169). New York: Springer.

Lee, G. R., & Whitbeck, L. B. (1987). Residential location and social relations among older persons. *Rural Sociology, 52,* 89–97.

Lichenstein, P., Gatz, M., Pedersen, N. L., Berg, S., & McClearn, G. E. (1996). A co-twin control study of response to widowhood. *Journals of Gerontology: Psychological Sciences, 51B,* 279–289.

Lowenthal, M., & Haven, C. (1968). Interaction and adaptation: Intimacy as a critical variable. *American Sociological Review, 33,* 20–30.

Macunovich, D. J., Easterlin, R. A., Crimmins, E. M., & Macdonald, C. (1993). Echoes of the baby boom and bust: Recent and prospective changes in living alone among elderly widows in the United States. *Demography, 32,* 17–28.

Manton, K. G. (1990). Mortality and morbidity. In R. H. Binstock & L. K. George (Eds.), *Handbook of aging and the social sciences*, 3d ed. (64–90). San Diego: Academic Press.

Moen, P. (1992). *Women's two roles: A contemporary dilemma.* Westport, CT: Greenwood Publishing.

Moen, P. (1996). A life course perspective on retirement, gender, and well-being. *Journal of Occupational Health Psychology, 1,* 131–144.

Moen, P. (1995). Gender, age and the life course. In R. H. Binstock & L. George (Eds.), *Handbook of aging and the social sciences*, 4th ed. (171–187). San Diego: Academic Press.

Olsen, T. (1992). "Tell Me a Riddle." In M. Kohn, C. Donley, & D. Wear (Eds.), *Literature and aging: An anthology* (153–183). Kent, OH: Kent State University Press.

Pillemer, K., Hegeman, C., Albright, B., & Henderson, C. (1998). Building bridges between families and nursing home staff: The partners in caregiving program. *The Gerontologist, 38,* 499–503.

Riley, M. W., Kahn, R. L., & Foner, A. (1994). *Age and structural lag.* New York: Wiley.

Rosow, I. (1967). *Social integration of the aged.* New York: Free Press.

Rowe, J. W., & Kahn, R. L. (1998). *Successful aging.* New York: Pantheon.

Stephens, M. A. P. (1990). Social relationships as coping resources in later-life families. In M. A. P. Stephens, J. H. Crowther, S. E. Hobfoll, & D. L. Tennenbaum (Eds.), *Stress and coping in later-life families* (1–20). New York: Hemisphere.

Umberson, D., Kessler, R. B., & Wortman, C. B. (1992). Widowhood and depression: Explaining long-term gender differences in vulnerability. *Journal of Health and Social Behavior, 33,* 10–24.

U.S. Bureau of the Census. (1993). Marital status and living arrangements: March 1992. *Current Population Reports,* Series P20–468. Washington, DC: U.S. Government Printing Office.

Wolf, D. A. (1995). Changes in the living arrangements of older women: An international study. *The Gerontologist, 35,* 724–731.

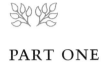

PART ONE

Overview of Major Issues and Approaches

CHAPTER ONE

Social Integration and Aging
Background and Trends

Karl Pillemer and Nina Glasgow

One of the towering themes in the history of modern social science has been the importance of social integration. For more than a century, scholars have grappled with such questions as, Are social institutions that tie individuals into meaningful communities breaking down? Are citizens of contemporary societies becoming isolated from one another? Does the atomization of individuals place them at risk of a host of problems, including antisocial behavior, physical illness, or poor mental health?

The thinker most responsible for calling attention to problems of social integration and disintegration was Emile Durkheim. In his famous theoretical and empirical work *Suicide* (1951), he proposed that suicide was inversely related to the degree of integration into society, including integration into the family, religion, and political institutions. Excessive individualism, according to Durkheim, was a direct cause of suicide. He noted that "egoistic suicide results from the fact that society is not sufficiently integrated at all points to keep all its members under control . . . society, weak and disturbed, lets too many persons escape too completely from its influence" (373).

Expanding on his study of the causes of suicide, Durkheim's assessment of modern society is somewhat gloomy. Writing at the turn of the century, he held that old, stable forms of social organization were being swept away but were not being replaced by new forms. Freed from intimate social involvement in these institutions, he claimed that people see nothing to which they can belong. Durkheim waxed poetic when he described the failure of society to integrate individuals who, "without mutual relationships tumble over one another like so many liquid molecules, encountering no central energy to retain, fix, and organize them" (389). As society disintegrates, the individuals detach themselves from social life; this phenomenon brings with it the tendency toward unhealthy and antisocial behavior.

Although the novelty of his methods and the clarity of his thinking made Durkheim uniquely adept at addressing the problem of social integration, the theme has remained a dominant one in the sociological tradition. Social thinkers investigating the upheavals of both the industrial revolution and the political revolution in France saw individuals becoming separated from communal structures as the old world of village and church disappeared. Ferdinand Toennies proposed his famous distinction between *Gemeinschaft*, or the old world of community and tradition, and *Gesellschaft*, the modern society based on individuals, industry, and contractual relationships. This theme has permeated social analysis ever since (Nisbet, 1966).

Cultural critics of the 1960s expanded this view. For example, in his bestseller *The Pursuit of Loneliness* Philip Slater (1970) argued that American culture deeply frustrates human desires for community, interdependence, and engagement. The best-known recent statement of the dangers of social disintegration is Robert Bellah and colleagues' *Habits of the Heart* (1996), which chronicled contemporary ambivalence about individualism and commitment. This book raised an alarm, arguing that "individualism . . . has marched inexorably through our history." Such individualism "may have grown cancerous," and "it may be threatening the survival of freedom itself" (vii). Society requires, in these authors' views, "a transition to a new level of social integration" (286).

The issue of social integration has recently become prominent again in the scholarly discussion of "civil society" (cf. Schudson, 1998; Fullinwider, 1999). A number of analysts have argued that American society is undergoing a process of civic disengagement, whereby volunteer activity, association membership, and social trust is declining. Robert Putnam, in his widely cited essay "Bowling Alone" (1995) identified the diminishing of communal structures in the recent history of the United States. Putnam points to an apparent decline in various civic associations and formal group activities (including the bowling leagues indicated in the title) to argue that both membership in civic associations and various kinds of informal connections are on the wane.

Beyond sociological theory and cultural critique, a concern with social integration has also permeated empirical research in social science over the past several decades. Studies of interpersonal ties, social networks, social support, and close relationships occupy a large number of researchers in the United States and around the world, and a variety of professional organizations and scholarly journals have emerged that deal exclusively with these issues. Along with perceived threats to social integration, intervention programs (such as support groups for nearly every human problem) have sprung up. Media reports on the loneliness, isolation, and disenfranchisement of various population groups appear regularly. The twin themes of integration and isolation remain of considerable interest within contemporary society.

SOCIAL INTEGRATION OF OLDER PERSONS

In this context, the social integration of older persons has also emerged as a topic of both scientific and public concern. Indeed, perhaps because the segregation of older individuals from the societal mainstream was so obvious to many analysts, gerontology echoed sociology in giving social integration and isolation of older persons a place of prominence. Key debates throughout the 1960s and 1970s within research on aging centered on the question, Is maintaining social integration a key problem for older persons? In this chapter, we will touch on several themes that form the starting point for our efforts.

Disengagement Theory: An Archetypal Debate

Although younger researchers on aging are unlikely to remember it as anything more than an historical footnote, the debate that began in the early 1960s over the question of the social disengagement of older persons encapsulates divergent views regarding social relations in later life. Disengagement theory (Cumming & Henry, 1961) begins with the observation that elderly people withdraw from social roles. This theory does not simply assume that such withdrawal occurs because the aged become infirm and disabled and therefore abandon social functions and associations. Instead, disengagement theory argues that the older person begins to disengage *before* it is absolutely necessary. This process removes people from vitally necessary social roles before they become incapable of performing them. Elders interact with fewer people and their role sets come to exclude roles considered vital to the larger society. Proponents of disengagement theory saw this process as natural, universal, and mutually satisfying to both society and elderly persons.

Criticism of disengagement theory began shortly after its conception (cf. Hochschild, 1975; Rose, 1965). Critics held that the theory was too simplistic and did not take account of the vast individual differences among elderly persons, some of whom clearly do not disengage. More important, "activity theorists" (Havighurst, 1964) mustered evidence that continued social engagement, rather than disengagement, predicted high morale among older persons. Finally, a point was made that is germane to this volume: the disengagement of those in later life may have more to do with a lack of *opportunity* for the performance of meaningful roles than with a universal functional process. This lack of opportunity is due to society's negative attitudes toward the old and to structural lag (Riley, Kahn, & Foner, 1994). Instead of accepting the universality of disengagement, critics have argued that institutional factors propelling elderly persons into disengagement should be changed.

Irving Rosow: Revisiting a Classic

Not long after the debate over disengagement had erupted and begun to die down, Irving Rosow published a skillful and compelling analysis of the social needs and relationships of older persons, entitled *Social Integration of the Aged* (1967). Rosow began the work with an insight that has stood the test of time: "Problems of old age are of two general kinds: those that older people actually have, and those that experts think they have" (1). In Rosow's view, the key problems of later life are not health care or economic well-being, as important as these may be. He argued that "the most significant problems of older people . . . are intrinsically social. The basic issue is that of social integration" (8).

Rosow pointed out that older people remain reasonably well integrated psychologically in terms of sharing the basic values and beliefs of society. However, he asserted that they do suffer from dramatic losses in two key areas: social roles and group memberships. This attrition begins around age 65 and accelerates after age 75. Roles are lost in the domains of employment, marital status, and income. Using extensive data from the 1950s and 1960s, Rosow also documented declining group membership in the family, in friend relationships, and in organizations.

These processes lead, according to Rosow, to alienation and isolation. One component of this alienation is role ambiguity in old age. Unlike other periods in the life course, in which old roles are replaced by new ones, the role of "old person" is unstructured; it is, Rosow asserts, "a basically empty role" (31). A second threat to social integration of older people is the systematic devaluation of them as a class. Younger people do not accept the old, and they view older persons stereotypically. Ironically, older persons themselves share these stereotypical beliefs, and thus have little incentive to change them (in the way that other minorities have striven to change public perceptions of their groups).

Rosow's summary of this general state of affairs bears repeating:

> [Older people] share the central beliefs of society and do not change these because they age. Hence, their integration does not suffer from holding distinctive deviant values. But their loss of social roles and group memberships does undermine their social integration. They become marginal participants, often ignored, rejected, and discriminated against by younger persons, and in extreme cases they are seriously isolated from the life around them. . . . Under these conditions, the social world of old people contracts. Their estrangement from previous roles and memberships deprives them of central group supports as well as responsibility, power, privilege, resources, and prestige. These deprivations are a distinctive discontinuity in life which they have little incentive to accept and for which they are not systematically prepared or socialized. (34–35)

Rosow did not conclude his book with optimistic predictions for the future or with concrete solutions. Although he noted that social participation differs to some degree among subgroups of the aged, it was his belief that older people as a class are deprived of primary and secondary group associations.

Despite the clarity of Rosow's message and the extensive research agenda he proposed, research on aging in ensuing years took a somewhat different turn. Rather than directly confronting the broadly conceived theme of social integration, investigators over the past several decades have generally focused their efforts on specific components of social integration. Thus, the themes raised by disengagement theory and by Rosow's work have continued to be explored, but more narrowly.

The 1970s and Beyond: Related Research Streams

Over the past two decades in particular, several streams of research in sociology, psychology, and anthropology have examined components of social integration. However, rather than focusing on the question of whether growing older compromises social integration, investigators have primarily focused on the degree to which social connectedness leads to positive outcomes. Two lines of research have been particularly dominant in social science research on this topic: social support and multiple roles. A plethora of studies in both areas has supported Durkheim's central insight—that greater social integration leads to physical and psychological well-being. We will touch only briefly on these topics here, as many of the following chapters treat them in detail.

Social Support. Compelling evidence for the benefits of social integration comes from the literature on social support and well-being. The overwhelming finding that social support serves as a buffer against stressful life events and chronic stressful conditions (Antonucci, 1990; Eckenrode & Gore, 1990; Wethington & Kessler, 1986) clearly applies to the older population (George, 1996).

A weak set of social relationships has been found to be related to psychological distress among older persons. Research on loneliness has produced similar findings; lonely older individuals are substantially more likely to experience mental illness, such as depression (Antonucci, 1990; Bowling & Farquhar, 1991; Mullins et al., 1989; Dugan & Kivett, 1994). Even more striking are findings relating to mortality, morbidity, and recovery from illness. Results from the famous Alameda County Study showed that the absence of social ties predicted mortality among elderly persons, even when controlling for social class, baseline health status, and health practices (Berkman, 1983). Other studies have found that socially isolated elderly persons are more likely to develop health problems (cf. Bosworth & Schaie, 1997; Seeman et al., 1996), and less likely to engage in good health behavior and the use of appropriate self-care during recovery (Mutran et al., 1995; Noburn et al., 1995; Oxman & Hull, 1997).

Multiple roles and well-being. Closely tied to the work on social support and its emphasis on relationships are studies of role occupancy. The past several decades have seen a host of studies showing that social integration in the form of involvement in multiple roles supports well-being. Multiple roles appear to promote psychological well-being at all stages of adulthood, providing social contacts, social identity, social status, and giving purpose, meaning, and guidance to life (Adelman, 1994; Hong & Seltzer, 1994; Moen et al., 1989, 1992; Thoits, 1992).

To cite just two examples, Thoits (1983, 1986) used panel data to analyze the effects of the acquisition or loss of roles over a two-year time period. Loss of important roles strongly predicted poorer mental health. Moen and colleagues (Moen et al., 1992; Moen et al., 1995) have drawn on data collected thirty years apart on a sample of women. They documented links between multiple role occupancy in middle and later adulthood and women's longevity, physical health, and psychological well-being. What Rose Coser (1991) termed a "plurality of life worlds" appears to foster health and longevity for both men and women in the second half of life.

In sum, the literature on social support and on multiple roles shows a degree of consensus unusual in social research: social integration does matter. Greater embeddedness in social roles and in networks of social support helps promote health and happiness in the second half of life. In the remainder of this chapter, we turn our attention to some indicators of social integration, asking to what extent older persons are integrated or isolated.

INDICATORS OF SOCIAL INTEGRATION AND ISOLATION

Recall that Rosow as well as others hold that the declining resources of older persons in such areas as health and income, as well as role loss, can lead to diminished social participation and to social isolation. However, it is important to ask: What does the evidence show? Are there data indicating that people in fact experience decreasing social integration as they age? Our reading of the literature indicates the need to differentiate among various indicators of social integration. In some areas, increasing age does not appear to lead to isolation, whereas in other cases older persons do seem to be at risk.

In the remainder of this chapter, we will shed light on these issues by reviewing the state of older persons' social integration in key areas.

In each of these domains, we address the question of whether older persons experience deficits in social integration, in comparison to younger groups in the population. We examine trends over time, although this has not been possible in every case. In some cases, we comment on variations among subgroups of the older population. It is important to state at the outset that there is limited evidence regarding several of the areas we wish to cover. Therefore, our goal is not to paint a definitive picture but rather to sketch the outlines of some major features of social integration in later life.

Marital Status and Living Arrangements

The marital status and living arrangements of older people are key determinants of their social integration. Married individuals provide companionship and emotional as well as instrumental support to their spouses. The overall result is a positive outcome for health and well-being. Research has shown that marriage is beneficial to one's health and well-being (see, for example, Berkman, 1983; Moen et al., 1989), that divorce in particular is detrimental to health status (Young & Glasgow, 1998), and even that mortality is lower among married than unmarried individuals (Berkman & Syme, 1979; Gove, 1973).

Starting with the 15–20 age group, Siegel (1993) found that the proportions of men and women who are married increase sharply between the ages of 25 and 30, reach a peak at about age 35 and plateau through about age 45, and subsequently decline steadily through the remainder of life. This pattern results from mortality trends: aging frequently is accompanied by widowhood. This trend, along with the growing prevalence of divorce, means that a large number of people grow older without a spouse.

The shift is especially dramatic for women (Table 1.1). Starting at about age 45, the proportion of men who are married increasingly exceeds the proportion of women who are married; age-related declines in the percentage married are steep for women but gradual for men over the remainder of the life course (Siegel, 1993). Almost half of all women aged 65 and older are widowed. Among the oldest old (aged 85 and above), the vast majority of women (81 percent) are widowed (Table 1.1). Women's greater longevity, their tendency to marry men somewhat older than themselves, and men's higher remarriage rates after divorce or widowhood all contribute to the gender differences in marital status. The net result is that older women are at greater risk of

Table 1.1. Marital Status, by Age and Gender, 1950, 1980, 1990, and 1998

Marital Status	Male (%)		Female (%)	
	Aged 65 and over	Aged 85 and over	Aged 65 and over	Aged 85 and over
1950				
Single	8.4	7.7	8.9	9.7
Married	65.7	33.6	35.7	7.0
Spouse present	62.1	30.4	33.2	5.3
Widowed	24.1	57.9	54.3	82.9
Divorced	1.9	0.8	1.1	0.4
1980				
Single	5.5	5.6	6.7	7.9
Married	76.3	48.4	37.5	8.4
Spouse present	72.5	41.1	35.0	6.1
Widowed	14.6	43.8	51.7	81.8
Divorced	3.6	2.1	4.2	2.0
1990				
Single	4.2	3.5	4.9	6.2
Married	76.5	51.1	41.4	10.6
Spouse present	74.2	46.9	39.7	10.1
Widowed	14.2	43.4	48.6	79.8
Divorced	5.0	2.0	5.1	3.4
1998				
Single	3.8	4.5	4.7	5.5
Married	75.1	49.9	42.9	13.4
Spouse present	72.6	45.6	40.7	10.9
Widowed	14.9	42.0	45.2	77.4
Divorced	6.1	3.6	7.1	3.7

Sources: Percentages for 1950 and 1980 were adapted from Table 6.2 in Jacob S. Siegel (1993), *A Generation of Change: A Profile of America's Older Population,* New York: Russell Sage Foundation. Siegel's sources were U.S. Bureau of the Census, 1950 and 1980, *U.S. Summary,* Series PC–D. Percentages for 1990 and 1998 were from the U.S. Bureau of the Census, Current Population Reports, Series P–20, No. 450, *Marital Status and Living Arrangements: March 1990 and March 1998, Update,* Washington D.C.: U.S. Government Printing Office, 1991, 1998.

becoming socially isolated because widowhood is also often accompanied by living alone (see also Bronfenbrenner et al., 1996).

Historical Trends. The marital composition of older men changed substantially between 1950 and 1990. Among men aged 65 and older, the proportion married rose from 66 percent in 1950 to 76 percent in

1990, while the proportion widowed declined from 24 percent to 14 percent (Table 1.1). During the same period, the proportion of married older women also increased while the proportion widowed declined, but the shifts for women were small by comparison to those for men. The increase in the proportion of older married men occurred despite the aging of the older male population, and it was accompanied by a decrease in the percentage widowed. These two trends resulted partly from higher marriage rates in the early twentieth century and the well-established increase in life span, which increased the chances of both partners surviving in the later decades of this century (Siegel, 1993). From 1990 to 1998, however, small increases occurred in the proportions of divorced women and men, with corresponding small declines in the proportions married. Over all, the opportunity for older men to be socially integrated through marriage has increased over time.

The living arrangements of individuals are closely linked to their marital status. Along with the greater likelihood of women to become widowed, they are also more likely than men to live alone (see also Bronfenbrenner et al., 1996). In 1990, three quarters of men aged 65 and older lived with a spouse, whereas little more than a third of older women did (Table 1.2). The tendency for older women to live alone has increased substantially over time (from 24% in 1960 to 42% in 1998), whereas the proportion of older men living alone increased only slightly during the same time period. Both men and women have become less likely over time to co-reside with relatives other than a spouse, but for women the change has meant an increased propensity to live alone; men are more likely to live in married-couple family households.

Subgroup variations. Changes in marital status and living arrangements with advancing age generally follow the same pattern for whites and African Americans, except that much higher proportions of elderly whites are married and much higher proportions of elderly African Americans are widowed (Siegel, 1993). Approximately one third of the white older population lives alone, compared to one half of older African Americans. To the extent that being married is beneficial to social support and social integration, African Americans are disadvantaged relative to whites. Other characteristics of more extended family support networks may offset potential disadvantages resulting from African Americans' marriage rates during old age, but we are not aware of studies that definitively address this issue.

Future trends. Projections of future prospects for the marital composition and living arrangements of older people foresee little change

Table 1.2.   Living Arrangements of the Population Aged 65 and Above, by Gender, 1960, 1985, 1990, and 1998 (Noninstitutional Population)

Living Arrangements	Both Sexes (%)	Males (%)	Females (%)
		1960	
Alone	18.6	12.1	24.1
With spouse	51.1	69.2	36.2
With other relative	24.8	13.9	33.9
With nonrelatives only	5.5	4.8	5.7
		1985	
Alone	30.2	14.7	41.1
With spouse	53.4	75.0	38.3
With other relative	13.9	7.5	18.4
With nonrelatives only	2.4	2.9	2.1
		1990	
Alone	31.9	16.6	42.8
With spouse	54.1	74.3	39.7
With other relative	12.6	7.7	16.2
With nonrelatives only	1.3	21.4	1.3
		1998	
Alone	31.9	18.4	41.7
With spouse	54.0	72.6	40.7
With other relative	12.7	7.0	16.8
With nonrelatives only	1.3	2.0	0.8

Sources: Percentages for 1960 and 1985 are adapted from Table 6.10 in Jacob S. Siegel (1993), *A Generation of Change: A Profile of America's Older Population,* New York: Russell Sage Foundation. Siegel's sources were U.S. Bureau of the Census, *Current Population Reports,* Series P–20, No. 410, 1996, and Census of Population, *Subject Reports,* PC(2)–4B, 1960. Date for 1990 and 1998 are from the U.S. Bureau of the Census, Current Population Reports, Series P–20, No. 450, *Marital Status and Living Arrangements: March 1990, March 1998 Update,* Washington, D.C.: U.S. Government Printing Office, 1991.

between 2000 and 2020 (Siegel, 1993). With the entry into old age of the baby-boom cohorts, however, the shares of single and divorced persons, especially single men and divorced women, are expected to rise sharply; the proportional shares of widowed men and women are expected to decline. Nonetheless, future trends in marital composition and living arrangements will be influenced by factors that make prediction difficult, including "the evolution of attitudes regarding marriage, divorce, and living together; future changes in the economic and social status of women; shifting attitudes toward living alone or with others; the prospects for the reduction of mortality, especially in late life; and, quite important, the prospects for convergence of male and female death rates" (Siegel, 1993: 325). Marital status trends among baby boomers suggest that they will be more at risk of social isolation during old age than current cohorts of older people.

Intergenerational Relationships

Although research suggests that spouses are the family members who provide the greatest amount of emotional and instrumental support to older persons, children are also a very important vehicle for social integration. Both high levels of contact and mutually supportive exchanges are reported by parents and by their adult children (Pillemer & Suitor, 1998; Suitor et al., 1995). Toward the end of the life course, adult children often provide needed care and support in situations where an older parent's spouse has predeceased him or her (see, for example, Silverstein & Angelelli, 1998).

In our examination of the changing nature of intergenerational relations, one major historical shift is worthy of note. Historical research has demonstrated that intergenerational co-residence in the late stages of life was common in earlier historical periods, particularly in the case of widows and the infirm. Specifically, older parents who became too ill to live by themselves saw living with their children as a primary option (Hareven, 1996). However, there has been a large decline in intergenerational co-residence since the beginning of this century, such that it can be characterized as one of the major demographic transitions of the century (Ruggles, 1994).

Regarding this major shift in age structuring and the life course, Kertzer and Laslett (1995) note that: "it has changed the life course of individuals along with the developmental cycle of the family and of the domestic group as a whole. The immemorial association in family time between the exit of the parental generation and the beginnings of the independent family life of the child generation has gone forever. The consequent proliferation and prolongation of the situation known as the empty nest stage, in which the parental couple stays together at home after the departure of their children, a situation so familiar in the contemporary West, are almost exclusively the result of aging" (43–44).

These changes are now established characteristics of contemporary society, which simply did not exist before. This shift has had major consequences for social integration of the aged. In past times, households rarely contained older people living alone but instead contained intergenerational families. Leaving questions of relationship quality aside, the continual presence of a child in the household certainly provided a connection and a source of assistance that older persons living alone are not guaranteed. The change away from co-residence between older and younger members of families places older women, in particular, at greater risk of social isolation now than in the past.

Moving to the present day, an important question is to what degree demographic trends will affect intergenerational relationships and thus the social integration of older persons. To answer this question, it is useful to look at the dynamics of the current generation of middle-aged adults (the so-called baby-boom generation) from two perspectives: as the *children* of aging parents and—at a future point—as the older *parents* of their own adult children.

Perhaps the most striking change in intergenerational relations among adults is the result of the dramatically lengthened lifespan. Family members will spend more time than ever before occupying intergenerational family roles. As adults, baby boomers can look forward to 30 or more years of shared lifetime with their parents. To illustrate this change, over the past 150 years the proportion of middle-aged and older women with one or more surviving parents increased dramatically. In 1800, a 60-year-old woman had about a 3 percent chance of having a living parent, but by 1980 her chances had increased to 60 percent (Watkins et al., 1987).

The lengthened lifespan can provide opportunities for positive involvement by older persons in the lives of younger generations. In this sense, the longer shared lifetime can be expected to increase opportunities for parent-child interaction and support in later life. However, parents of the baby boomers will benefit to a greater degree than their children, owing to the high fertility of the postwar generation: the parents of the boomers have, on average, three children surviving until age 40 per each ever-married female. However, for the baby boomers themselves, this figure is projected to be under two for each ever-married female (Easterlin, 1996). Thus, the boomers' contacts with their own children may be less socially integrating, given findings that the number of offspring is positively related to the total support received from children (Uhlenberg, 1993).

Parent-child relations will also be affected by the trends in marriage discussed earlier. In contrast to their parents, the baby boomers have had less frequent marriage than other cohorts. In addition, the boomers have much higher rates of marital dissolution owing to divorce than do their parents. When today's older parents married, a very large majority could assume that they would live with their partners until they were parted by death. This is quite different for the baby boomers. From the 1950s through the late 1980s, the divorce rate rose to the point at which baby-boomer children are almost equally likely to have their marriages terminated by divorce as death (Easterlin, 1996). Their high divorce rate may impair the boomers' relationships with their adult offspring. Both older men and older women who have divorced report a decline in the strength of intergenerational ties, including lower contact and less emotional support (Uhlenberg & Miner, 1996). Most people who divorce do eventually remarry, and in that way some lost ties are replaced. But divorce and remarriage negatively affect intergenerational exchanges and relationships between older parents and their adult children (Pezzin & Schone, 1999).

The outcome of these trends may be a higher risk of social isolation in later life for the baby boomers than for the current older population. The baby boomers share several characteristics that predict a large proportion of them will live alone: lower numbers of adult children, higher marital dissolution, and better health at retirement. It is estimated that fully a third of the leading edge of the baby boom will live alone by age 65, compared to between one fifth and one quarter of their parents' generation (Easterlin, 1996). It may be more of a challenge for their offspring to provide emotional and instrumental support under these conditions.

In sum, it is likely that the social integration provided by intergenerational relationships will go through two major phases over the coming decades. The current older cohorts appear to have large resources for family support, including relatively large numbers of living children and greater likelihood of an intact marriage. Societal preparations for the baby-boom generation as it enters old age must take a different set of circumstances into account: larger numbers of persons living alone without the benefits conferred by a spouse and with fewer offspring. Given the projected increase in the aged population overall, a shortage of caregiving resources in both the formal and the informal sectors may result.

Geographic Mobility

Geographic proximity has been shown in prior research to be the strongest predictor of frequency of contact between older parents and their non-co-resident adult children (Dewit et al., 1988; Krout, 1988; Rossi & Rossi, 1990; Spitze & Logan, 1991). A high rate of geographic mobility among either younger or older age groups thus would be an important factor in reducing kin support and social integration of older people. Contrary to the perception that geographic mobility has increased over time, however, both Siegel (1993) and Uhlenberg (1993) demonstrate that geographic mobility among both younger and older age groups has declined over time in the United States. Using data from the 1987 to 1988 National Survey of Families and Households, Uhlenberg (1993) estimates that 74 percent of older people have an adult child living within a 25-mile radius of them.

Although overall rates of geographic mobility have diminished during the past few decades, to the extent that migration does occur, it tends to be selectively channeled. The migration of people considered to be of the prime working ages is most often motivated by a search for job opportunities. This has resulted in historic out-migration of young adults from farming areas of the Plains states in the middle section of the country. A large number of rural counties in those states have disproportionately high concentrations of older people (Glasgow, 1988). In essence, the older people have been left behind.

Indeed, a few local-area studies have shown that older urban residents are more likely than their rural counterparts to live near their adult offspring (Bultena, 1969; Krout, 1984; Youmans, 1963). Lee et al. (1990) used data from the National Long-Term Care Survey to examine place of residence differences in the likelihood of impaired older persons to co-reside with an adult child or live within one-half hour's travel time to an adult child. Their study found that residents of large cities were more likely than any other residence group to co-reside with an adult child. Large-city and farm residents were more likely than small-city (under 50,000 population) and rural non-farm residents to live near an adult child. Most likely, an analysis conducted with a representative sample of all older people would show such rural-urban differences by region in the likelihood of living proximate to adult children.

Among older people, migration of the "young-old" is primarily to destinations in the Sunbelt, such as Florida and Arizona; those areas are distinguished by a high concentration of older persons who tend to have low probabilities of contact with their adult children (Siegel, 1993). After age 75, and with mounting health problems, older people who migrate tend to move to metropolitan areas, presumably to be nearer their adult children or better health care services (Glasgow, 1988; Longino, 1990). Therefore, although geographic mobility rates have declined over time, regional and place of residence differences in the risk of social isolation among older people do exist. In particular, migration trends are likely to produce pockets of older persons who do not have close relatives nearby.

Social Network Participation

Do people decrease their participation in social networks as they age? To the extent that resources become more constrained in later life, the social network could contract. It is argued that health is one such resource: good health allows us to engage in social activities and to maintain friendship ties. Similarly, income promotes social integration, for example, by allowing people to travel to visit others, to use the telephone freely, and to entertain in their homes. Further, the exit from key roles, such as that of worker, can reduce the frequency of ties to others (Morgan, 1988; see also Chapter 3, this volume). The death of a spouse can reduce the number of active contacts an older person has, because the former spouse's network members may not continue their involvement with the survivor. This is especially the case of widowers, because older husbands tend to rely on wives for their social contacts.

Several studies indicate that this hypothesized state of affairs may in fact be the case, at least as far as network size is concerned. Using General Social Survey (GSS) data for 1985, David Morgan (1988) examined differences in participation in social networks as a function of age. His analysis demonstrated that older respondents indeed reported attenuation of their social networks: "The network of people with whom they discuss important matters is smaller, contains fewer roles, and provides less frequent contacts" (S135). The average size of the social network drops precipitously between the ages of 60 and 65, possibly representing the impact of the loss of the work role. A second decline occurs around age 75, which may be related to the onset of health problems. Morgan found that much of the variance in these declines is explained by the availability of resources. Declining income was particularly responsible for the negative effect. In a study that also used the GSS data, Marsden (1987) similarly found a decline in network size with increasing age, and Campbell and Barrett (1992) found that in comparison to adults in middle age, older adults had smaller network sizes.

These findings are limited, however, because of their cross-sectional nature. In a nationally representative longitudinal study of persons aged 65 and over, Krause (1999) examined changes in social support between two survey administrations (1992–93 and 1996–97). Contact with friends declined significantly during this period. Almost half of the respondents (49%) reported a decline in contact with friends, whereas only 14 percent noted an increase (with 37% reporting no change).

Thus, some evidence indicates that network size shrinks with age. Since network size can be conceptualized as the resource pool from which people draw social support, we might expect that social support would also decline with age. However, several studies indicate that this network change does not necessarily translate into a decrease in social support. Antonucci and Akiyama (1987), in a national random sample of adults aged 50 and above, found no age differences in the amount of support received from network members. Levitt et al. (1993) also found no overall differences across three generations of women in either network size or the amount of support provided by the network. However, they uncovered an age-related shift in the content of the network: younger women included fewer family members and more friends in their networks, whereas older women reported the reverse (a finding that echoes Marsden, 1987).

Similarly, Lynch (1998) examined the way in which age affects variations in social support, using the second wave of the Americans' Changing Lives data set for individuals aged 31 and over. Lynch found a high level of positive support among all age groups, with no marked decline among late middle-aged and older persons. In fact, positive support from children was found to increase with age. Interestingly, an indicator of negative social support—the "demandingness" of network members—was found to be lower among the older respondents. In Krause's (1999) longitudinal study, older persons reported receiving increasing social support over time.

Thus, the impact of decreasing network size, which could lead to isolation of older persons, may be mitigated by the sustained social support of the remaining network members and, in particular, by kin.

The shift toward greater family versus friend involvement could be problematic, however, given the repeated finding that support and interaction with friends is more predictive of psychological well-being than is that which comes from family members. Although the basic support needs of the aged appear to be met, the life-enhancing aspects of weaker ties may be lost, which in turn might threaten social integration.

Additional light is shed on this issue by considering possible variations in social support within the older population. Two dimensions in particular have been highlighted in the literature: gender and health status. Despite the general findings regarding the robustness of support among older age groups, it is clear that subgroups of the older population suffer deficits in social network integration, and two groups in particular—men and persons with serious health problems.

Gender. It is clear that the degree of social support varies by gender. Gender differences in support, which appear to begin in adolescence (Miller & Lane, 1991; O'Conner, 1990), are maintained in adulthood. Women have larger networks of confidants and receive higher levels of social support from friends and relatives than do men (cf. Harrison et al., 1995; Okun & Keith, 1998; Turner & Marino, 1994). Further, there is evidence that gender differences in support become more marked across the adult life course. Fischer and Oliker (1983) reported that men were less likely than women to replace friendships that were lost in the later years, which is consistent with Field and Minkler's (1988) finding that women's contact with associates remained relatively stable over fourteen years while men's declined. Similarly, both Wister and Strain (1986) and Matt and Dean (1993) found greater gender differences in interaction patterns among older than middle-aged adults, with women having more frequent interaction.

Health. Second, social network size declines markedly among impaired older persons. It is noteworthy that all of the social support studies reviewed above rely on respondents who are capable of responding to survey questions. Persons with severe chronic disabilities, such as Alzheimer's disease, have been found to experience precipitous declines in contact with significant others, especially non-family members (see Chapter 5, this volume). Similarly, psychologically distressed older persons suffer reductions in support from friends, especially those in the oldest age group (Matt & Dean, 1993). Further, nursing home placement—which has been estimated to affect between 25 and 50 percent of the older population at some point in their lives (although only 5 percent at any one time)—characteristically leads to the severance of many or most social relationships outside of the facility (Siegel, 1993). For these reasons, ill and institutionalized older persons are far more apt to report severe loneliness than are persons without those problems (Wenger et al., 1996).

Older Persons Are Likely to Exit the Work Role

Two trends regarding employment are having a significant impact on the social integration of persons in late midlife and beyond. As noted earlier, average life expectancy has increased to an impressive degree, with Americans living longer than ever before. At the same time, however, public and private sector retirement policies have encouraged early exit from the work force among American male workers, who have been retiring from full-time involvement in the labor force at progressively earlier ages (Burkhauser & Quinn, 1990). At the beginning of the twentieth century, the majority (63%) of men aged 65 and over were active workers. By 1995, however, only about one in six (16%) of older men were employed. Over the same period, a small but constant proportion of women aged 65 and older was employed (about 8%). Middle-aged women's employment in the labor force, in contrast to the experience of men, has increased over time.

Most retiring Americans go from full-time, continuous employment to full-time, continuous leisure. However, many workers in the 50–64 age range report they would like to continue working longer if their employers offered to train them for new positions, offered them part-time work, or provided jobs with more flexible hours. Instead, older workers are left with few alternative pathways (such as phased retirement in the form of part-time or part-year jobs) and little assistance in developing life plans for the next three decades (or more) of their lives (Moen, 1996).

These two trends—increased longevity and earlier retirement—are producing an expanding "third age" of life (Laslett, 1991). This stage follows retirement but is prior to the onset of serious health problems or disability. Social scientists have repeatedly characterized this stage as one that provides few socially defined roles and opportunities, in contrast to earlier periods of the life course (see Chapter 3, this volume). In fact, the post-retirement years are often cast as postproductive years, a period in which adults with few family obligations have discharged their "work" obligations along with departure from their career jobs.

In this period of comparative "rolelessness" individuals can be especially at risk of experiencing social isolation. For many adults, paid work is a major, if not the principal, source of purposive activity, social relations, independence, identity, and self-respect. Employment is the way that we become integrated and acknowledged as members of the larger community. Thus, the loss of the work role can reduce social integration. Although many retirees plan for and enjoy retirement, it nevertheless represents an exit from a highly valued role—that of paid employee—and, in many cases, the loss of most work relationships. If new, meaningful roles are not found, retirement can represent a serious break in social integration.

Volunteering Declines Late in Life

In recent years, increasing attention has been paid to volunteer activity among older persons. This is in part encouraged by the perceived value of such unpaid labor to society. In a time of shrinking public resources, agencies hope to fill service gaps with volunteer labor (Janoski, 1998) and see older persons as a particularly promising group of potential volunteers because of their greater available leisure time (Musick et al., 1999). Conversely, it is asserted that volunteering provides important benefits for older persons. Specifically, volunteering may facilitate social integration by providing new, meaningful roles precisely when previous roles are being lost.

Although the measurement of "volunteering" has varied greatly from study to study, there is indeed evidence that this form of social participation provides benefits for persons in later life. Particularly striking are findings indicating that engaging in moderate volunteer activity can reduce the risk of mortality. In a thirty-year longitudinal study, Moen and colleagues (1992) found that membership in voluntary associations substantially reduced mortality risk. And in a recent large-scale study, Musick and colleagues (1999) also found volunteer work to have a protective effect on mortality. In addition to reducing the risk of death, voluntary social participation also appears to have positive effects on a variety of physical and mental health outcomes (see Young & Glasgow, 1998, for a recent review).

Thus, volunteer work appears to be a highly important vehicle for the social integration of older persons and one that leads to positive outcomes both for society and for individuals. To what extent do persons in later life avail themselves of the opportunities for enhanced social integration that volunteerism provides? Unfortunately, existing data are too scanty to be considered definitive. However, there is at least suggestive evidence on the questions, Has the extent of volunteering by older persons changed over time? Do older persons volunteer more or less than younger groups?

Chambré (1993), who examined data from thirteen surveys conducted between 1965 and 1990, presented the most comprehensive review of existing research on volunteerism by persons aged 65 and older. Her findings indicate that volunteer activity does diminish somewhat in the older age groups. The highest rates of volunteering occur in early midlife (ages 25 to 44), when nearly two thirds volunteer. This rate declines to 47 percent among those aged 65 to 74, and to 32 percent among persons 75 and over. Other data sources indicate that volunteering among the "oldest-old" declines even further; for example, among those aged 80 and over, 27 percent reported volunteering (Chambré, 1993). As with other areas we have discussed, the most likely reason for the decline in the oldest age groups is health problems that limit both mobility and the ability to undertake strenuous volunteer activity (Herzog et al., 1989).

However, there appears to be a trend toward an increase in volunteerism among older people. Chambré (1993) notes that although a clear link exists between age and the propensity to volunteer, this negative relationship has become more muted in recent years. Reasons for this increase include a rise in public and media attention to community service by older persons; changing demographics that have led to a better-educated older population (who are in turn more likely to volunteer); and a rise in government-sponsored programs and private sector initiatives promoting volunteerism in later life (Chambré, 1993).

DISCUSSION

The goal of this chapter was to set the stage for the empirical and theoretical discussions that follow. At the outset, we noted that social scientists have by and large moved beyond the "great debate" over the integration of older persons. Instead of characterizing the later years as ones of role loss, devaluation, and anomie, it is clear that we must examine the paired themes of integration and isolation in specific contexts. Rather than making global pronouncements regarding the status of older persons, we see it as the task of the sociology of the life course to examine *who* is integrated, *when*, and *under what circumstances*. It is necessary wherever possible to examine life-course patterns of social integration, as well as social contexts that either promote or hinder integration.

Perhaps a final reference to Durkheim can help clarify our perspective. In *Suicide*, Durkheim argues that because the tendency toward egotism is a general societal trend, it must be met with sweeping, society-wide measures. This is the theme of the works by Rosow and others up to the present day. In contrast, we view the older population as consisting of subgroups of individuals, some of whom, because of these subgroup characteristics, are at greater risk of isolation, while others receive special protection. What is critically needed is attention to individual and subgroup differences rather than global societal critique.

Thus, based on our review of the evidence above, some subgroups of older persons may be at risk of a lack of social integration. Further, this disadvantage may be cumulative. Several key points we made in this chapter are the following:

— Older men's marriage rates have increased over time relative to that of women, which suggests an increase in older men's social integration and other benefits that marriage confers.

— A higher proportion of older women live alone today than in the past, owing primarily to a decrease in co-residence with adult children after becoming widowed or experiencing poor health.

— The baby-boom generation may be at risk of social isolation because of lower marriage rates, higher rates of divorce, and smaller numbers of offspring.

— Geographic mobility rates have declined in the United States among both younger and older adults. However, this finding does not appear to be true of rural areas, in which an outflow of young people is taking place. This outflow decreases the probability that older rural parents will receive support in times of need.

— Social network size shrinks during old age compared to younger ages, often concomitant with the loss of the work role, increasing health problems, and declining income.

— The trend toward earlier retirement, along with increased longevity and better health status of older people, has created a relatively long period of comparative "rolelessness."
— With increasing age, volunteer activity declines.

Emerging from this summary are profiles of persons who may experience deficits in social integration in later life. We would, for example, expect a widowed, retired woman, who is over age 75 and in poor health, to be at risk of isolation. Further, such a person residing in a rural area might be particularly at risk. However, a healthy 65-year-old man, still in the workforce and married, is substantially less likely to experience problems with social integration (although the passage of time may increase his risk).

In conclusion, is social integration a theme of major importance in the second half of life? In our view, the answer is indisputably yes. Is social integration threatened for all older persons, as a *class* of people? We would give this question a qualified "no"; qualified because ageism continues to be pervasive in our society and may lead to prejudice and stereotyping of older persons. However, there is ample evidence (including that presented in later chapters of this book) that many persons are highly integrated in later life, such that we do not see this as the most useful approach. Finally, is social integration compromised at some points in the life course for certain types of individuals? Emphatically yes. The following chapters explore both the problems and the prospects of social integration in a number of key domains in the second half of life.

REFERENCES

Adelman, P. K. (1994). Multiple roles and psychological well-being in a national sample of older adults. *Journals of Gerontology: Social Sciences, 49*, S277–S285.

Antonucci, T. C. (1990). Social supports and relationships. In R. H. Binstock & L. K. George (Eds.), *Handbook of aging and the social sciences*, 3d ed. (205–226). New York: Academic Press.

Antonucci, T. C., & Akiyama, H. (1987). Social networks in adult life and a preliminary examination of the convoy model. *Journals of Gerontology, 42*, 519–527.

Bellah, R., Madsen, R., Sullivan, W. M., Swidler, A., & Tipton, S. M. (1996).

Habits of the heart: Individualism and commitment in American life.
Berkeley: University of California Press.

Berkman, L. F. (1983). The assessment of social networks and social support in the elderly. *Journal of American Geriatrics Society, 3,* 743–749.

Berkman, L. F., & Syme, S. L. (1979). Social networks, host resistance, and mortality: A nine-year follow-up study of Alameda County residents. *American Journal of Epidemiology, 100,* 186–204.

Bosworth, H. D., & Schaie, K. W. (1997). The relationship of social environment, social networks, and health outcomes in the Seattle Longitudinal Study. *Journals of Gerontology: Psychological Sciences, 52,* P197–205.

Bowling, A., & Farquhar, M. (1991). Associations with social networks, social support, health status and psychiatric morbidity in three samples of elderly people. *Social Psychiatry and Psychiatric Epidemiology, 26,* 115–126.

Bronfenbrenner, U., McClelland, P., Wethington, E., Moen, P., & Ceci, S. J. (1996). *The state of Americans.* New York: Free Press.

Bultena, G. L. (1969). Rural-urban differences in the familial interaction of the aged. *Rural Sociology, 34,* 5–15.

Burkhauser, R. V., & Quinn, J. F. (1990). Economic incentives and the labor force participation of older workers. *Research in Labor Economics, 11,* 159–179.

Campbell, K. E., & Barrett, A. L. (1992). Sources of personal neighbor networks: Social integration, need, or time? *Social Forces, 70,* 1077–1100.

Chambré, S. M. (1993). Volunteerism by elders: Past traditions and future prospects. *The Gerontologist, 33,* 221–228.

Coser, R. L. (1991) *In defense of modernity: Role complexity and individual autonomy.* Stanford, CA: Stanford University Press.

Cumming, E., & Henry, W. (1961). *Growing old: The process of disengagement.* New York: Basic Books.

Dewit, D. J., Wister, A. V., & Burch, T. K. (1988). Physical distance and social contact between elders and their adult children. *Research on Aging, 10,* 56–80.

Dugan, E., & Kivett, V. R. (1994). The importance of emotional and social isolation to loneliness among very old rural adults. *The Gerontologist, 34,* 340–346.

Durkheim, E. (1951). *Suicide: A study in sociology.* J. A. Spaulding & G. Simpson (Trans.). New York: Free Press.

Easterlin, R. A. (1996). Economic and social implications of demographic patterns. In R. H. Binstock & L. K. George (Eds.), *Handbook of aging and the social sciences,* 4th ed. (73–93). San Diego: Academic Press.

Eckenrode, J., & Gore, S. (1990). *Stress between work and family.* New York: Plenum.

Field, D., & Minkler, M. (1988). Continuity and change in social support between young-old and old-old or very-old age. *Journals of Gerontology: Psychological Sciences, 43,* 100–106.

Fischer, C. S., & Oliker, S. J. (1983). A research note on friendship, gender, and the life cycle. *Social Forces, 62,* 124–133.

Fullinwider, R. K. (Ed.) (1999). *Civil society, democracy, and civic renewal.* Lanham, MD: Rowman and Littlefield.

George, L. K. (1996). Social factors and illness. In R. H. Binstock & L. K. George (Eds.), *Handbook of aging and the social sciences,* 4th ed. (229–252). San Diego: Academic Press.

Glasgow, N. (1988). The nonmetro elderly: Economic and demographic status. *Economic Research Service, Rural Development Research Report No. 70.* Washington, DC: U.S. Department of Agriculture.

Gove, W. R. (1973). Sex, marital status, and mortality. *American Journal of Sociology, 79,* 45–67.

Hareven, T. K. (1996). The impact of the historical study of the family and the life course paradigm on sociology. *Comparative Sociological Research, Supplement 2,* 185–205.

Harrison, J., Maguire, P., & Pitceathly, C. (1995). Confiding in crisis: Gender differences in pattern of confiding among cancer patients. *Social Science and Medicine, 41,* 1255–1260.

Havighurst, R. (1964). Changing status and roles during the adult life cycle: Significance for adult education. In H. W. Burns (Ed.), *Social Backgrounds of Adult Education* (17–38). Boston: Center for the Study of Liberal Education for Adults.

Herzog, A. R., Kahn, R. L., Morgan, J. N., Jackson, J. S., & Antonucci, T. C. (1989). Age differences in productive activities. *Journals of Gerontology: Social Sciences, 44,* 129–138.

Hochschild, A. R. (1975). Disengagement theory: A critique and proposal. *American Sociological Review, 40,* 553–569.

Hong, J., & Seltzer, M. M. (1994). Psychological consequences of multiple roles: The nonnormative case. *Journal of Health and Social Behavior, 36,* 386–398.

Janoski, T. (1998). Being volunteered: The impact of social partners and pro-social attitudes on volunteering. *Sociological Forum, 13,* 495–519.

Kertzer, D., & Laslett, P. (1995). *Aging in the past: Demography, society, and old age.* Berkeley: University of California Press.

Krause, N. (1999). Stress and the devaluation of highly salient roles in late life. *Journals of Gerontology: Psychological Sciences, 54b,* S99–S108.

Krout, J. A. (1984). The utilization of formal and informal support of the aged: Rural versus urban differences. NY: Unpublished final report to the AARP Andrus Foundation.

Krout, J. A. (1988). Rural versus urban differences in elderly parents' contact with their children. *The Gerontologist, 28,* 198–203.

Laslett, P. (1991). *A fresh map of life: The emergence of the third age.* Cambridge: Harvard University Press.

Lee, G. R., Dwyer, J. W., & Coward, R. T. (1990). Residential location and proximity to children among impaired elderly patients. *Rural Sociology, 55(4),* 579–589.

Levitt, M. J., Weber, R. A., & Guacci, N. (1993). Convoys of social support: An intergenerational analysis. *Psychology and Aging, 8,* 323–326.

Longino, C. F., Jr. (1990). Geographical distribution & migration. In R. H. Binstock and L. K. George (Eds.), *Handbook of aging and the social sciences,* 3d ed. (45–63). San Diego: Academic Press.

Lynch, J. A. (1998). The role of life stress, social support, and self-actualization in adapting to a disability: The experience of hospitalized older adults. *Dissertation Abstracts International, Section B,* 1371.

Marsden, P. V. (1987). Core discussion networks of Americans. *American Sociological Review, 52,* 122–131.

Matt, G. E., & Dean, A. (1993). Social support from friends and psychological distress among elderly persons: Moderator effects of age. *Journal of Health and Social Behavior, 34,* 187–200.

Miller, J. B., & Lane, M. (1991). Relations between young adults and their parents. *Journal of Adolescence, 14,* 179–194.

Moen, P. (1996). Changing age trends: The pyramid upside down? In U. Bronfenbrenner, P. McClelland, E. Wethington, P. Moen & S. J. Ceci (Eds.), *The changing state of Americans* (208–258). New York: Free Press.

Moen, P., Dempster-McClain, D., & Williams, R. M., Jr. (1989). Social integration and longevity: An event history analysis of women's roles and resilience. *American Sociological Review, 54,* 635–647.

Moen, P., Dempster-McClain, D., & Williams, R. M. (1992). Successful aging: A life course perspective on women's roles and health. *American Journal of Sociology, 97,* 1612–1638.

Moen, P., Robison, J., & Dempster-McClain, D. (1995). Caregiving and women's well-being: A life course approach. *Journal of Health and Social Behavior, 36,* 259–273.

Morgan, D. L. (1988). Age differences in social network participation. *Journals of Gerontology: Social Sciences, 43,* S129–S137.

Mullins, L. G., Longino, C. F., Jr., Marshall, V., & Tucker, R. (1989). An examination of loneliness and social isolation among elderly Canadian seasonal migrants in Florida. *Journals of Gerontology: Social Sciences, 44,* S580–S586.

Musick, M. A., Herzog, A. R., & House, J. S. (1999). Volunteering and mortality among older adults: Findings from a national sample. *Journals of Gerontology: Social Sciences, 54,* S173–S180.

Mutran, E., Reitzes, D. C., Mossey, J., & Fernandez, M. E. (1995). Social support, depression, and the recovery of walking ability following hip fracture surgery. *Journals of Gerontology: Social Sciences, 50B,* S354–S361.

Nisbet, R. A. (1966). *The sociological tradition.* New York: Basic Books.

Noburn, J. E., et al. (1995). Self-care assistance from others in coping with functional status limitations among a national sample of older adults. *Journals of Gerontology: Social Sciences, 50B,* 101–109.

O'Conner, P. (1990). The adult mother/daughter relationship: A uniquely and universally close relationship? *Sociological Review, 38,* 293–323.

Okun, M. A., & Keith, V. M. (1998). Effect of positive and negative social exchanges with various sources on depressive symptoms in younger and older adults. *Journals of Gerontology: Psychological Sciences, 53B,* 4–20.

Oxman, T. E., & Hull, J. G. (1997). Social support, depression, and activities of daily living in older heart surgery patients. *Journals of Gerontology: Psychological Sciences, 52B,* 1–14.

Pezzin, L. E., & Schone, B. S. (1999). Parental marital disruption and intergenerational transfers: An analysis of lone elderly parents and their children. *Demography, 36,* 287–297.

Pillemer, K., & Suitor, J. (1998). Baby boom families: Relations with aging parents. *Generations, 23,* 65–70.

Putnam, R. (1995). Bowling alone: America's declining social capital. *Journal of Democracy, 6,* 65–78.

Riley, M. W., Kahn, R. L., & Foner, A. (1994). *Age and structural lag.* New York: Wiley.

Rose, A. M. (1965). Group consciousness among the aged. In A. M. Rose and W. A. Peterson (Eds.), *Older people and their social world.* Philadelphia: F. A. Davis.

Rosow, I. (1967). *Social Integration of the Aged.* New York: Free Press.

Rossi, A. S., & Rossi, P. H. (1990). *Of human bonding: Parent-child relations across the life course.* New York: Aldine de Gruyter.

Ruggles, S. (1994). The transformation of American family structure. *American Historical Review, 99,* 103–128.

Schudson, M. (1998). *The good citizen: A history of American civic life.* New York: Free Press.

Seeman, T. E., Bruce, M. L., & McAvay, G. J. (1996). Social network characteristics and onset of ADL disability: MacArthur studies of successful aging. *Journals of Gerontology: Social Sciences, B51B,* 191–200.

Siegel, J. S. (1993). *A generation of change: A profile of America's older population.* New York: Russell Sage Foundation.

Silverstein, M., & Angelelli, J. J. (1998). Older parents' expectations of moving closer to their children. *Journals of Gerontology: Social Sciences, 53,* S153–S163.

Slater, P. (1970). *The pursuit of loneliness: American culture at the breaking point.* Boston: Beacon Press.

Spitze, G., & Logan, J. R. (1991). Sibling structure and intergenerational relations. *Journal of Marriage and the Family, 5,* 871–884.

Suitor, J. J., Pillemer, K., Keeton, S., & Robison, J. (1995). Aged parents and aging children: Determinants of relationship quality. In R. Blieszner & V. H. Bedford (Eds.), *Aging and the family: Theory and research* (223–250). Westport, CT: Praeger.

Thoits, P. A. (1983). Multiple identities and psychological well-being: A reformulation and test of the social isolation hypothesis. *American Sociological Review, 48,* 174–187.

Thoits, P. A. (1986). Multiple identities: Examining gender and marital status differences in distress. *American Sociological Review, 51,* 259–272.

Thoits, P. A. (1992). Identity structures and psychological well-being: Gender and marital status comparisons. *Social Psychology Quarterly, 55,* 236–256.

Turner, R. J., & Marino, F. (1994). Social support and social structure: A descriptive epidemiology. *Journal of Health and Social Behavior, 35,* 193–212.

Uhlenberg, P. (1993). Demographic change and kin relationships in later life. In G. L. Maddox and M. P. Lawton (Eds.), *Annual review of gerontology and geriatrics: Kinship, aging, and social change, Vol. 13* (219–238). New York: Springer.

Uhlenberg, P., & Miner, S. (1996). Life course and aging: A cohort perspective. In R. H. Binstock & L. K. George (Eds.), *Handbook of aging and the social sciences,* 4th ed. (208–228). San Diego: Academic Press.

Watkins, S. C., Menken, J. A., & Bongaarts, J. (1987). Demographic foundations of family change. *American Sociological Review, 52,* 346–58.

Wenger, C. G., Davies, R., Shahtahmasebi, S., & Scott, A. (1996). Social isolation and loneliness in old age: Review and model. *Aging and Society, 16*, 333–358.

Wethington, E., & Kessler, R. (1986). Perceived support, received support, and adjustment to stressful life events. *Journal of Health and Social Behavior, 27*, 78–89.

Wister, A. V., & Strain, L. (1986). Social support and well-being: A comparison of older widows and widowers. *Canadian Journal on Aging, 5*, 205–220.

Youmans, E. G. (1963). *Aging patterns in a rural and an urban area of Kentucky.* Bulletin No. 681. Lexington, KY: Agricultural Experiment Station.

Young, F. W., & Glasgow, N. (1998). Voluntary social participation and health. *Research on Aging, 20*, 339–362.

CHAPTER TWO

Multiple Roles, Social Integration, and Health

Elaine Wethington, Phyllis Moen, Nina Glasgow, and Karl Pillemer

Many studies have shown that the quality and quantity of social relationships are positively related to health. In Chapter 1, we reviewed a long research tradition that links social integration, in the form of social support and participation in multiple life roles, to good health and well-being among older people (cf. Lowenthal & Haven, 1968; George, 1996a; Moen et al., 1992). The extensive knowledge base about social integration has clear implications for promoting productive social involvement, as well as health and well-being, through the later years of life.

Less clear, however, are the mechanisms by which social integration, social participation, and social support improve health and well-being in later life. Relatively few studies have attempted to specify the particular pathways by which social relationships enhance or protect health. We believe that this issue is critically important to understanding the causes and consequences of social integration in later life. In this chapter, our approach is to link several theoretical approaches to social integration and social support with the life-course perspective on human development (George, 1993). We incorporate the social psychological perspective on social support (Wethington & Kessler, 1986; Cutrona et al., 1990; Sarason, Sarason, & Pierce, 1990) and research on the functional mechanisms underlying the support process (Coriell & Cohen, 1995; Cutrona, 1986; Harlow & Cantor, 1995).

Our approach builds upon the work of earlier investigators in three ways. First, we focus on *direct* rather than indirect measures of the mechanisms of social integration (cf. Bolger & Eckenrode, 1991). Second, we examine *mechanisms* specific to particular health outcomes (e.g., Fawzy et al., 1995; Seeman et al., 1996). And third, we conceive of various health outcomes as both *interdependent and as unfolding over time* (George, 1996a).

We believe that such increased theoretical and methodological sophistication will enable researchers to specify *social selection* effects in models relating social factors to health. The phenomenon of social selection presents a conundrum to researchers who wish to argue that social integration leads to well-being: that is, the inverse possibility that healthy people are more likely to be engaged in multiple roles and multifaceted social networks precisely *because* they are healthier. Thus it is not clear which comes first—health or social relationships. In this chapter, we develop a framework to assist researchers in untangling this issue.

Further, most theoretical reviews of research on social support, social integration, and participation and their relationships to health also point to problems regarding underlying measures of social support (cf. House et al., 1988; Thoits, 1995). In this chapter we address these concerns about measurement. We discuss both conventional and less common measures (including semi-structured narrative interviewing techniques) that have been used to collect information about the ways in which people undergoing life transitions experience social support. These transitions are likely to entail changes in social networks and in the way people are socially integrated into their communities and neighborhoods. We argue that wider use and understanding of contextual measures of social integration, participation, and support will encourage a leap forward in the sophistication of models and methods in research on individuals' roles, relationships, and well-being.

To summarize our approach, throughout this chapter we develop three major themes. The first theme is the need for integration of theoretical perspectives on multiple roles, social support, and social integration theory. Such integration is necessary to uncover the complexity of social relationships in later life. The second theme relates to the use of contextual measures to elaborate the connection between source of support and function, as a way to integrate the two theoretical perspectives. The third theme involves innovative research designs we believe are most appropriate for future analyses of social integration and social support in midlife and beyond.

Integrating Research on Multiple Roles, Social Integration, and Health

The simplest and most traditional way to examine the relationship between social roles and health has been to view involvement in roles as indicators of social integration (Durkheim, 1951). Social integration, in this context, is defined as social cohesion with the larger society. Using this approach, researchers typically have attempted to specify mechanisms that promote the positive consequences of social integration in particular research contexts and in regard to a particular health outcome. This approach reflects the belief that role involvement and social support both maintain health and well-being as well as buffer the effects of stress.

Other theoretical perspectives have taken a more complex view of the relationship between integration and health outcomes; below, we describe several of these. Focusing on the relationship of role involvement to well-being, we review the contrasting role enhancement and role strain perspectives. Using the integrated approach outlined above, we attempt to unravel this particular confusion regarding roles.

Role Enhancement and Role Strain

Both the Introduction and Chapter 1 of this book propose that involvement in meaningful roles promotes well-being. This view, termed the *role enhancement* perspective, suggests that men and women engaging in multiple roles should experience higher levels of physical and emotional health than those with fewer roles, regardless of their age. A key assumption of this perspective is that the accumulation of social identities or roles benefits individuals (e.g., Sieber, 1974). Social integration, in the form of multiple roles, is presumed to increase power, prestige, resources, and emotional gratification, including social recognition and a heightened sense of identity. Assuming a causal role for social participation, considerable research indicates that multiple roles do, in fact, foster health and longevity for both men and women (Moen, 1997: 91; Moen et al., 1989, 1992; Moen et al., 1994; Thoits, 1986).

An alternative argument, the *role strain* perspective, emphasizes the costs rather than the benefits of multiple roles (Goode, 1960). This perspective is typically employed when discussing the interplay between work and family roles. It has guided many of the studies examining the impacts of employment on women's lives, especially for those women who are also wives and mothers. It assumes a fixed quantity of time, energy, and commitment available for family and non-family role responsibilities. The role strain perspective has guided much research on work stress in the social and medical sciences, as well (Lepore, 1995).

Role enhancement and role strain perspectives, although useful in their day, are in the midst of major theoretical revision. Most important, advances in research and measurement utilizing them have encouraged the field to adopt more complex measurements of the component mechanisms of these perspectives (e.g., Carr, 1998). Research on the importance of social relationships to health, and on mechanisms of roles and social integration have increased the interdisciplinary nature of this work, uniting the fields of medicine, public health, and psychology.

Further, studies contrasting the predictive power of enhancement and strain perspectives (Wethington & Kessler, 1989; Bolger et al., 1990; O'Neil & Greenberger, 1994; Moen, 1992) have found that neither perspective fully explains the patterns of mental and physical health associated with the number and the quality of roles. For example, a *role context* approach (Moen et al., 1992) points to the importance of locating role involvements in particular circumstances. Clearly, there is a need for a more fully articulated perspective linking health and social integration that still features the concept of roles but also integrates research from several disciplines and places roles in context.

Age, Life-Course Stage, and Birth Cohort: Benefits of a Life-Course Perspective

Research using the role enhancement and role strain perspectives has been limited because it rarely explicitly addresses possible contextual distinctions by age, life-course stage, or birth cohort. In our view, these issues can be illuminated by a life-course perspective (and the use of longitudinal data), linking social integration with physical health and psychological well-being. A life-course perspective considers not only whether men and women occupy multiple roles in the later years of adulthood but also the timing and duration of role occupancy *throughout* adulthood (Giele & Elder, 1998). This perspective holds that the impacts of earlier resources and life pathways cannot be understood without reference to issues of timing, trajectories, and transitions.

Role Trajectories. Research is now beginning to focus on the concept of role trajectories. A role trajectory is defined as the history of commitment and participation in a given social role across time, such as that of paid work. (Career commitment and development is a well-known example of a role trajectory.) The role trajectory concept refocuses and raises new research questions about the nature and impact of social integration on health. For example, it refocuses questions, such as whether particular role conditions—for example, working more than forty hours a week—are more conducive (or detrimental) to well-being and social integration later in life than cutting back on work hours. The trajectory concept also raises the possibility that patterns of role participation over time, rather than current role involvement, affect health and functioning (Moen et al., 1992). For example, how does the patterning of men's and women's involvement in different aspects of family life throughout adulthood affect their health in later adulthood?

One further consideration raised by the trajectory concept is history of past role participation. It is well known that marriage is positively related to health and well-being. But does the emotional and physical detriment of not being married hold true for the person who has been divorced or widowed over a quarter of a century as well as for the person divorced or widowed in the last six months? Given the age stratification and role allocation systems in our society, older individuals typically experience role loss as they move into the later years of adulthood (Riley et al., 1994). Does the loss of a role in late adulthood have the same negative effect on health as its loss in middle adulthood, when loss is less normative or expected?

Social Selection versus Social Causation. Applying the life-course perspective reframes the strategy for dealing with problems of causal ordering in research on multiple roles and health. When measuring both at the same time we simply cannot determine whether multiple role occupancy is a contributor to rather than a consequence of health and well-being. Indeed, most findings linking health with social integration are ambiguous because the causal direction of effects is unclear (House et al., 1988). As Verbrugge (1983) pointed out, the issue is one of social causation versus social selection.

Social causation assumes that social integration influences health. By contrast, social selection assumes that healthy people are the ones more likely to take on and maintain multiple social roles. But the choice between the social causation and the social selection argument is less crucial than gaining an understanding of the pathways to health and social integration in later adulthood. Causation and selection probably operate simultaneously and interactively in a dynamic cascade of events over the life course. Successful aging encompasses both social integration (multiple roles) and health in the later years of life. What is required is a dynamic approach to health and social integration, one that considers the extent to which experiences throughout the life course shape roles and well-being later in life.

Consider, for example, the evidence regarding the relationship between the role of employee and women's physical health. This evidence is simultaneously straightforward and ambiguous. The fact that employed women are typically more healthy than non-employed women, regardless of their age or the year in which they are studied, is very straightforward. At every age level, employed women report fewer chronic conditions and less short- or long-term disability than do fulltime homemakers. Women who are simultaneously wives, mothers, and wage earners have higher levels of physical well-being than nonemployed mothers, single mothers, and employed childless wives (Verbrugge, 1983). However, the ambiguity arises when we attempt to establish causation. Whether married working mothers are more healthy *because* of their multiple roles or whether healthy individuals are more likely to adopt multiple roles remains unclear. Both interpretations are likely to be true: (1) Healthy women are active in a number of roles, including paid work; and (2) being active does promote better health.

To resolve this dilemma, it is necessary to focus on specific configurations of roles in specific contexts. To provide one example, some types of employment, when combined with marriage and motherhood, may be related to coronary disease. One ten-year study showed that married mothers who had three or more children and who were employed in clerical occupations were more vulnerable to heart disease (Haynes & Feinlieb, 1980). An early study by Welch and Booth (1977) added to our understanding of the employment-health link. They found that married women who had been employed for more than one year were healthier than those who had worked for only a short period of time. To be sure, both groups were healthy enough to work. But because those employed longer were healthier, it may be that the positive relationship typically found between employment and health is not due simply to healthy women choosing to work but to the effects of their work experience as well.

Accumulation of Advantage or Disadvantage. A life-course perspective suggests that prior experiences, including the occupancy and patterning of roles in early adulthood, can affect subsequent well-being. This view leads to the question of whether *role biography* or *current role repertoire* is more conducive to personal feelings of well-being in later adulthood. In other words, knowing something about individuals' past experiences would help to account for differences in psychological well-being later in life. A more dynamic, longitudinal, and contextual view of the relationship between health and well-being is necessary. It may not be role occupancy alone but rather the timing, sequencing, duration, or number of spells in particular roles that is consequential for both social integration and emotional well-being (Moen et al., 1992). If studies included measures of all these aspects of roles, it would be possible to show whether the experience of particular roles, their timing in the life course, or their persistence affects the physical and psychological well-being of older men and women. It is also imperative to look beyond employment to other roles that are important in older people's lives, such as non-paid work, organizational and religious involvements, and family roles, including caregiving (see Chapter 3, this volume).

We do not know whether taking on community, volunteer, or organizational roles in late adulthood can compensate for the transition out of family and occupational roles. Roles may have different impacts at different stages of the life course and in different contexts, especially regarding transitions in later life; little is known about the import of family and non-family roles beyond the normative years of retirement. As Chapter 1 in this book indicated, both men and women experience a decline in family and non-family roles in later years as children leave home, marriages end, and careers come to an end. Because earlier experiences shape health and well-being later in life there is likely to be a certain "cumulativeness" to the effects of social integration, with those socially connected in earlier adulthood the most likely to remain socially connected in their later years.

In sum, we believe that the life-course perspective can assist greatly in untangling the relationship between occupying multiple roles and positive physical and mental health outcomes. Next, we turn our attention to the relationship between social support and these outcomes.

A MODEL OF THE RELATIONSHIP BETWEEN SOCIAL SUPPORT AND HEALTH OUTCOMES

There is a great deal of theoretical as well as empirical work supporting a distinction between the health-promoting aspects of social integration and functional support. The theoretical model we use to guide our discussion is presented in Figure 2.1.

For our purposes here, in the model we focus on one aspect of social integration (as defined in the Introduction): network structure. For ease of presentation, we grouped this component of social integration into two levels: the close network (family and friends), and the meso-network (institutional memberships and participation, including work, group memberships, and religious participation). Figure 2.1 portrays these levels in dynamic relation with one another through the course of life and in daily interaction (see Messeri et al., 1993). Gains in one level of the network may compensate or substitute for losses in the other. In this schema, family and friends, as well as participation in the meso-network, are hypothesized to provide social support to maintain the emotional and practical functions of daily living.

Both dimensions are critical to our understanding of this issue.

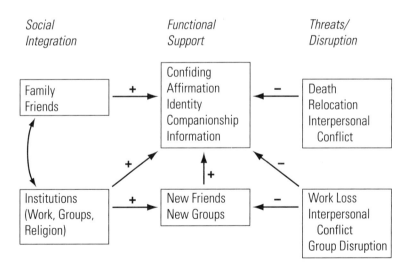

Figure 2.1   Theoretical Scheme for Dynamic Relationships among Social Integration, Functional Social Support, and Threats/Disruption to Social Support.

Specifically, one's close network of family and friends is an important source of social support, fulfilling such functions as confiding, affirmation, identity-maintenance, companionship, and information provision. But also important are institutional sources and settings for support (Rook, 1995) that contribute both to perceptions of the availability of support (such as a sense of cohesion contributing to identity) as well as to actual provision of support (e.g., sources of information). The institutional context also helps maintain stable levels of social support through the generation of new contacts over time, who replace (substitute for) family and friends lost through close network disruption (Rook & Schuster, 1996). Community-level resources also contribute more directly to well-being through the sense of identity and cohesiveness they give to their members.

At both levels, the dynamics of social integration may be positive as well as negative. Threats to and disruption of social integration and social support occur among both family and friends, and in community structures. The experiences of separation and loss such as death, relocation, and interpersonal conflict, threaten adequate levels of functional social support. In this theoretical schema, new friends and contacts from the meso-network are hypothesized to compensate for losses in the close network. Disruptions in the meso-network (that is, the institutional setting) also pose threats to the maintenance of social support, either directly through the loss of identity or provision of information, or indirectly by weakening an individual's ability to substitute for losses in the closer network.

Empirically, social integration is directly related to health, including mortality: socially integrated individuals live longer than those who are not socially integrated (Berkman & Syme, 1979; Moen et al., 1989). The theoretical support for this association ranges from psychological theory on personality formation, such as Bowlby's theory of attachment (Bowlby, 1969) to sociological theory on the health-promoting functions of different types of ties (cf. Messeri et al., 1993). Much work on this topic assumes that social integration wields its major impact on health through functional social support (Thoits, 1995). Still needed is empirical work showing how changes in social provisions are related to group membership, new family formation, or transformation in intimate relationships over the life course.

Another gap in both theory and empirical research is that the exact mechanisms through which social integration affects health have not yet been linked to direct provision of social support (Thoits, 1995).

Indeed, social integration has not been shown, when measured as the *number* of social ties, to buffer the impact of stressors on mental or physical health (House et al., 1988; Kessler & McLeod, 1985; Thoits, 1995). This finding implies that crisis support may not be the most powerful pathway through which social integration contributes to health and mental health. Social integration may operate more as a resource for everyday support and interaction that maintains health, encourages positive health behavior, or facilitates the use of medical care (Vilhjalmsson, 1993).

For example, the presence of a sexual partner who is also a confidant has been found to buffer the effects of severe stressors on mental health (Brown & Harris, 1978). Research evidence (Wethington & Kessler, 1986) documents that *perceived* social support, rather than actual support received during a crisis, buffers the impact of stress on health. Taken together, research suggests that social integration serves more as a resource maintaining health and functioning (a "main effect"). As yet, the means by which it has positive impacts are not well delineated.

THE NEED FOR CONTEXTUAL MEASURES

How should researchers on later life address this complexity in the relationship between social integration, social support, and well-being? One answer, in our opinion, lies in the development of more sensitive measures. Specifically, we believe that the *contextual measurement approach* provides a basis for developing a more comprehensive analysis of social integration and health, when combined with social-psychological and life-course perspectives.

Contextual measures assess change in relationships and relationship functioning over time (Brown & Harris, 1989) by classifying descriptive narratives of social interaction and use of support. Contextual measures allow researchers to address many interesting questions that are difficult to approach using conventional measures. Some transitions in the social network and roles can be recast as "dependent variables"—that is, products of changes in other domains. For example, life transitions in the later adult years can involve gaining new relationships (creating new opportunities for social integration), losing relationships (creating a threat to current levels of social integration), or transforming participation in a current social setting (changing the source or character of social integration). When attempting to map out the impact of "supporter change" on social integration as a dependent variable, it becomes clear that prior relationship or role functioning predicts present functioning and has an impact on how well people navigate transitional states.

Thoits (1995) recommended that researchers begin integrating narrative reports of social support transactions with standard questionnaire assessments of social support to enrich the meaning of reports. Such conceptual specification will be useful for advancing research and practice using social support, including intervention research. Most of our knowledge of how social support and social integration operate is not fine-tuned enough to design targeted interventions for groups in need, especially for the most socially isolated members of society (see also Link & Phelan, 1995).

Mechanisms of Functional Social Support

Social scientists traditionally take a functional approach toward defining and measuring the benefits and risks of social integration. Social integration is presumed to provide (1) access to social support; (2) stable alliance with others in like-minded groups; (3) social control and socialization; (4) identity maintenance processes; and (5) information exchange relevant to health behavior and maintenance. It is worthwhile to review these key functions, which may take on special importance in later life.

First, most research has focused on how roles and networks provide access to social support. Positive social support, specifically *instrumental assistance and emotional sustenance,* is hypothesized to promote positive physical and psychological health, thus constituting an important benefit of social integration (House et al., 1988; Umberson et al., 1996). A second, less studied mechanism is the provision of *stable alliance,* that is, the power of the group augmenting the power of the individual. This can be either objective, as in group leadership or participation promoting individual interest, or subjective/symbolic, as in the perception of support from related others (Wethington & Kessler, 1986) or attachment (Parkes & Weiss, 1983).

The third mechanism, *social control and socialization,* is often overlooked as a mechanism of social integration in the literature on role involvement. It is, however, among the most powerful in its lifelong impact. Roles expose one to and demand discipline through activities regulated by ritual, by institutional expectations, and by processes of learning (Umberson, 1987).

The fourth mechanism is the contribution of role involvement to a sense of *meaning, purpose in life,* and *group and individual identity.* The notion of "multiple identities" (Thoits, 1986) refers to the function of multiple roles for providing a variety of sources of behavioral appraisal. More rewarding roles are hypothesized to compensate for the negative feedback from more troublesome roles (Linville, 1987). The availability of positive feedback is believed to underlie a sense of efficacy and confidence. The availability of multiple sources of feedback also may underlie the perception of choice and freedom (Sieber, 1974).

The final mechanism is the *exchange of health information and facilitation* for maintaining mental and physical health (Coriell & Cohen, 1995; Cutrona et al., 1990; Rook, 1995). Network theorists have emphasized how access to multiple sources of information facilitates health through direct information and assistance. This mechanism is one of the best specified in the research literature, and it is the most integrated into research on physical health and illness.

Taking Account of "Outcome"

A life-course approach to multiple roles, social integration, and health also implies another important point: researchers should take care to differentiate theory, predictions, and measurement across various outcomes. The concept of "health" can be measured in a variety of different ways, as a disease state, as a state of positive social or psychological functioning, or as self-perceived wellness.

From a practical standpoint, it makes sense to consider whether a change in role involvement is likely to have a specific impact on psychological health, physical health, or both. Do particular changes in roles or social networks produce short-term changes in health (e.g., susceptibility to infectious disease) or long-term changes in health (e.g., progression in cardiovascular disease)? The period over which such disease develops leads to different predictions about how much role change is necessary before a change in health status should be expected. Researchers also should decide in advance whether to measure objective or subjective effects on health. For example, jobs high in physical demands may have more long-term objective impacts on health over time, while jobs low in mental demands may have more long-term subjective impacts on health.

A further issue related to outcomes was noted earlier; namely, that social integration in the form of social values and relationships is not only beneficial but may also generate stress. Social relationships and roles inevitably entail the possibility of interpersonal conflict, disappointment, dashed expectations, excessive demands, and conflicts of interests and commitments. Katz and Kahn (1978) developed one of the classic research formulations of this observation, applying it to the work setting. They pointed out that occupational integration carries the risk of overload (too much work), conflict (interpersonal conflict and expectational conflict), and ambiguity (lack of clarity in direction, or confusion). Some of these stresses result from "over-integration," as when an individual is subject to too many demands, too many expectations, or entrapment in an inappropriate role (Thoits, 1995). Research on providing care to aged and infirm relatives also highlights how role participation does not always lead to positive health outcomes (Moen et al., 1994).

In sum, these stresses flow from the truism that individual and group interests are often not the same. Role partners and constituent groups are not necessarily neutral in disputes or free of conflicting interest. Role partners are not always in egalitarian relationships. Role partners are sometimes not effective at communicating expectations and demands and sometimes not informed in their advice (Lehman et al., 1986). Social integration can thus result in negative outcomes.

METHODS FOR A NEW RESEARCH AGENDA

We hope that the discussion thus far has convinced readers that these issues are highly complex and present intriguing challenges for empirical investigators. In our view, the most fruitful path for advancing research on multiple roles, social integration, and health in later life is to combine the insights of qualitative research with data derived from empirically rigorous quantitative designs and analytic strategies (see also Thoits, 1995). We now turn to four empirical strategies for taking account of health-related selection when assessing the relationship between roles, social integration, and health. We examine the relative strengths and shortcomings of (1) collecting life history data relating to role participation and health; (2) the use of daily diary techniques; (3) quasi-experimental or "natural experiment" research; and (4) experimental interventions designed to improve social integration.

Retrospective Life History Data

The use of life history data may be particularly helpful for specifying the complex role of selection processes that channel the less mentally or physically healthy into fewer productive or less prestigious social roles. Researchers would be served best by using a blend of quantitative and qualitative techniques for such endeavors.

Large, multivariate retrospective quantitative life history surveys are particularly helpful in identifying patterns or sequences of social role trajectories over time. Large surveys such as these have identified particular combinations of roles over time that are associated with choices and decisions in later life and affect social integration (Moen, 1997; Moen et al., 1992). Retrospective research of this type can identify and describe patterns that are indicative of social selection. However, such research is not likely to identify the underlying causes of selecting one trajectory over another. Although respondents to such surveys can reliably recall major events and transitions (Kessler & Wethington, 1991), even from the relatively distant past (Brown & Harris, 1982), such recall applies only to *objective* events. Subjective states and aspects are most likely affected by recall or recency bias (Herbert & Cohen, 1996). They are also affected by selective processes in autobiographical memory (Rubin et al., 1998) and in the search for cause, or meaning, in past events (Ross & Newby-Clark, 1998). Thus, the data generated may be limited in important ways. Further research is needed on how autobiographical memory affects the recall of life history—an especially important issue for respondents in later life, who may be asked to recall much earlier events.

Longitudinal Data

Acknowledging the limitations of studying such a dynamic process as social integration in retrospective designs, researchers typically turn to longitudinal studies. Longitudinal studies are particularly useful when they are focused on groups predicted to be at very high risk of low social integration. One such group would be older workers nearing retirement during an economic downturn. Such workers are more likely to retire earlier than they anticipated or wished.

Longitudinal studies are particularly effective if they have collected data over a very long time from the same individuals. Multiple-year panel surveys are more likely to observe long-term changes in people's lives. They are also more likely to capture relatively rare role transitions, for example, divorce, remarriage, and widowhood for most individuals. A challenge for users of long-term studies, however, is that relatively few studies contain information that reflects more contemporary research questions on social integration and health.

Longitudinal studies can effectively address some questions regarding health and role participation, if the studies have useful measures addressing the causes of social selection. Using a control variable approach, researchers typically assume that by controlling for an earlier value of the psychological outcome they can adjust for initial differences between subjects who subsequently changed roles versus those who have not, thus obtaining an unbiased estimate of the impact of the role change (Wethington & Kessler, 1989). This procedure does not guarantee that selection bias is eliminated or reduced. It only eliminates bias under very restricted conditions, which are not often achieved.

In particular, these conditions are not achieved when examining role changes involving work or other relationships, where chronic role stress or poor relationship quality is associated with changes in role enactment (Thoits, 1994). A history of chronic difficulties poses a challenge to researchers: in such situations, stress and relationship problems cannot be assumed to be taking place independent of *prior* emotional health or ease of social interaction in general. There is considerable evidence that relationship difficulties and poor health in adulthood emanate from a history of relationship disorder (Mickelson et al., 1997). In other words, exposure to the conditions that cause role change may not be random with respect to the health outcome under investigation.

Longitudinal study of relationships across the life course would be enhanced if relationships rather than individuals were studied over time and from the point of view of more than one person in the relationship. The relationship, multiple-informant design is most common for studies of married couples, but it could be extended to include other dyadic or triadic relationships. Multiple-informant designs can be used to help overcome some of the difficulties that arise from memory bias, such as forgetting events (e.g., Kessler & Wethington, 1991).

Another strategy is to use the "catch up" sample, that is, re-interviewing respondents years later who were in a cross-sectional survey (see, for example, Moen et al., 1989). Other useful new designs for longitudinal studies of relationships are daily diary and experience-sampling methods of data collection (Eckenrode & Bolger, 1995). Both types of designs allow investigators to collect data on naturally occurring interactions in the environment, across time for the same individuals. Stress researchers have used these designs most extensively, but they are also well suited for studying short-term fluctuations in social support and participation patterns (Larson & Almeida, 1999).

Quasi-Experimental Designs

Although the use of the life history or daily diary approaches are likely to result in gathering much useful qualitative and quantitative naturalistic data on roles, stress, and health, these approaches are still inadequate in several important ways. To make strong arguments that role participation *per se* promotes social integration, a researcher needs to be able to establish that role participation is a "random" event. However, the trouble derives from the standard selection problem discussed throughout this chapter. Highly "integrated" people are given greater opportunity or acquire more skill to acquire productive and prestigious roles—from which, role theory suggests, people receive the most benefits. The concepts of "accumulation of disadvantage" and "healthy worker," although useful, theoretically coherent, and defensible ways of describing the reality of selection, do not readily yield to simultaneous statistical testing with role theory formulations. As has been described above in regard to retrospective life history data, the statistical issues surrounding endogeneity do not disappear. Role gain and loss that is "random" with respect to previous characteristics is hard to approximate even in the longitudinal survey.

An example of the difficulty relates to the interconnection of family roles and work roles across the life course. Women (and men) to some extent select the level of work-family stress to which they expose themselves. Selection into occupation is not a random event and depends in part on the skills acquired through education and family modeling (Kohn & Schooler, 1983). Nor is the selection of social relationships in adulthood random. For example, the acquisition of a demanding job may lead to foregoing parenthood altogether, and even marriage. Attitudes toward the relative importance of work versus family may have an impact on career or relationship trajectory (Gerson, 1985). Selecting a marital partner who supports the career, and would even shoulder the burden of family for a period of time, is critical to combining two careers in a household (Bielby & Bielby, 1992). Thus, a statistical control strategy would be inadequate in the face of such complexity. Suggestive answers would emerge from carefully analyzed data, but hard proof would still be lacking.

In the eyes of medically inclined researchers, the "gold standard" for assessing the impact of social integration on health lies in quasi-experimental studies. The two types considered here are natural experiments (matched comparisons) and intervention studies.

Natural Experiments. Natural experiments take advantage of a random event occurring to a group of people. The standard design includes a control group selected for demographic similarity to those who underwent the event. The success of this strategy depends upon the assumption of random exposure to the event. Thus the members of the control group should have been equally likely to experience the event as were members of the "treatment" group (or victims).

The major difficulty with the natural experiment is assuring that the condition of random exposure is met. For example, auto insurance rates indicate that young single males in urban areas tend to pay higher rates. This signals that the distribution of auto accidents is not random with respect to age, gender, region, and marital status. It may also indicate that auto theft is not random in respect to victim, a situation that may reflect the parallel tastes of young, single men and car thieves for particular car models.

The point is that selection processes can be very complicated, and that changes involving social integration probably cluster with the more complicated problems. Chapter 8 of this volume provides an example of a natural experiment in residential change, involving a longitudinal study of the social integration of community and retirement facility-dwelling older people. Participants were interviewed both before and after moving into the retirement facility.

The researchers (see Chapter 8) found that moving had an impact on social integration but that previous levels of social integration conditioned direction of the impact. Those persons with larger pre-existing social networks reported an increase in social participation, measured as the number of social roles in which the respondent reported some activity. Those with small pre-existing networks reported a decrease. Thus, the study points to a previously unknown selection factor that conditions change in the network, although it cannot identify precisely whether pre-existing attitudinal, behavioral, or situational factors matter most. Without the discovery of the selection factor, the researchers might have concluded that the "treatment" (moving into the facility) had no impact on levels of social participation and that moving had no more potential impact than staying in place.

Intervention Studies. Another design strategy to counter selection bias is experimental manipulation. Some researchers have successfully demonstrated that social support can have a positive impact on quality and length of life, even among the sickest patients (cf. Fawzy et al., 1995). Other supportive interventions, most particularly those to alleviate the suffering of end-of-life care, report more discouraging findings.

One explanation for the conflicting results is that social support interventions must provide content that is appropriate for the task and for the person being supported (Thoits, 1995). Most social support interventions to enhance health, however, provide a cafeteria of support options and provisions (Fawzy et al., 1995). As a group they are effective, but it is difficult to assess which of the many mini-interventions worked. (For a discussion of this issue, see Chapter 11, this volume.)

The major problem with making sweeping generalizations about the efficacy of different types of support interventions is that support is not randomly accepted and used. Accepting help is sometimes a difficult process that may threaten self-esteem and independence (Eckenrode & Wethington, 1990). If the support strategies in the intervention involve making use of available external assistance, and if respondents are randomly assigned, then one might accurately assess the impact of those strategies on health. If, however, the question is about more internally driven phenomena—such as whether the participant adopts different decision-making and affect-control strategies— then the impact might be to a great degree unobservable.

Thus, the evaluation of the relationship between social integration and health may, for the most part, rest upon non-observable activities. To evaluate the efficacy of social integration on health, policy makers and researchers may have to rely on less strict standards of proof than the experimental model.

CONCLUSION

In this chapter we identified several theoretical and empirical areas where measures of social integration, social support, and social and role participation require additional development. We also discussed research methods that, if more widely applied, might lead to substantial progress in assessing the relationship between social integration and health. Theory and research should move in tandem, by applying stronger research designs to test the implications of theory.

For example, Thoits (1995) called for researchers to make stronger differentiation between positive aspects of relationships (social support) and negative aspects (interpersonal difficulties). Contextual measures of social support, modeled on contextual measures of life events and difficulties (Brown & Harris, 1989), hold promise for advancing measurement in this area.

House and colleagues (1988) and Thoits (1995) also encouraged researchers to seek better theoretical understanding of how different functions of social support match to individual and situational needs. Contextual measures of social support provide a useful *exploratory* tool for building new theory relating the provision of support to health. However, researchers must follow this exploratory research with more scientifically rigorous experimental and intervention research.

Numerous theorists (e.g., House et al., 1988; Seeman et al., 1996; Thoits, 1995) have also called for the "reintegration" of individual-level social support theory with more traditional sociological research on how group or organizational involvement may promote the receipt of support or perceptions of available support in the environment. Longitudinal research based on the life-course perspective holds out the prospect of breaking new ground in this area. Research focused on relationships and groups over time, rather than solely on individuals, will also be an important tool in advancing theory.

REFERENCES

Almeida, D. M., Wethington, E., & Chandler, A. (1999). Daily transmission of tensions between marital dyads and parent-child dyads. *Journal of Marriage and the Family, 61*, 49–61.

Berkman, L., & Syme, L. (1979). Social networks, host resistance, and mortality: A nine-year follow-up study of Alameda County residents. *American Journal of Epidemiology, 109*, 186–204.

Bielby, W. T., & Bielby, D. (1992). I will follow him: Family ties, gender-role beliefs, and reluctance to relocate for a better job. *American Journal of Sociology, 97,* 1241–1267.

Bolger, N., DeLongis, A., Kessler, R. C., & Wethington, E. (1990). The microstructure of daily role-related stress in married couples. In J. Eckenrode & S. Gore (Eds.), *Stress between work and family* (95–115). New York: Plenum.

Bolger, N., & Eckenrode, J. (1991). Social relationships, personality, and anxiety during a major stressful event. *Journal of Personality and Social Psychology, 61,* 440–449.

Bowlby, J. (1969). *Attachment and loss.* New York: Basic.

Brown, G. W., & Harris, T. O. (1978). *Social origins of depression: A study of psychiatric disorder in women.* New York: Free Press.

Brown, G. W., & Harris, T. O. (1982). Fall-off in the reporting of life events. *Social Psychiatry, 17,* 23–28.

Brown, G. W., & Harris, T. O. (1989). *Life events and illness.* New York: Guilford.

Carr, D. (1998). The fulfillment of career dreams at midlife: Does it matter for women's mental health? *Journal of Health and Social Behavior, 38,* 331–344.

Coriell, M., & Cohen, S. (1995). Concordance in the face of a stressful event: When do members of a dyad agree that one person supported the other? *Journal of Personality and Social Psychology, 69,* 289–299.

Cutrona, C. E. (1986). Behavioral manifestations of social support: A microanalytic investigation. *Journal of Personality and Social Psychology, 51,* 201–208.

Cutrona, C. E., Cohen, B., & Ingram, S. (1990). Contextual determinants of the perceived supportedness of helping behaviors. *Journal of Social and Personal Relationships, 7,* 553–562.

Durkheim, E. (1951). *Suicide: A study in sociology.* J. A. Spaulding & G. Simpson (Trans.) New York: Free Press.

Eckenrode, J. E., & Bolger, N. (1995). Daily and within-day event measurement. In S. Cohen, R. C. Kessler, & L. U. Gordon (Eds.), *Measuring stress: A guide for health and social scientists* (80–101). New York: Oxford University Press.

Eckenrode, J., & Wethington, E. (1990). The process of mobilizing social support. In S. Duck & R. Silver (Eds.), *Personal relationships and social support* (83–103). Beverly Hills: Sage.

Fawzy, F. I., Fawzy, N., Arndt, L., & Pasnau, R. O. (1995). Critical review of psychosocial interventions in cancer care. *Archives of General Psychiatry, 52,* 100–113.

George, L. K. (1993). Sociological perspectives on life transitions. *Annual Review of Sociology, 19,* 353–373.

George, L. K. (1996a). Social factors and illness. In R. H. Binstock & L. K. George (Eds.), *Handbook of aging and the social sciences,* 4th ed. (229–252). San Diego: Academic Press.

George, L. K. (1996b). Missing links: The case for a social psychology of the life course. *The Gerontologist, 36,* 248–255.

Gerson, K. (1985). *Hard choices: How women decide about work, career, and motherhood.* Berkeley: University of California Press.

Giele, J. K., & Elder, G. H., Jr. (1998). *Methods of life course research: Qualitative and quantitative approaches.* Thousand Oaks, CA: Sage.

Goode, W. R. (1960). A theory of role strain. *American Sociological Review, 25,* 483–495.

Harlow, R. E., & Cantor, N. (1995). To whom do people turn when things go poorly? Task orientation and functional social contacts. *Journal of Personality and Social Psychology, 69,* 329–340.

Haynes, S. G., & Feinlieb, M. (1980). Women, work, and coronary heart disease: Prospective findings from the Framingham Heart Study. *American Journal of Public Health, 70,* 133–141.

Herbert, T., & Cohen, S. (1996). Measurement issues in research on psychosocial stress. In H. B. Kaplan (Ed.), *Psychosocial stress: Perspectives on structure, theory, life course, and methods* (295–332). New York: Academic Press.

House, J. S., Umberson, D., & Landis, K. R. (1988). Structures and processes of social support. *Annual Review of Sociology, 14,* 293–318.

Katz, D., & Kahn, R. L. (1978). *The social psychology of organizations.* New York: Wiley.

Kessler, R. C., & McLeod, J. D. (1985). Social support and mental health in community samples. In S. Cohen & L. Syme (Eds.), *Social support and health* (219–240). New York: Academic Press.

Kessler, R. C., & Wethington, E. (1991). The reliability of life event reports in a community survey. *Psychological Medicine, 21,* 723–738.

Kohn, M. L., & Schooler, C. (1983). *Work and personality: An inquiry into the impact of social stratification.* Norwood, NJ: Ablex Publishing.

Larson, R. D., & Almeida, D. M. (1999). Emotional transmission in the daily lives of families: A new paradigm for studying family process. *Journal of Marriage and the Family, 61,* 5–20.

Lehman, D. R., Ellard, J. H., & Wortman, C. B. (1986). Social support for the bereaved: Recipients' and providers' perspectives on what is helpful. *Journal of Consulting and Clinical Psychology, 54,* 438–446.

Lepore, S. (1995). Measurement of chronic stressors. In S. Cohen, R. C. Kessler, & L. U. Gordon (Eds.), *Measuring stress: A guide for health and social scientists* (102–120). New York: Oxford University Press.

Link, B. G., & Phelan, J. (1995). Social conditions as fundamental causes of disease. *Journal of Health and Social Behavior, Extra Issue,* 80–94.

Linville, P. W. (1987). Self-complexity as a cognitive buffer against stress-related illness and depression. *Journal of Personality and Social Psychology, 52,* 663–676.

Lowenthal, M. F., & Haven, C. (1968). Interaction and adaptation: Intimacy as a critical variable. *American Sociological Review, 33,* 20–30.

Messeri, P., Silverstein, M., & Litwak, E. (1993). Choosing optimal support groups: A review and reformulation. *Journal of Health and Social Behavior, 34,* 122–137.

Mickelson, K. D., Kessler, R. C., & Shaver, P. R. (1997). Adult attachment in a nationally representative sample. *Journal of Personality and Social Psychology, 73,* 1092–1106.

Moen, P. (1992). *Women's two roles: A contemporary dilemma.* Dover, MA: Auburn House.

Moen, P. (1997). Women's roles and resilience: Trajectories of advantage or turning points? In I. H. Gotlib & B. Wheaton (Eds.), *Stress and adversity over the life course: Trajectories and turning points* (133–156). New York: Cambridge University Press.

Moen, P., Dempster-McClain, D. I., & Williams, R. M. (1989). Social integration and longevity: An event history analysis of women's roles and resilience. *American Sociological Review, 54,* 635–647.

Moen, P., Dempster-McClain, D. I., & Williams, R. M. (1992). Successful aging: A life course perspective on women's roles and health. *American Journal of Sociology, 97,* 1612–1638.

Moen, P., Robison, J., & Fields, V. (1994). Women's work and caregiving roles: A life course approach. *Journals of Gerontology: Social Sciences, 49,* S176–S186.

Moen, P., & Wethington, E. (1992). The concept of family adaptive strategies. *Annual Review of Sociology, 18,* 233–251.

O'Neil, R., & Greenberger, E. (1994). Patterns of commitment to work and parenting: Implications for role strain. *Journal of Marriage and the Family, 56,* 101–118.

Parkes, C. T., & Weiss, R. S. (1983). *Recovery from bereavement.* New York: Basic.

Riley, M. W., Kahn, R. L., & Foner, A. (1994). *Aging and structural lag: Society's failure to provide meaningful opportunities in work, family, and leisure.* New York: Wiley.

Rook, K. S., & Schuster. T. L. (1996). Compensatory processes in the social networks of older adults. In G. R. Pierce, B. R. Sarason, & I. G. Sarason (Eds.), *Handbook of social support and the family* (219–248). New York: Plenum.

Ross, M., & Newby-Clark, I. (1998). Construing the past and the future. *Social Cognition, 16,* 133–150.

Rubin, D., Rahal, T. A., & Poon, L. W. (1998). Things remembered in early adulthood are remembered best. *Memory and Cognition, 26,* 3–19.

Sarason, B. A., Sarason, I. G., & Pierce, G. R. (1990). *Social support: An interactional view.* New York: Wiley.

Seeman, T. E., Bruce, M. L., & McAvay, G. J. (1996). Social network characteristics and onset of ADL disability: MacArthur studies of successful aging. *Journals of Gerontology: Social Sciences, 51B,* S191–S200.

Sieber, S. (1974). Toward a theory of role accumulation. *American Sociological Review, 39,* 567–578.

Thoits, P. A. (1986). Multiple identities: Examining gender and marital status differences in distress. *American Sociological Review, 51,* 259–272.

Thoits, P. A. (1994). Stressors and problem-solving: The individual as psychological activist. *Journal of Health and Social Behavior, 35,* 143–160.

Thoits, P. A. (1995). Stress, coping, and social support processes: Where are we? What next? *Journal of Health and Social Behavior, Extra Issue,* 53–79.

Umberson, D. (1987). Family status and health behaviors: Social control as a dimension of social integration. *Journal of Health and Social Behavior, 28,* 306–319.

Umberson, D., Chen, M. D., House, J. S., Hopkins, K., & Slaten, E. (1996). The effect of social relationships on psychological well-being: Are men and women really so different? *American Sociological Review, 61,* 837–857.

Verbrugge, L. (1983). Multiple roles and the physical health of men and women. *Journal of Health and Social Behavior, 24,* 16–30.

Vilhjalmsson, R. (1993). Life stress, social support, and clinical depression: A reanalysis of the literature. *Social Science and Medicine, 37,* 331–342.

Welch, S., & Booth, A. (1977). Employment and health among married women with children. *Sex Roles, 3,* 385–397.

Wethington, E., & Kessler, R. C. (1986). Perceived support, received support, and adjustment to stressful life events. *Journal of Health and Social Behavior, 27,* 78–89.

Wethington, E., & Kessler, R. C. (1989). Employment, parenting responsibility, and psychological distress: A longitudinal study of married women. *Journal of Family Issues, 10,* 527–546.

Wethington, E., & Kessler, R. C. (1993). Neglected methodological issues in employment stress. In B. Long & S. Kahn (Eds.), *Women, work and coping: A multidisciplinary approach to workplace stress* (269–295). Montreal: McGill-Queens.

PART TWO

SOCIAL INTEGRATION IN MAJOR DOMAINS OF LATER LIFE

A Life-Course Approach to Retirement and Social Integration

Phyllis Moen, Vivian Fields, Heather E. Quick, and Heather Hofmeister

In this chapter we use a life-course approach to analyze social integration following the transition to retirement. Retirement is an interesting case through which to view social integration, since it is a key status transition, one that underscores the dynamic processes of development and change in social roles over the life span. In fact, one useful way of depicting the life course is as a series of movements in and out of various roles (Elder et al., 1996), with retirement representing later-life withdrawal from the work force. Increasingly, scholars define retirement as leaving one's primary career job (although, as we discuss later in this chapter, it may be accompanied by post-retirement employment at another job). Does this role exit mean that the new retiree is in danger of social isolation, or do other role involvements replace that of not-yet-retired worker?

With age, formal institutional roles (such as that of career employee) decline, whereas ambiguous and informal roles become prominent. Retirement is just such an informal tenuous role, with no clear social functions (Rosow, 1985). Does being retired have a deleterious effect on psychological well-being? By drawing on a life-course perspective, we focus on pathways of social integration, considering the community participation of both older (not-yet-retired) workers and retirees, and the influences of social context, timing, and the process of change for social integration and well-being in the retirement years. Missing in many studies of well-being in the second half of life is any focus on unpaid social participation in volunteer work and in community organizations. Such participation in clubs and volunteer work may replace paid employment as a key means of social integration in retirement.

We first discuss important life-course themes, including the need to conceptualize *pathways* to social integration following retirement, going on to conceptualize both social integration and the nature of the retirement status passage. Then we draw on data from the *Cornell Retirement and Well-Being Study* to provide insights into the implications of the retirement transition for social integration for those who are retired in the 1990s.

LIFE-COURSE THEMES

Three life-course themes are crucial for understanding the interplay between social integration, retirement, and the links between the two: *process, timing,* and *context.*

Process

"Process" refers to the various pathways that lead to change; it concerns the multiple ways we can get from point A to point B. Specifically, retirement is a series of role transitions rather than a single event. Neither is retirement necessarily a one-way exit from the labor force; it may mean entering a second or third career in either paid or unpaid work (Han & Moen, 1999; Moen, 1998a, b). And it may or may not be accompanied by lifestyle changes in activities, routines, and well-being.

Process draws attention to role *trajectories,* the ways roles are played out over the life course. For example, the family life cycle reflects a blend of continuity and change in roles, resources, relationships, and relevant identities over the life course and across the transition to retirement. Moreover, this blend is frequently different for men and women. An important proposition of life-course analysis is that an understanding of one life phase (such as retirement) requires it to be placed in the larger context of life pathways. And being male or female shapes the nature, organization, and patterning of family, work, and community roles throughout life (Moen, 2000). Do men's and women's prior role biographies or current family roles affect their community integration in retirement?

A life-course formulation suggests that early experiences matter, that to understand life in retirement requires knowledge of the prior life course. But in some cases, what may matter most is *current*, not *past*, resources and relationships. For example, does knowing about the job individuals retired from help in estimating the likelihood of post-retirement employment, membership in clubs, or volunteer participation? Or do current circumstances (such as age, health, marital status, income, and whether there are children at home) explain levels of paid and unpaid social participation?

Process points to the interdependency between work, family, and community attachments, as well as the interdependency between the lives of different family members. Thus, individuals have lives that are, more often than not, *linked lives*, across time and across generations (Elder et al., 1996; Moen 2000). Retirement, family roles, community participation, and occupational careers are typically examined exclusive of other social roles and of each other. What we do not know is how work and family experiences shape life after retirement.

Timing

The life-course perspective emphasizes the importance of timing, of looking beyond simply *whether* or not a transition occurs, to *when* transitions (such as retirement) occur (Elder et al., 1996). Role entries or exits that are "off time" (i.e., earlier or later than is socially prescribed) may be more stressful or disruptive than "on-time" role transitions (George, 1993). Thus those who retire "early" or "late" may experience retirement very differently from those who retire closer to the traditional retirement age norm.

How long individuals have been retired may also have important implications for their activities, perceptions, and well-being. Someone who just retired may have very different experiences than someone who has been retired for many years.

The literature on aging and the life course (Elder et al., 1996; Moen, 1996a, 2000; Riley et al., 1988) has sensitized researchers to the multiple meanings of age. First, age is an indicator of changes in biological and psychological functioning that set limits on social behavior. Changes in older workers' health, for example, can affect both the timing of their retirement and their ability to engage in family, social, and community activities.

Second, age is an important determinant of people's social roles, independent of their capacities and preferences, and is reflected in what Riley (1987) refers to as the *age stratification system*. For example, culturally grounded norms and frames shape individual expectations and beliefs about the "right" time to retire (Hagestad & Neugarten, 1985; Neugarten et al., 1965; Rook et al., 1989) and about "appropriate" activities in retirement.

Third, at a given time, age is an indicator of birth-cohort membership and of life experiences shared with other members of that cohort (Ryder, 1965). The retirement experiences of each generation are always unique, leading to different goals, expectations, and lifestyles in retirement.

Context

Context refers to the unique environment that shapes the individual life course, including the retirement experience. The personal circumstances of retirees—whether they graduated from college, whether they are married, whether they have children at home, as well as the employment and health status of their spouses—may have important implications for their social integration in retirement.

Gender is a key variable setting the context of lives, reflecting not only physiological differences but also unique family, occupational, and historical circumstances (Moen, 1995, 1996a, b, 2000). For example, traditional gender roles, which allocate the informal caregiving of our society to women as wives, mothers, and daughters, mean that because women take time out for family responsibilities, they are less advantaged than men in terms of pensions, social security, and other financial resources in retirement (Quadagno, 1995). They are also apt to be caregiving for ailing relatives (Moen et al., 1994). One would anticipate men's and women's markedly different expectations, obligations, and opportunities throughout their lives as well as in their later years to shape their social integration in retirement.

Unanticipated and crisis events, such as widowhood or a major illness, may render retirees particularly vulnerable to social isolation. Even planned events, such as retirement itself, can have wide-ranging and unexpected impacts.

CONCEPTUALIZING PATHWAYS TO SOCIAL INTEGRATION IN THE RETIREMENT YEARS

A life-course approach to retirement and social integration requires the fleshing out of the various dimensions embodied in the notion of occupational "career" that culminates in the retirement transition. Career pathways can be conceptualized in a variety of ways (Barley, 1989; Pavalko et al., 1993). One way is in terms of a *series of positions,* an orderly and hierarchical progression (Slocum, 1967). Individuals experiencing uneven or downward pathways as employees may be focused more on their family and social roles, smoothing the way for life after retirement.

A second way of viewing career trajectories is in terms of their relative *continuity.* Thus, individuals may move in and out of the labor force, in and out of various types of jobs in the years prior to retirement. Women who started their careers in mid-life after raising their families may be less happy with retiring from the work world than are men who have worked throughout adulthood. Men may want to leave their jobs, whereas women may feel they have more yet to contribute.

A third career dimension has to do with the *objective conditions of work.* Professionals or managers often hold jobs offering a great deal of intrinsic satisfaction (in the form of autonomy, for example). At the same time, such high status occupations are frequently "greedy" occupations, requiring extensive time and emotional commitments, thus potentially limiting social involvement throughout life. Research has shown that the opportunities for challenging work, as well as occupational uncertainty, affect workers' values, abilities, and outlook for themselves and their children (Kohn, 1995). Do work characteristics spill over into retirement, affecting the likelihood of social involvement following retirement?

Yet a fourth dimension involves *subjective expectations,* for example, the implicit "contracts" between employers and employees, as well as between family members regarding division of labor (at home and at work), job security, and job progression. These "contracts" may shape the retirement experience. For example, retirees who were forced to retire earlier than they had expected to may be more isolated in retirement.

These four (interrelated) dimensions of occupational careers have analogues in *family* careers. In families, individuals fill a *series of positions* over the life course; they experience *continuity* in their relationships under specific *objective conditions,* such as the presence of children at home, whether the spouse is in or out of the labor force, and the pre-retirement division of household labor. Individuals are also influenced by *subjective expectations* within their families, such as gender role attitudes, ideas about the appropriate timing of family events, and marital quality. Both family and work characteristics affect social involvement throughout life, including the degree and kind of social participation in retirement.

Education may also shape life in retirement. Educational credentials, status in the occupational hierarchy, and family status are central components of *cultural capital,* affecting habits, choices, preferences, and strategies of action (Bourdieu, 1984; Breiger, 1995) and consequently the "tool kit" (Swidler, 1986) of skills and strategies brought to the retirement years.

ADAPTING TO THE "CRISIS" OF RETIREMENT

A *crisis* has been defined as a sudden and frequently unexpected gap between claims (or needs) and resources (Elder, 1974; Moen et al., 1983). Retirement, for some, is just such a crisis, especially for those "downsized" in their fifties. And even for those who retire in their sixties, facing the next thirty years with no clear road map to other forms of productive engagement can be daunting, in part because of the structural lag in institutionalized roles for retirees (Riley et al., 1994). The discrepancy between what is required, expected, or counted on, on the one hand, and the realities of situational and structural exigencies, on the other, can produce a stressful environment fostering emotional tensions and strain. This stress can be reduced either by reducing claims and/or changing available options and resources; social integration may be a crucial piece of this puzzle. What is key is that retirees have both objective resources available to them and a subjective sense of control.

Retirement involves a range of strategies and adaptations. These can be categorized as (a) changes in the *family economy,* (b) alterations in *roles* and *relationships,* and (c) efforts to cope with *tensions* and *strains.*

Changes in the Family Economy

The notion of the family economy is crucial to understanding decision-making regarding retirement (Moen & Wethington, 1992); choices about retirement—and life after retirement—are made in light of family resources and subjective assessments. Retirement is both an individual and a family transition (Kim & Moen, 2000a, b; Moen et al., 2000; Smith & Moen, 1998). Whether or not an individual retires is related to a number of family contingencies, such as household income, family members' health, and the ages of husbands, wives, and children. But family roles and relationships are shaped by gender. Given their historically more tangential and interrupted ties to the workforce (Brinton, 1988; Moen, 1992; Tomaskovic-Devey, 1993; Wolf & Fligstein, 1979), women may be both less likely to have experienced an "orderly" career progression (along the four dimensions described above) and more likely to have put family ahead of their careers (Han & Moen 1999; Moen 1998a). It is not clear how men's and women's distinctive life paths affect their social integration in retirement.

Health and age are other key considerations, affecting both the timing of retirement and the likelihood of working as a contract worker or in a second career after retirement (Burkhauser & Quinn, 1989, 1990; Chirikos & Nestel, 1989; DeViney & O'Rand, 1988; Palmore et al., 1985). Caregiving for an ill or infirm relative may provide incentive for a retiree to retire early, while still having children in the home may delay retirement. Health, age, and caregiving responsibilities may also affect social integration following retirement.

Following the retirement transition, retirees may change their expenditure patterns, move to other homes or areas of the country, or seek other jobs. Their spouses may also change the amount of time they put in on the job or may themselves retire (Moen et al., 2000). Whether family members take on or leave paid work may be triggered by changes in health or financial circumstances or lifestyle changes. Thus, adaptations to retirement typically reflect a series of strategies, a process unfolding over time, rather than a single event.

Alterations in Roles and Relationships

Since changes in employment and unemployment have been shown to alter decision-making power and patterns of family interaction (Moen et al., 1983; Turner et al., 1995), it is logical to expect that the retirement transition would similarly affect relationships with family members, friends, and neighbors as well as one's community participation. Retirement increases the time the retired spouse spends at home, changes couples' expectations about the household division of labor, and (usually temporarily) causes frustration until new roles are established (Ekerdt & Vinick, 1991).

Although contact with coworkers is apt to be markedly curtailed, other social ties may increase following retirement. Within the family unit, one possibility is that other family members also change their roles, with, for example, one's spouse retiring as well. Retirees may also increase their time and emotional investment in their neighbors, church, or community, strengthening or creating social ties that they did not have time or energy for prior to retirement. The job one retires from may also affect subsequent social relationships, such as participation in retiree clubs and other organizations. We know very little about the continuity and change in relations with friends and former coworkers. In the *Cornell Retirement and Well-Being Study*, described below, we found that "missing coworkers" was, by far, the most often cited disadvantage of retirement. Fully 72 percent of retired respondents mentioned this as a concern. Family members, friends, and coworkers have been described as "a convoy of social support" (Antonucci, 1994), moving through life together, but it is not clear how this "convoy" changes when one or both spouses retire. Neither do we know whether participation in clubs and organizations or in volunteer work become substitutes for paid work following retirement.

Coping with Tensions and Strains

Whether changes in roles or relationships accompanying the retirement transition are stressful depends on their centrality and meaning (Thoits, 1995; Wheaton, 1990). Whether retirement affects a person's sense of psychological self-worth and well-being may well depend on the degree of planning regarding the retirement transition, its timing, and the reasons why the individual is retiring. It also may depend on the degree of social integration following retirement. Research has shown that psychological well-being in the retirement years is associated with the social, psychological, and economic resources that individuals bring to the retirement transition (Moen et al., 1992; Moen, 1997).

For example, economic capital matters. When retirement brings a major drop in income and little savings, one could expect an increase in ambiguity and apprehension concerning the future. Similarly, social capital—personal resources gained from social experiences and connections—is important as well. Those retirees who are involved in clubs and volunteer work may well be the most self-reliant individuals. A logical adaptive response for those retiring from an unsatisfactory job might be to disengage from the work role, placing greater emphasis on community ties as a source of emotional support.

Others may "cope" with any strains generated by retirement by seeking relief in hobbies, exercise, or other forms of leisure activity. We know little about the styles of coping adopted by retirees, but we do know that those who are most isolated are the most vulnerable to psychological distress in their retirement years, pointing to the importance of social integration.

ILLUSTRATIVE EXAMPLES

In the remainder of this chapter we draw on data from the *Cornell Retirement and Well-Being Study* to examine (1) the nature of social integration in retirement, (2) pathways to social integration, and (3) implications of social integration for the well-being of those retiring in the 1980s and 1990s. We consider the interrelationship of retirement, integration, and well-being in terms of gender as well as in the context of retirement timing and choice, past experiences (especially career trajectory and the characteristics of the job one is retiring from), subjective meanings and definitions, and situational exigencies and possibilities.

The *Cornell Retirement and Well-Being Study* investigates factors that promote productive lives following retirement. Respondents were drawn from six large employers in upstate New York: two Fortune 500 firms, a university, two hospitals, and a public utility. The sample includes 762 men and women, aged 50–72, from all occupational levels. Sixty percent of the participants were already retired from their career jobs at the time of the first interview in 1994–95. The average age of the retirees is 62, and the average age of the not-yet-retired group is 56. Respondents were asked about their health, their work and volunteer activities, as well as relationships with family, friends, and the community.

We draw on these data to look at the relationships between social integration, retirement, and well-being. First, speaking to the assumption that men and women who are retired are in greater danger of social isolation than are men and women who are actively employed (Rosow, 1974, 1985), we ask, *Are retired men and women less socially integrated than employed men and women in the same age group?*

Second, vulnerability and risk factors are not evenly distributed. Prior research has documented the importance of location in the social structure for psychological vulnerability (e.g., Thoits 1986). Accordingly, we ask, *Who is socially integrated? What family and background characteristics are associated with community participation in retirement?*

Third, we investigate the relationship between social integration and *psychological* integration: *Do retired men and women with family, social, and community role involvements perceive themselves as less isolated?* And finally, what is the impact of social integration and perceptions on later life quality? Evidence suggests that most men and women *enjoy* their retirement years (Quick & Moen, 1998; Secombe & Lee, 1986; Jewson, 1982). Is this due to their continuing social integration? *What is the relationship between both social integration and psychological integration and well-being in retirement?*

Does Being Retired Mean Less Integration?

From the perspective of age stratification (Riley et al., 1994) and role theory (Ebaugh, 1988; Merton, 1968; Rosow, 1967), the retirement transition is less a transition *to* than a transition *from*, with the leaving of one's career job a central and consequential role exit in terms of both identity and status. Is it also inevitably correlated with reduced social participation in the broader community? Baltes and Baltes (1990) describe the process of aging as one of *selective accommodation*, with certain activities and behaviors gaining new prominence even as others fade. But we know very little about the selective accommodation following retirement (Featherman et al., 1990). Do family roles take on new significance in the face of retirement from career jobs? Does community participation in clubs and organizations or in volunteering replace employment following retirement? Were retirees in the 1990s likely to take on second or third careers following their retirement? What is the relative adjustment of men and women to retirement? Given their traditional focus on family roles and relationships, is retirement from the career job "easier" for women than men? Using

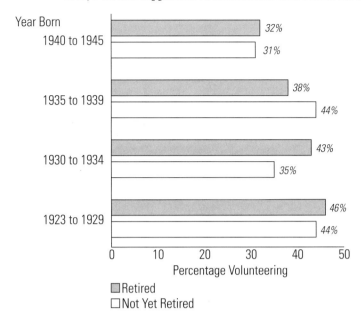

Figure 3.1   Volunteering by Birth Cohort and Retirement Status. *Source: Cornell Retirement and Well-Being Study,* Wave 1 (1994–1995), N = 762. *Note:* Differences by retirement status only, p = .08; differences by cohort only: p = .03.

data from the *Cornell Retirement and Well-Being Study,* we attempt to shed light on these questions.

Volunteerism. One potentially important role in retirement is that of community volunteer. In our sample, volunteering actually increases with age (see Figure 3.1). Retirees in the *Cornell Retirement and Well-Being Study* in their sixties and early seventies are more likely to be volunteering than retirees in their fifties. (Because the data we are using are cross-sectional, we cannot draw conclusions about whether these differences are true retirement age differences or are, in fact, cohort differences. It may be that the differing historical contexts that each cohort experienced have differential impacts upon attitudes toward volunteerism. Alternatively, people may be more likely to volunteer as the newness of retirement wears off and they feel the need to include more productive activity in their lives.)

Although there is a tendency for retirees in our sample to volunteer more than those who are not yet retired (37% vs. 43%; p = .08), the real difference between the two groups is in the amount of time spent volunteering. Those who are not yet retired typically volunteer about twelve hours per month, while retirees average about twenty-one hours per month (p = .002).

Are there any differences in volunteer participation by gender? Herzog and colleagues (1989) found that older women were slightly more likely than older men to participate in volunteer work. They found the greatest divergence in the 55–64 age group, with two fifths (40.3%) of women volunteering compared to only a third (33%) of men. About equal proportions of men and women in their 65–74 age group sample reported volunteering (39.1% to 39.8%), with 27 percent of women over 75 in their sample volunteering, compared to 25.4 percent of men. In our *Cornell Retirement and Well-Being Study* we have not found such gender differences in volunteering among those in their fifties, sixties, and early seventies, possibly because our sample represents men and women who are more similar in that both have held or are currently holding full-time jobs. (Thus women who are primarily housewives are, by definition, not in this sample.)

We also investigated participation in religion as another form of formal social integration. In our Cornell study, looking first at men, we observe nearly identical rates of religious participation among retirees and those not yet retired; in the sample of women, we find that retirees attend church significantly more than those who are not yet retired (57% vs. 46%). The proportion of retired women who feel religion is "very important" to their lives also tends to be higher (60%) than it is for the not-yet-retired women (52%; p = .097).

Men and women retirees in our sample do not differ significantly in rates of club membership from those who are not yet retired. In retirement, however, men are more apt to be members of clubs and organizations than are women (62% vs. 52%).

Though fewer retirees than those who are not-yet-retired describe themselves as "very busy" (43% vs. 63%), they do not necessarily use the extra time they have available in community involvement.

Paid Work. Whether or not retirees are engaged in paid work following their retirement depends on their age. Almost half (49%) of 50–59 year old males are employed after retirement from their career jobs. Among women in their fifties, the figure is lower but still amounts to 39 percent. However, even among this relatively young group of retirees, only one fourth of the men and about a fifth of the women are working full time.

When we look at retirees aged 60–72, the employment levels drop considerably. While more than one quarter (27%) of the men and one-fifth (20%) of the women in this age group are still working for pay, very few (just 11% of the men and only 5% of the women in their sixties and early seventies) are working full time. This prevalence of part-time employment among retirees suggests that those who work for pay following their "formal" retirement from their primary career jobs experience a change in the subjective experience of the role of worker.

Some employed post retirement are working as consultants or have temporary employment. Others have taken jobs with less economic and social prestige than their career employment offered. (One former engineer opened up a hot dog stand.) The majority of retirees lose the important role of paid full-time worker, whether they work after retirement or not. Is this loss of role accompanied by a diminishment in other roles? For example, does the retired individual tend to disengage from social participation in their communities, or does the retiree compensate for the loss of their career jobs by substituting other forms of social involvement?

Informal and Family Roles. Gender is a key factor in shaping family experiences of older adults. For example, only 58 percent of the women retirees in our sample are married, compared to 88 percent of the men retirees. Those men and women who are not retired are more apt to be married (89% of the men and 65% of the women). Higher survival rates among older women, combined with the greater likelihood that men marry younger women and are more apt to remarry, means that fewer women than men are married during this stage of life. Retired women are also significantly more likely to be widowed than their not-yet-retired counterparts.

Retirees are less likely than the not yet retired to have children living at home (19.5% vs. 36.5%), even after controlling for age. It may well be that older workers with children still at home have financial obligations that prevent them from retiring. There are gender differences in the parenting role as well, with men (both older workers and retirees) more likely than women to have children at home. Only 23 percent of retired men and 15 percent of retired women have children at home (as opposed to 42% of not-yet-retired men, and 32% of women who are not yet retired). This is both because men in this sample have their children at a later age than do the women ($p = .000$), and those who remarry are more likely than women in this age group to start new families.

There is no significant difference by retirement status in the percentage of the sample involved in caregiving for aged or infirm relatives. Among retirees, women provide care at higher rates (29%) than do retired men (17%), and women are much more likely to be caring for a spouse (5.2%) than are men (.4%). Retired women are also involved in intensive caregiving (defined as caregiving for 10 hours or more per week) at three times the rate of retired men (10% of the women vs. 3.3% of the men; p = .004). Among not-yet-retired men and women, there is no significant difference in intensive caregiving. Our data reinforce the findings of other research that older women are more likely than older men to be active in caregiving and to have caregiving impact their work lives (Allen, 1990; Brody, 1985, 1989; Horowitz, 1985; Moen et al., 1994; Pavalko & Artis, 1997; Qureshi & Walker, 1989).

Retirees in our sample are more apt to be grandparents than those not yet retired (76% vs. 51%; p = .000), which is not surprising given their age. What is surprising is that among both men and women in their fifties, retirees are more apt to be grandparents (59%) than are those in the same age category who are not yet retired (46%).

Retired women in our sample are more involved in a number of informal and family-related roles than are those who are not yet retired. Retired women are more likely to visit relatives regularly (75% vs. 65%; p = .03) and to be caregivers for spouses than their non-retired counterparts (5% vs. 1.2%; p = .04). Retired women are also more likely than the not yet retired to frequently visit their neighbors (65% to 50%; p = .004).

In terms of multiple roles (worker, volunteer, club member, neighbor, etc.), men are more apt to occupy more social roles whether they are not yet retired (on average, 6.06 roles for men to 5.54 roles for women) or retired (on average, retired men hold 5.97 roles compared to 5.36 for women). Though some roles are lost with retirement, overall retired men and women do not seem to be suffering from social isolation.

Who Is Likely to Be Integrated in Retirement?

A life-course focus on the retirement transition suggests that we must look beyond simply whether retirement is associated with less social integration to the more complex question of mapping the *pathways* to social integration among the retired. In looking at women who were wives and mothers in the 1950s, Moen et al. (1992) found that both social integration and prior psychological resources promoted subsequent integration thirty years later (see also Moen, 1997). Here we investigate the factors promoting social integration in the retirement years, considering especially health, educational level, and characteristics of the "career" job. In addition to family ties, there is a long history (beginning with Durkheim) emphasizing the importance of social participation in the broader community. Accordingly, we draw on the *Cornell Retirement and Well-Being Study* to assess the pathways to such participation in the form of post-retirement work, volunteer work, club membership, and social hobbies.

Retirement and Health

First, health is an important component of a positive retirement experience (Quick & Moen, 1998; Martin Matthews & Brown, 1988; Atchley, 1976). Though poor health is frequently a reason for retiring (Anderson & Burkhauser, 1985; Bound, 1991; Chirikos & Nestel, 1989; Palmore et al., 1985), most of the existing research literature has shown that retirement per se is not directly related to early mortality or health decline. An early longitudinal study (Streib & Schneider, 1971) found that retirement had no impact on health. In fact, retired individuals sometimes report improvements in their health status following retirement. Most early research on retirement suggests that being retired has no deleterious effects on either physical or psychological health; most retirees say they are satisfied with their retirement, and some even report better health (Atchley, 1976; Barfield & Morgan, 1969). Other research finds that retired individuals may engage in healthy behaviors such as exercising more often.

In the *Cornell Retirement and Well-Being Study* we find that those who cited "poor health" as part of their reason for retirement are, in fact, less likely to participate in the community than those who indicated that poor health was "not at all important" in their retirement decisions. Those retirees who cited health problems as having an effect on their decision to retire are significantly less likely to be working (20% to 31%; $p = .032$), to be participating actively in religious institutions (42% to 56%; $p = .019$) or to be members of clubs (47% vs. 57%; $p = .031$). But while poor health has a deleterious effect on participation, even those who retired because of "poor health" participate at relatively high levels.

Past and Current Roles and Resources

Do we see a cumulation of advantage or disadvantage by social status, in the sense that retirees having more education or retiring from high status jobs are more apt to remain fully involved in their communities? Or are those retiring from low status, less engaging work the most likely to have developed community ties? This issue relates to the whole life-course question of the impact of earlier life experiences on subsequent integration. To address whether prior circumstances and interests matter, we draw on two types of data: (1) the factors associated with post-retirement employment, volunteering, club or organizational membership, and social hobbies; and (2) the implications of role salience and reasons for retirement for subsequent integration.

We do see evidence of a cumulation of advantage with regard to education. Those retirees with college degrees are more apt to be employed, volunteering, and club or organization members following retirement.

In fact, the only role that is higher for those with less education is being a grandparent, with 85 percent of retirees with only a high school education having grandchildren, compared to only 64 percent of retirees holding college degrees. In examining the data from the *Cornell Retirement and Well-Being Study,* Quick and Moen (1998) found a number of factors affecting social participation. First, both education and having held a professional job are important correlates to employment following retirement and, for men, to unpaid volunteer work as well. For women, having had a professional occupation is positively related to all forms of post-retirement social participation: paid work, unpaid volunteering, belonging to a club, engaging in social hobbies. For men, but not women, good health is also key to post-retirement employment. And good health matters for participation in social hobbies, regardless of gender.

Although retirement does not seem to be related to fewer family involvements, in some cases they may inhibit social participation in the broader community. For example, being a grandparent, living near grandchildren, visiting relatives often, and enjoying time with their family are all *negatively* related to men's working for pay following retirement. Having children still living at home is negatively related to retired women's engagement in social hobbies, and grandmothers are less likely to volunteer than are women who do not have grandchildren. These family involvements might actually be experienced as constraints on time and energy that would be needed for social participation outside of the home. Thus, retirement may foster two alternative paths to social integration—one focusing on family ties, and one focusing on community participation, with individuals typically investing in family *or* community roles in retirement, but not both.

Preparation and Timing

Pre-retirement planning and preparation seem to have a different relationship to retired men's and women's social participation. First, men who planned for retirement are less likely to be working after retirement. Men who discussed their plans with family or friends are *less* likely to be working, whereas women who did so are *more* likely to be working after retirement. Developing hobbies in preparation for retirement is similarly negatively related to post-retirement employment for men but is positively related to participation in social hobbies and club involvement for women.

As noted earlier, both men and women who retire early (prior to age 60) are more likely to take on a post-retirement job than are those retiring later. Recent retirees seem to be somewhat more involved as well. Men who have retired within the past four years are more likely to be engaged in social hobbies, and women who retired within the past four years are more likely to be working post-retirement.

Are the Socially Integrated More Likely to Experience Psychological Integration?

Perceptions of Involvement versus Isolation. Another form of integration can be gauged by subjective perceptions. About one in five retirees in our sample describe themselves as feeling bored, and about one in four (27.9% of men and 23.1% of women) see themselves as unproductive. Retired women are less likely to report that they feel lonely (despite their greater likelihood of being widowed) than women who have not yet retired; this is true even after controlling for age. One in five (20.6%) retired women feels lonely, a number significantly *less* than the almost three in ten (27.8%) of the not-yet-retired women in our sample who feel lonely. This difference remains significant even after controlling for age. Men are less apt to feel lonely, whether they are still in their career jobs (10%) or retired (13%). Fewer retired men and women feel "very busy" (43.4%) compared with those who have not yet retired (63.2%).

We see a strong link between actual experience and perceptions of involvement. Those who are socially integrated are less likely to feel isolated. For example, men and women who are married feel less lonely than do those who are widowed. Mothers and grandmothers are more likely than those women without children or grandchildren to feel "very busy." Fathers and grandfathers, in contrast, are less likely to report feeling very busy than are men with no children or grandchildren.

Also, men who report that time spent with their family is one of the better aspects of retirement are *more* likely to indicate feelings of loneliness, while women who enjoy spending time with their families feel *less* lonely. Not surprisingly, the often burdensome role of care-giving is positively associated with feelings of "busyness" for both men and women.

Post-retirement employment is negatively related to feelings of isolation, especially for men. Working men are less likely to report feelings of loneliness, boredom, and lack of productivity. Working women are also less likely to report feeling unproductive and, in fact, are more likely to report that they feel "very busy." Being involved with social hobbies is associated with less loneliness for men. Visiting neighbors seems to be important for women's perceptions; women who visit with their neighbors at least twice per month are less likely to report that they feel lonely. Furthermore, men who attend religious services regularly and who have multiple role involvements are less likely to feel unproductive or less useful than they might have been prior to retirement. It is interesting to note that feeling very busy is not associated with any measures of social participation for men, but for women, working for pay, being a club member, attending religious services, and having multiple role involvements are all associated with feelings of "busyness."

Marriage as a Form of Social and Psychological Integration. Husbands or wives who retire may find that being married eases the retirement transition, with their spouse an important source of social support. For others, however, being married may be an additional source of stress, particularly if retirement creates a disjuncture in roles and expectations between spouses. Marital quality has been shown to be a key emotional resource, promoting psychological integration. Using data from the *Cornell Retirement and Well-Being Study*, two studies (Kim

& Moen, 2000; Moen et al., 2000) show that employment and retirement patterns of couples are related to marital quality and satisfaction.

They found that retirement was positively associated with marital quality. Specifically, husbands and wives who are both retired are more satisfied with their marriages than husbands and wives in couples where neither has retired (see Figure 3.2). Conversely, husbands and wives undergoing the actual retirement transition report the most conflict in their marriages. And regardless of whether they themselves are in or out of the labor force, the husbands of wives who have been full-time homemakers, in a traditional marriage arrangement, report the highest quality of marital life.

What can we conclude about the ties between married life and

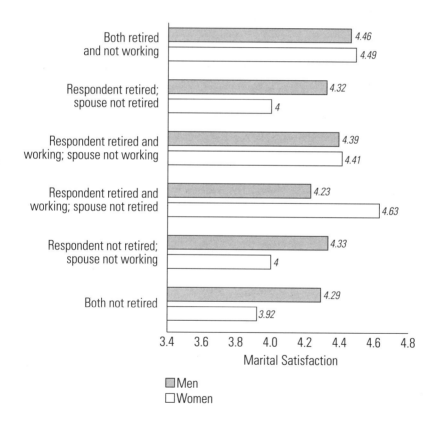

Figure 3.2 Couples' Work Status and Marital Satisfaction. *Note:* Couples' work status, p = .003; gender, p = .052. Interaction, p = .076.

couples' work lives as they approach and experience the retirement transition? Subjective dispositions apparently play a large role in fostering marital quality. Those respondents who are satisfied with retirement, or consider those years the best of their lives, report the healthiest marriages, despite what they actually are doing. Knowing whether a person is retired or not is less informative than knowing their spouse's labor force status and the configuration of the two. How respondents feel about their employment or retirement status and their feelings about their actual roles may well shape marital quality. The lower marital quality of husbands and wives who are in non-traditional marriages (with the wife not yet retired while the husband has already left the workforce) suggest that the perception of role appropriateness may be an important factor for marital quality.

Social Integration in the First Five Years of Retirement. Moen et al. (2000) report that the initial transition from career to retirement increases marital conflict, but being retired over the long term reduces conflict. Richardson and Kilty (1991) also find that well-being fluctuates in the initial stages of retirement, reflecting an adjustment period within the first year or two in which men and women may develop coping strategies or find social activities to compensate for the loss of their career jobs. By focusing on those who have retired recently, we can get a glimpse of the process of adjustment to retirement. There are 311 men (183) and women (128) in the *Cornell Retirement and Well-Being Study* sample who retired within the five years preceding our survey.

For men in this recently retired subsample, post-retirement employment differs by duration of retirement. Those who are currently re-employed have been "retired" an average of 2.28 years, whereas the men who are not employed have been retired longer—an average of 2.86 years (p = .004). Although men approaching the end of their third year of retirement are less likely to be employed, women's involvements are higher. Women in this recently retired subsample who are volunteering have been retired, on average, 2.97 years (as compared to the non-volunteers who have been retired only 2.30 years; p = .01). Similarly, women who attend religious services on a regular basis have been in retirement longer (2.77 years as compared to 2.26 years; p = .047).

Although we see a pattern of involvement for men within their first five years of retirement, only differences in post-retirement employment are statistically significant. Other forms of social participation are also higher until the end of the third year, and then are lower by the end of the fourth year. Men most likely to report that the retirement years are better have been retired between three and four years. For women, the pattern is less clear, although there is a slight increase in the proportion volunteering and attending religious services with years since retirement.

DOES SOCIAL INTEGRATION PROMOTE WELL-BEING IN RETIREMENT?

Thus far we have discussed the characteristics of those who are *socially integrated*. In this section we assess whether those retirees who are socially integrated are also the most psychologically *advantaged*.

Paid Work

Not surprisingly, retirees in the *Cornell Retirement and Well-Being Study* who are employed following retirement report higher levels of health and energy than do those who are not working for pay, but this finding could represent some degree of selection (with those less healthy either leaving or not taking on jobs). Men and women holding post-retirement jobs are also more likely to see their retirement years as better than their pre-retirement years.

We see striking differences by gender in the links between post-retirement employment and well-being. When we examine the relationship between post-retirement work and well-being by gender, we find that retired men who are re-employed report fewer depressive symptoms, a higher sense of mastery, more self-esteem, and a higher general level of satisfaction with life than do their non-working counterparts (see also Kim & Moen, 2000b). Retired women who are re-employed, on the other hand, report *more* depressive symptoms, a lower sense of mastery, less life satisfaction, and about the same sense of self-esteem compared to those not employed. Men may hold a job in retirement because they want to be in the workforce; retired women may be employed because they need the extra income. Women and men who are not employed after retirement have similar scores on measures of mastery, self-esteem, general satisfaction, health, illness, and depression. The only significant difference we find between non-employed retired men and women is in their reported level of energy, with women reporting significantly lower (p = .02) levels of energy than men.

Club Membership and Volunteer Work

Researchers have begun to investigate the health consequences of involvement in *unpaid* volunteer activities (see Chambré, 1984, 1987; Fischer & Schaffer, 1993; Moen & Fields, 2000; Moen et al., 1989, 1992, 1994; Okun et al., 1984; Young & Glasgow, 1998). Still, participation in voluntary associations, or in volunteering activities generally, is vastly under researched. We examine both volunteer participation and participation in clubs and organizations, finding both to be positively related to psychological health. Retirees active in clubs or organizations report fewer depressive symptoms, higher mastery and self-esteem, more energy, higher life satisfaction, and greater satisfaction with retirement. Those who are volunteering also report higher self-esteem, greater life satisfaction, and more energy. These findings hold regardless of gender.

Religious Participation

There is some evidence that church membership and frequency of religious attendance is inversely related to mortality, after controlling for a range of risk factors (Berkman & Breslow, 1983; House et al., 1986). And frequent church attendance has been associated with less psychological distress (see Ellison, 1991). In the *Cornell Retirement and Well-Being Study* we find gender differences in the links between religious involvement and various measures of psychological health. Men who regularly attend religious services report a higher sense of mastery, higher happiness, and greater life satisfaction compared to men who do not. But women who attend religious services report a *lower* sense of mastery, happiness, and satisfaction as opposed to those who do not; they are also less likely to report that life is better in retirement. It may be that these women are feeling a lack of connection and attend services more frequently in hopes of making that connection.

Family Participation

Particular family contingencies can either promote or hamper well-being following retirement. The impact of caregiving on well-being in the second half of life—for children, for spouses, for parents or other infirm relatives—has not been systematically investigated. However, we do know that women involved in caregiving are more likely than men to experience strain (Moen et al., 1994; Young & Kahana, 1989; Zarit et al., 1986). Antonucci (1994) suggests that women not only have more close ties, but they are also more burdened by these intimate relationships than are men.

In the *Cornell Retirement and Well-Being Study* we explore the differential effects of caregiving on men and women. Retired women who are caregiving ten hours a week or more have higher average scores on scales measuring self-esteem and willingness to accept a challenge than do women who are caregiving for fewer hours or not at all. We find that retired men who provide care for more than ten hours a week seem to show more psychological stress than women in that position. Retired men who are caregiving intensively tend to have lower self-esteem, a lower sense of mastery, and tend to be less accepting of new challenges than those who are not involved in intensive caregiving. Men may find the role of intensive caregiver to be unfamiliar. Note, however, that these deleterious relationships are not evident in men who are involved in lower levels of caregiving.

Psychological Integration

Volunteering, being a member of a club or organization, or working for pay are objective measures of community involvement or integration. But integration also has cognitive and emotional aspects. These subjective components of integration are strongly associated with measures of well-being showing that men and women who *feel* more connected are more content with their retirement years. Feeling lonely, feeling bored, and feeling unproductive are all inversely associated with both men's and women's reports of retirement quality. Retired men and women who report having felt lonely at least one day in the past week report a lower sense of mastery, lower self-esteem, and less energy as compared to those who are not lonely. Similarly, men and women who report that boredom or feeling unproductive are negative aspects of their retirement have a lower sense of mastery, lower self-esteem, more depressive symptoms, and less energy overall. Conversely, men and women who report that they are "very busy" have, on average, higher self-esteem and feel more energetic than those who feel less busy. And for men, the "very busy" also have higher mastery.

Multiple Forms of Community Participation

It may not be particular roles but multiple role involvements that are related to well-being in retirement. The general consensus is that occupying multiple roles may be more beneficial to men's rather than women's psychological well-being (Barnett & Baruch, 1985; Menaghan, 1989; Thoits, 1986), but whether this is the case for older men and women is not known. We turn first to role *combinations*, looking at three key non-family forms of social capital: post-retirement employment, volunteer participation, and club/organizational participation. More than one in five (22.5%) of our sample are not involved in any of these activities. The same proportion (22.5%) is formally volunteering (in connection with membership in clubs/organizations) but not working for pay. Almost a fifth (19.2%) are active members of clubs or other social organizations (typically, such groups as bridge or garden clubs) but not in volunteer participation. Each of the other work/club/volunteer role combinations includes fewer than 10 percent of our sample of retirees.

There is a significant gender difference in these forms of engagement, with more retired men than women involved in all three (11.1% to 5.2%), and more women than men engaged in none of the three (27.7% to 18%) (see Figure 3.3).

There is also a difference by age (not shown). Retirees in their fifties are more apt than those in their sixties or early seventies to be engaged in all three roles (13.7% to 6.9%) or to be involved just in paid work (16.8% to 6.4%). Older retirees, in contrast, are more apt to be participating in formal volunteer work in their communities (25.1% to 12.6%) or in none of these activities (23.5% to 18.9%).

Those who experienced a serious illness in the past year are the least apt to be engaged in any of these activities (17.1 % to 30.9%), to be involved in only paid work (4.6% to 11.1%), to be both employed and club members (4.6% to 7.9%), or to be engaged in work, volunteerism, and club activities (6.3% to 9.3%). However, retirees who have had a serious illness are about equally likely to be participating exclusively as informal volunteers (7.9% to 7.5%), as formal community volunteers (20.4% and 23.9%), and as both workers and informal volunteers (5.3% to 4.3%). Participants in religious activities are more likely to be engaged in formal volunteering in an organizational setting compared to those who do not participate in religious activities (30.9% to 13.1%).

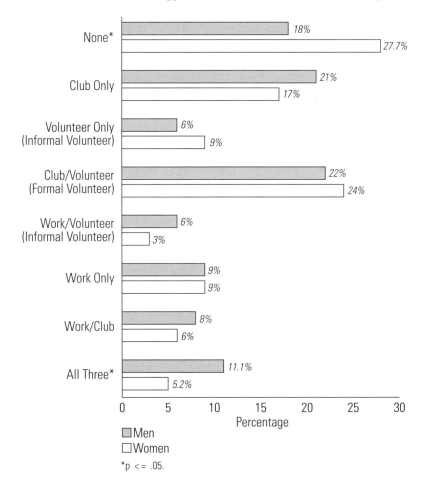

Figure 3.3 Retirees' Work, Club Membership, and Volunteer Role Combinations by Gender. *Source: Cornell Retirement and Well-Being Study,* Wave 1 (1994–95), N = 457.

There appears to be a cumulation of social capital by educated retirees. Those with college degrees are more apt to be involved in all these roles (14.7%), compared to those with some college (7.9%) or those who have at most a high school degree (4.8%). Three in ten (30.8%) retired high school graduates are neither workers nor volunteers nor club members, compared to two in ten (21.1%) of those with some college and only one in ten (10.0%) of college graduates. Moreover, those with less education are more apt to be exclusively club or organization members (high school = 21.6%; some college = 25.0%; college degree = 12.0%).

What are the implications of these various combinations of roles for retirees' well-being? The highest levels of mastery are reported by those who are simultaneously working, volunteering, and active in clubs and organizations (x = 3.26), as well as those who are engaged in formal volunteering (x = 3.25). (Formal community participation includes activities such as working for the League of Women Voters or the Volunteer Fire Department.) The lowest levels of mastery are reported by those who are only informal volunteers (occasionally "helping out," not as part of a community group; x = 2.99) or those who neither work, volunteer, nor belong to any clubs or organizations (x = 3.03). Those who report the highest energy levels are those who are working, volunteering, and active in clubs and organizations (x = 8.22); those reporting the lowest levels are not involved in any of these three activities (x = 6.86). Retirees who report the highest levels of self-esteem are retirees who are involved in formal volunteering but who are not working (x = 3.50). Those with the lowest self-esteem do not work or belong to clubs and organizations (x = 3.21 for those who informally volunteer, and x = 3.27 for those who do not).

CONCLUSIONS

Life changes, such as retirement, can be both beneficial and detrimental to individual development (Cooper, 1990). Since jobs provide routines, rituals, and role identity, retirement from one's career job restructures not only life patterns but also self-conceptions and meanings. For many individuals, the retirement transition is a time of uncertainty, when the meaning and purpose of life is open to new interpretation (Moen, 1998a). Part of the difficulty in gauging the impact of the retirement transition on social integration and well-being is that it constitutes both a positive and negative change, and is both voluntary and involuntary. Thus, how individuals perceive their retirement becomes extremely consequential. In the Cornell study of the retirement transition we have found that some workers are literally counting the days until they can retire, much as military draftees used to mark off the days until their discharge. Others become defensive when queried about the timing of their retirement, claiming adamantly that they will "never" retire, that they will be carried off their jobs in a coffin. One important consideration is whether individuals see themselves as moving to new opportunities and challenges or simply from employment.

The meaning of work for most individuals is the opportunity it provides to participate fully in society. Retirement from paid work can cut individuals off from that participation, as well as the identity and sense of community it provides. Mature adulthood has been characterized as vital involvement in life's generative activities (Erikson et al., 1986). Social participation in meaningful activities and roles in the later years of adulthood can promote both psychological and physical health (Butler & Gleason, 1985; Moen, 1995, 1997). We have found retirees who are actively integrated into their communities—those who take on paid work and participate in formal community volunteer work—are the best off in terms of life quality. The retirement transition can offer an occasion for the development of a new identity and can foster ongoing engagement in various forms of paid and unpaid activities. But existing structural arrangements, policies, norms, and practices often fail to provide the opportunities, roles, and challenges that can fully exploit the possibilities of life—and health—after retirement.

REFERENCES

Allen, J. (1990). Caring work and gender equity in an aging society. In J. Allen & A. Pifer (Eds.), *Women on the front lines: Meeting the challenge of an aging America* (221–240). Washington, DC: Urban Institute.

Anderson, K. H., & Burkhauser, R. V. (1985). The retirement-health nexus: A new measure of an old puzzle. *Journal of Human Resources, 20,* 315–330.

Antonucci, T. C. (1994). A lifespan view of women's social relations. In B. F. Turner & L. E. Troll (Eds.), *Women growing older: Psychological perspectives* (239–269). Thousand Oaks, CA: Sage.

Atchley, R. C. (1976). *The sociology of retirement.* New York: Schenkman.

Baltes, P. B., & Baltes, M. M. (1990). *Successful aging: Perspectives from the behavioral sciences.* Cambridge, UK: Cambridge University Press.

Barfield, R., & Morgan, J. N. (1969). *Early retirement: The decision and the experience.* Ann Arbor: Survey Research Center, University of Michigan.

Barley, S. R. (1989). Careers, identities, and institutions: The legacy of the Chicago School of Sociology. In M. B. Arthur, D. T. Hall & B. S. Lawrence (Eds.), *Handbook of career theory* (41–65). New York: Cambridge University Press.

Barnett, R. C., & Baruch, G. K. (1985). Women's involvement in multiple roles and psychological distress. *Journal of Personality and Social Psychology, 49,* 135–145.

Berkman, L. F., & Breslow, L. (1983). *Health and ways of living: The Alameda County study.* New York: Oxford University Press.

Bound, J. (1991). Self-reported objective measures of health in retirement models. *Journal of Human Resources, 26,* 108–137.

Bourdieu, P. (1984). *Distinction.* Cambridge: Harvard University Press.

Breiger, R. (1995). Social structure and the phenomenology of attainment. *Annual Review of Sociology, 21,* 155–236.

Brinton, M. (1988). The social-institutional bases of gender stratification: Japan as an illustrative case. *American Journal of Sociology, 94,* 300–334.

Brody, E. M. (1985). Parent care as a normative family stress. *The Gerontologist, 25,* 19–29.

Brody, E. M. (1989). Caregiving daughters and their local siblings: Perceptions, strains, and interactions. *The Gerontologist, 29,* 529–538.

Burkhauser, R. V., & Quinn, J. F. (1989). American patterns of work and retirement. In W. Schmall (Ed.), *Redefining the process of retirement: An international perspective* (91–114). Berlin: Springer-Verlag.

Burkhauser, R. V., & Quinn, J. F. (1990). Economic incentives and the labor force participation of older workers. In L. Bassi & D. Crawford (Eds.), *Research in labor economics, Vol. 11* (159–179). New York: JAI Press.

Butler, R. N., & Gleason, H. P. (1985). *Productive aging: Enhancing vitality in old age.* New York: Springer.

Chambré, S. M. (1984). Is volunteering a substitute for role loss in old age: An empirical test of activity theory. *The Gerontologist, 24,* 294–295.

Chambré, S. M. (1987). *Good deeds in old age: Volunteering by the new leisure class.* Lexington, MA: Lexington Books.

Chirikos, T. N., & Nestel, G. (1989). Occupation, impaired health, and the functional capacity of men to continue working. *Research on Aging, 11,* 174–205.

DeViney, S., & O'Rand, A. M. (1988). Age, gender, cohort succession and labor force participation of older workers, 1951–1984. *Sociologist Quarterly, 29,* 525–540.

Durkheim, E. [1897] (1951). *Suicide: A study in sociology.* J. A. Spaulding & G. Simpson (Trans.). Glencoe, IL: Free Press.

Ebaugh, H. R. F. (1988). *Becoming an ex: The process of role exit.* Chicago: University of Chicago Press.

Ekerdt, D. J., & Vinick, B. H. (1991). Marital complaints in husband-working and husband-retired couples. *Research on Aging, 13,* 364–382.

Elder, G. H., Jr. (1974). *Children of the Great Depression: Social change in life experience.* Chicago: University of Chicago Press.

Elder, G. H., Jr., George, L. K., & Shanahan, M. J. (1996). Psychosocial stress over the life course. In H. B. Kaplan (Ed.), *Psychosocial stress: Perspectives on structure, theory, life course, and methods* (247–292). Orlando, FL: Academic Press.

Ellison, C. G. (1991). Religious involvement and subjective well-being. *Journal of Health and Social Behavior, 32,* 80–99.

Erikson, E. H., Erikson, J. M., & Kivnick, H. Q. (1986). *Vital involvement in old age.* New York: Norton.

Featherman, D. L., Smith, J., & Peterson, J. G. (1990). Successful aging in a post-retired society. In P. Baltes & M. M. Baltes (Eds.), *Successful aging: Perspectives from the behavioral sciences* (50–93). New York: Cambridge University Press.

Fischer, L. R., & Schaffer, K. B. (1993). *Older volunteers: A guide to research and practice.* Newbury Park, CA: Sage.

George, L. K. (1993). Sociological perspectives on life transitions. *Annual Review of Sociology, 19,* 353–373.

Gove, W. R., & Hughes, M. (1979). Possible causes of the apparent sex differences in physical health: An empirical investigation. *American Sociological Review, 44,* 126–146.

Hagestad, G. O., & Neugarten, B. L. (1985). Age and the life course. In R. Binstock & E. Shanas (Eds.), *Handbook of aging and the social sciences,* 2d ed. (35–61). New York: Van Nostrand Reinhold.

Han, S.-K., & Moen, P. (1999). Clocking out: Temporal patterning of retirement. *American Journal of Sociology, 105,* 191–236.

Herzog, A. R., Kahn, R. L., Morgan, J. N., Jackson, J. S., & Antonucci, T. C. (1989). Age differences in productive activities. *Journal of Gerontology: Social Sciences, 44,* 129–138.

Horowitz, A. (1985). Sons and daughters as caregiver to older parents: Differences in role performances. *The Gerontologist, 25,* 612–617.

House, J. S., Strecher, V., Metzner, H. L., & Robbins, C. A. (1986). Occupational stress and health among men and women in the Tecumseh community health study. *Journal of Health and Social Behavior, 27,* 62–77.

Jewson, R. H. (1982). After retirement: An exploratory study of the professional women. In M. Szinovacz (Ed.), *Women's retirement: Policy implications of current research* (169–181). Beverly Hills, CA: Sage.

Kim, J., & Moen, P. (2000a). Late midlife work status and transitions. In M. Lachman (Ed.), *Handbook of midlife development* (in press). New York: Wiley.

Kim, J., & Moen, P. (2000b). Work/retirement transitions and psychological well-being in late midlife. Unpublished manuscript.

Kohn, M. L. (1995). Social structure and personality through time and space. In P. Moen, G. H. Elder, Jr., & K. Lüscher (Eds.), *Examining lives in context: Perspectives on the ecology of human development* (141–168). Washington, DC: American Psychological Association.

Kohn, M. L., & Schooler, C. (1983). *Work and personality: An inquiry into the impact of social stratification.* Norwood, NJ: Ablex.

Martin Matthews, A., & Brown, K. H. (1988). Retirement as a critical life event: The differential experiences of men and women. *Research on Aging, 9*, 548–557.

Menaghan, E. G. (1989). Role changes and psychological well-being: Variations in effects by gender and role repertoire. *Social Forces, 67*, 696–714.

Merton, R. K. (1968). The Matthew Effect in Science. *Science, 159*, 56–63.

Moen, P. (1992). *Women's two roles: A contemporary dilemma.* Westport, CT: Greenwood Publishing.

Moen, P. (1995). A life course approach to postretirement roles and well-being. In L. A. Bond, S. J. Cutler, & A. Grams (Eds.), *Promoting successful and productive aging* (230–257). Thousand Oaks, CA: Sage.

Moen, P. (1996a). Gender, Age and the Life Course. In R. H. Binstock & L. George (Eds.), *Handbook of aging and the social sciences*, 4th ed. (171–187). San Diego: Academic Press, Inc.

Moen, P. (1996b). A life course perspective on retirement, gender, and well-being. *Journal of Occupational Health Psychology, 1*, 131–144.

Moen, P. (1997). Women's roles and resilience: Trajectories of advantage or turning points? In I. H. Gotlib & B. Wheaton (Eds.), *Stress and adversity over the life course: Trajectories and turning points* (133–156). New York: Cambridge University Press.

Moen, P. (1998a). Recasting careers: Changing reference groups, risks, and realities. *Generations, 22*, 40–45.

Moen, P. (1998b). Aging and women's life course. In E. A. Blechman & K. D. Brownell (Eds.), *Behavioral medicine & women: A comprehensive handbook* (87–92). New York: Guilford Press.

Moen, P. (2000). The Gendered Life Course. In R. H. Binstock & L. George

(Eds.), *Handbook of aging and the social sciences*, 5th ed. San Diego: Academic Press (in press).

Moen, P., Dempster-McClain, D., & Williams, R. M., Jr. (1989). Social integration and longevity: An event history analysis of women's roles and resilience. *American Sociological Review, 54,* 635–647.

Moen, P., Dempster-McClain, D., & Williams, R. M., Jr. (1992). Successful aging: A life course perspective on women's roles and health. *American Journal of Sociology, 97,* 1612–1638.

Moen, P., & Fields, V. (2000). Retirement and well-being: Does community participation replace paid work? Unpublished manuscript.

Moen, P., Kain, E. L., & Elder, G. H., Jr. (1983). Economic conditions and family life: Contemporary and historical perspectives. In R. R. Helson & F. Skidmore (Eds.), *The high costs of living: Economic and demographic conditions in American families* (213–259). Washington, DC: National Academy Press.

Moen, P., Kim, J., & Hofmeister, H. (2001). Couples' work/retirement transitions, gender, and marital quality. *Social Psychology Quarterly,* forthcoming.

Moen, P., Robison, J., & Fields, V. (1994). Women's work and caregiving roles: A life course approach. *Journal of Gerontology: Social Sciences, 49,* 176–186.

Moen, P., & Smith, K. R. (1986). Women at work: Commitment and behavior over the life course. *Sociological Forum, 1,* 450–475.

Moen, P., & Wethington, E. (1992). The concept of family adaptive strategies. *Annual Review of Sociology, 18,* 233–251.

Neugarten, B. L., Moore, J. W., & Lowe, J. C. (1965). Age norms, age constraints, and adult socialization. *American Journal of Sociology, 70,* 710–717.

Okun, M. A., Stock, W. A., Haring, M. J., & Witter, R. A. (1984). The social activity/subjective well-being relation: A quantitative synthesis. *Research on Aging, 6,* 45–65.

Palmore, E. B., Burchett, B. M., Filenbaum, G. G., George, L. K., & Wallman, L. M. (1985). *Retirement: Causes and consequences.* New York: Springer.

Pavalko, E. K., & Artis, J. E. (1997). Women's caregiving and paid work: Causal relationships in late mid-life. *Journal of Gerontology: Social Sciences, 52B,* S1–S10.

Pavalko, E. K., Elder, G. H., Jr., & Clipp, E. C. (1993). Work lives and longevity: Insights from a life course perspective. *Journal of Health and Social Behavior, 34,* 363–380.

Quadagno, Jill. (1995). The welfare state and the reproduction of gender: Making good girls and boys in the job corps. *Social Problems, 42*, 171–190.

Quick, H., & Moen, P. (1998). Gender, employment, and retirement quality: A life course approach to the differential experiences of men and women. *Journal of Occupational Health Psychology, 3*, 44–64.

Qureshi, H., & Walker, A. (1989). *The caring relationship.* Philadelphia: Temple University Press.

Richardson, V., & Kilty, K. M. (1991). Adjustment to retirement: Continuity vs. discontinuity. *International Journal of Aging and Human Development, 33*, 151–169.

Riley, M. W. (1987). On the significance of age in sociology. *American Sociological Review, 52*, 1–14.

Riley, M. W., Foner, A., & Waring, J. (1988). Sociology of age. In N. H. Smelser (Ed.), *Handbook of sociology* (243–290). Newbury Park, CA: Sage.

Riley, M. W., Kahn, R. L., & Foner, A. (Eds.) (1994). *Age and structural lag.* New York: Wiley.

Rook, K. S., Catalano, R., & Dooley, D. (1989). The timing of major life events: Effects of departing from the social clock. *American Journal of Community Psychology, 17*, 233–258.

Rosow, I. (1967). *Social integration of the aged.* New York: Free Press.

Rosow, I. (1974). *Socialization to old age.* Berkeley: University of California Press.

Rosow, I. (1985). Status and role change through the life cycle. In R. Binstock & E. Shanas (Eds.), *Handbook of aging and the social sciences* (62–93). New York: Van Nostrand Reinhold.

Ryder, N. B. (1965). The cohort as a concept in the study of social change. *American Sociological Review, 30*, 843–861.

Secombe, K., & Lee, G. R. 1986. Gender differences in retirement satisfaction and its antecedents. *Research on Aging, 8*, 426–440.

Slocum, W. L. (1967). *Occupational careers: A sociological perspective.* Chicago: Aldine.

Smith, D. B., & Moen, P. (1998). Spouse's influence on the retirement decision: His, her, and their perceptions. *Journal of Marriage and the Family, 60*, 734–744.

Streib, G. F., & Schneider, C. J. (1971). *Retirement in American Society.* Ithaca: Cornell University Press.

Swidler, A. (1986). Culture in action: Symbols and strategies. *American Sociological Review, 51*, 273–286.

Thoits, P. A. (1986). Multiple identities: Examining gender and marital status differences in distress. *American Psychological Review, 51,* 259–272.

Thoits, P. A. (1995). Stress, coping, and social support processes: Where are we? What next? *Journal of Health and Social Behavior, extra issue,* 53–79.

Tomaskovic-Devey, D. (1993). Labor-process inequality and the gender and race composition of jobs. *Research in Social Stratification and Mobility, 12,* 215–247.

Turner, R. J., Wheaton, B., & Lloyd, K. (1995). The epidemiology of social stress. *American Sociological Review, 60,* 104–125.

Veroff, J., Douvan, E., & Kulka, R. A. (1981). *The inner American.* New York: Basic.

Wheaton, B. (1990). Life transitions, role histories, and mental health. *American Sociological Review, 55,* 209–223.

Wolf, W., & Fligstein, N. (1979). Sex and authority in the workplace: The causes of inequality. *Annual Sociological Review, 44,* 235–252.

Young, F. W., & Glasgow, N. (1998). Voluntary social participation and health. *Research on Aging, 20,* 339–362.

Young, R., & Kahana, E. (1989). Specifying caregiver outcomes: Gender and relationship aspects of caregiving strain. *The Gerontologist, 29,* 660–666.

Zarit, S., Todd, P., & Zarit, J. (1986). Subjective burden of husbands and wives as caregivers: A longitudinal study. *The Gerontologist, 26,* 260–266.

CHAPTER FOUR

Transportation Transitions and Social Integration of Nonmetropolitan Older Persons

Nina Glasgow

This chapter explores effective transportation arrangements as a facilitator of social integration among older people, especially older rural residents. It also focuses on the relinquishment of driving as a key life-course transition in old age, one with profound consequences for the personal mobility and quality of life of all older people, and especially those in rural communities.

Transportation enables the individual to maintain social ties, participate in the community, and have access to goods and services. Effective transportation can be seen as a key link promoting older individuals' social integration, especially people who live in rural communities with dispersed patterns of settlement. By contrast, inadequate transportation can contribute to social isolation. Previous studies have assumed that transportation is important to maintaining ties to the larger community (e.g., Burkhardt & Berger, 1997; National Eldercare Institute on Transportation, 1994). Past research has not, however, examined the extent to which and how transportation affects the social integration of older people. Further, studies of the consequences of older persons' transportation arrangements for quality of life have largely been conducted in urban areas (e.g., Carp, 1971, 1972, 1988).

The *Cornell Transportation and Social Integration of Nonmetropolitan Older Persons Study*, analyzed in this chapter, focuses on the transportation mobility and social integration of rural older people and thus addresses a neglected area of research. Using a life-course perspective, we examine the *timing, context,* and *process* of transitions and trajectories in the use of different modes of transportation.

Different means of transportation include one's personal automobile; rides from others in the household; rides from informal helpers outside the household (e.g., family, friends, neighbors, or paid helpers); formal transportation services; and combinations of these. Not everyone has the functional capacity to use, the preference for, or access to all transportation options at all times.

Driving one's car is the means of personal mobility for most people in the United States. Driving is the preferred means of transportation among Americans of all ages. In the media and in the wider culture, driving symbolizes freedom, independence, and self-reliance (Eisenhandler, 1990). Adults in later life, however, are likely eventually to experience temporary or permanent loss of their driving ability—a loss often viewed by older persons and those around them as a critical life-course event and transition. Just as getting a driver's license is an important marker in adolescence of the move into adulthood, so too is the loss of driving a marker of the realities of old age. Becoming unable to use certain other types of transportation may also signal an important mobility transition for an older person. For example, reliance on public buses and on walking suggest that a person is functionally capable of getting around without needing much assistance.

This chapter establishes how older rural people construct their transportation arrangements, examines personal and contextual characteristics associated with different transportation statuses, and the consequences of older persons' transportation statuses for their social integration and quality of life. Because of the strong preference for driving, a major focus of the analysis is on drivers versus non-drivers (non-drivers, by implication, having to make other transportation arrangements).

A LIFE-COURSE PERSPECTIVE ON TRANSPORTATION TRANSITIONS AND SOCIAL INTEGRATION

Older people may continue to drive or have friends and relatives who are able and willing to drive them. They may also use formal means of transportation such as buses, taxis, or transportation provided by social service agencies. Still, a significant segment of the older population is transportation disadvantaged. This disadvantage is thought to result from the interplay between personal or household characteristics and attributes of the communities in which older persons live. Transportation disadvantage increases over the life course as older persons age, experience the onset of illness and disability, and lose members of their social networks (Iutcovich & Iutcovich, 1988).

Timing

Advancing age and the frequently accompanying increases in health problems and disability are key factors in the timing of loss of driving ability. In 1990, among a nationally representative sample of older people, more than 90 percent of men and approximately 75 percent of women between the ages of 65 and 74 were licensed drivers (Burkhardt et al., 1996). Among those aged 85 and older, only 55 percent of men and an even smaller proportion of women (25%) were licensed to drive. Older individuals with mounting frailties, slowed reaction times, and increased disability may also be unable to use public buses because public transit systems are usually designed for speed and adherence to fairly strict schedules (Revis & Revis, 1978).

Certain personal characteristics correspond to a lifetime of cumulative advantage or disadvantage (see, e.g., Moen, 1995), and such characteristics relate to types of transportation used and the timing of transportation transitions. Women, frail, and low-income older people are those most at risk of experiencing transportation difficulties (Marottoli et al., 1993; Patton, 1975; Revis & Revis, 1978; Richardson, 1987). For example, older women are less likely than older men to drive; they drive less frequently for fewer miles and are less likely to drive under adverse road conditions than men (Glasgow & Brown, 1997). Thus, the gender context of lives is an important influence on the timing of reduction in or cessation of driving.

Moreover, characteristics suggesting disadvantage tend to accumulate. Older women have lower incomes and are more likely to live in poverty than older men (see, e.g., Glasgow & Brown, 1998). Further, a low income makes owning and operating an automobile less affordable, regardless of driving ability. The prevalence of chronic illness and disability is greater among women than men (Holden, 1987), and health and disability affect driving status. Young-old, healthy males, on the other hand, have few transportation difficulties (Marottoli et al., 1993).

In our study, both focus group and survey respondents who were still driving were strongly negatively disposed to the possibility of eventually having to give up driving, a finding consistent with Carp's (1971) findings among older residents of San Antonio, Texas. In the Cornell study, former drivers (primarily the old-old) and the small number of respondents who had never driven relied on family or friends as their primary means of transportation. However, the timing of the transition from driving to reliance on informal networks for transportation (rides) was postponed as long as possible.

Context and Transportation Arrangements

Within a life-course framework, context can refer to residential environment or to personal characteristics, such as gender and marital status, that set the context of individuals' lives. We have discussed how the gender context of lives affects the timing of the transition from driver to non-driver. Here, we explore the association between gender and use of other means of transportation, as well as how geographic context affects older individuals' transportation.

Gender Context. Who in the social network is sought for assistance with transportation when older individuals have stopped driving or have never started? Carp (1972) found gender differences in getting rides, with older men more likely to use family sources and older women depending on both family and friend networks. Like older women in general (see Chapter 1), nonmetropolitan older women are disadvantaged compared to their male counterparts in the availability of a spouse (Glasgow, 1988). Women are more likely to be widowed and to live alone. Thus, older men are likely to have spouses available to provide rides should they have to relinquish driving. Women, in contrast, are less likely to have a spouse, which may be why they are more likely than men to depend on both family and friends for rides. A few studies have shown that informal social networks play an important role in providing transportation to rural older persons (Coward, 1987; Iutcovich & Iutcovich, 1988). But reliance on members of one's informal network for rides is limiting. It may also imperil the social integration of older people, should something happen to network members who provide rides.

Focus group data collected in conjunction with the *Cornell Transportation and Social Integration Study* suggested both positive and negative outcomes of relying on family and friends for rides (Glasgow

& Blakely, 2000). Older women who were getting rides from family members felt their families cared about them. Those who were getting rides from friends valued the social interaction and the feelings of inter-group reliance and reciprocity the experience engendered. Some men and women, however, expressed reluctance to ask family or friends for rides, citing the desire not to impose on others and their feelings of lost independence. The older men in the focus groups were especially likely to express the opinion that using public buses is more independence-enhancing than relying on members of one's informal network for rides. Carp's (1972) study of transportation among older residents of San Antonio reported similar drawbacks to getting rides from members of informal networks.

Geographic Context. Maintaining access to adequate levels of transportation is especially problematic among rural older persons (Cordes, 1985; Revis & Revis, 1978; Rosenbloom, 1988; Youmans, 1977). There are at least two reasons why rural older people are particularly vulnerable to becoming transportation disadvantaged.

First, rural older people risk greater social isolation than metropolitan older residents owing to the low population density and scattered nature of rural settlement. Rosenbloom (1988) has argued that the low-density settlement patterns of both rural and suburban areas of the United States pose environmental barriers to getting around by means other than a personal automobile. Rural and suburban areas often lack sidewalks, presenting a physical barrier that makes walking to activities difficult. Even when sidewalks are available, the distances from home to community services and activities prohibit many older people from walking to them. Distances to friends' and relatives' homes may also be too great to permit older people to walk for social visits.

Second, past research has shown that public transportation in rural areas is limited or lacking. Low population densities and scattered rural settlement patterns make public transportation difficult and costly to provide, and many rural communities do not have public transportation systems. Only 12 percent of communities with populations of less than 2,500 had public transportation (Talbot, 1985). Only 10 percent of rural communities had taxi service, and intercity bus lines served only 15 percent of places with lower than 2,500 population (Cordes, 1985). Passenger rail service is available in even fewer rural communities. Taietz and Milton (1979) showed that community complexity is an important determinant of the array of formally provided services. Rural communities thus have fewer services, including public transit and social service agency provided transportation for older and other special needs populations (Coward et al., 1994). Older individuals' use of public transit varies across metropolitan places as well, depending on the quality and convenience of different cities' transit systems (Carp, 1980).

The disproportionately heavy reliance among nonmetropolitan older people on personal automobiles as the primary means of transportation is reflected in high rates of vehicle ownership. Nationally, 67 percent of nonmetropolitan people aged 60–74 years owned their own vehicles, compared to only 34 percent of metropolitan older people of the same age group (Glasgow & Beale, 1985). Only 9 percent and 25 percent, respectively, of metropolitan and nonmetropolitan residents aged 75 or older owned their own vehicles. Such findings suggest that many older rural and small town residents relinquish their personal automobiles as they advance in age, but the findings may also reflect cohort differences in the propensity to own motor vehicles. Very little is known from past research about rural older persons' adaptations to the cessation of driving in low-density contexts where access to public transportation alternatives is limited.

The Process of Adaptation to Changes in Transportation Arrangements

Carp (1988) has argued that transportation is a key determinant of the "person-environment fit," or the fit between individual needs and community resources. Rural older people presumably continue to drive as long as possible to maintain access to goods, services, and facilities, and to participate in social support networks, community activities, and social roles. In other words, the person-environment fit is enhanced—and, presumably, social integration—among older rural residents who are able to drive. But what types of adaptations do older people make as they reduce or stop driving? Just how older rural residents adapt to the general deficit in formal transportation services has not been explored in depth in previous research.

Research has contradicted the myth that rural older people have more intimate and more extensive informal support networks than urban older people (Coward & Cutler, 1989; Lee & Cassidy, 1985; Lee & Whitbeck, 1987). In declining rural communities, informal social support networks may even shrink to such an extent that they are ineffective at the same time that services and institutions disappear from communities (Bylund & Crawford, 1987; Scheidt & Norris-Baker, 1990). Rural areas are characterized by diversity, however, and not all are declining in population or services. Regardless, most older people are likely to experience declines in their own or their spouses' driving ability as they age, and informal networks are likely to shrink as family, friends, and neighbors migrate, become incapacitated, or die. As noted above, this situation is exacerbated in rural communities, which often have a smaller base of publicly provided services than urban communities.

Burkhardt and Berger (1997) found that the transition from driver to former driver is a watershed event in the lives of older people, which is often accompanied by dissonance and denial. They identified stages of driving cessation, which include (1) limited driving, (2) cessation of driving, (3) adaptation to a new status, and (4) acceptance of not driving again. During the transition process, some older people learned about and even used transportation alternatives, but others resisted planning for the cessation of driving. Respondents in the Cornell study who participated in an educational workshop series held in the fall of 1996 were similarly resistant to planning for a future without driving (see Chapter 9). Such findings suggest that the process of driving cessation occurs gradually and that older people view the transition as a crisis in their lives.

According to Burkhardt and Berger (1997), adaptation to the cessation of driving is more successful when older individuals (1) have spouses who drive, (2) children living with or near them, (3) the financial resources to purchase alternative modes of transportation, (4) participate in religious institutions, (5) reside in areas with viable transportation alternatives, (6) are physically able to use public transportation, and (7) reduce their activities and their expectations to fit new circumstances. This last mechanism of adaptation suggests the potential for increased social isolation among those who stop driving. Burkhardt and Berger's findings also suggest that the cessation of driving may be particularly problematic for rural older people, because they live in areas with limited public transportation. Their research cannot be considered definitive because the number of respondents was small, and they were not randomly selected. It provides insights, however, into the transition process and the subsequent adaptations of older former drivers. More broadly based research is needed in order to confirm the validity of their findings.

Transportation and Social Integration: Survey Findings

The *Cornell Transportation and Social Integration of Nonmetropolitan Older Persons Study* collected data in 1995 from a representative sample of 737 persons aged 65 or older living in Cortland and Seneca Counties in upstate New York. Both counties are officially designated as nonmetropolitan, and respondents' residences range from open-country rural to villages and small towns to small cities. The city of Cortland is the largest place in the two counties, with a 1990 census population of 19,801. Seneca Falls, the largest town in Seneca County, had a 1990 census population of 9,384. The data were collected through a telephone survey, and 75.8 percent of eligible respondents participated.

The purpose of the survey was to determine the modes of transportation, driving and pedestrian behavior, participation in community activities and social networks, and the health status and sociodemographic characteristics of older respondents. The cross-sectional data used for the present analysis cannot fully capture the dynamic nature of transitions from driver to non-driver and the use of other means of transportation. We can, however, identify the transportation situations of older respondents, their life stage, and other characteristics that affect their transportation status.

In our analysis we examine the premise that transportation is a vital link enabling older persons to be and to remain socially integrated. Our purpose is to determine how older people living in a variety of relatively rural places organize their transportation and, subsequently, whether different transportation arrangements contribute to social integration and social well-being.

Modes of Transportation

Older persons may depend on a wide range of formal and informal arrangements for personal transportation. Formal modes are provided by public and private sector institutions. These modes include bus, taxi, and not-for-profit service, such as senior citizens' vans and rides provided by public agencies. Informal arrangements can be subdivided into transportation provided by one's household and that provided by friends, neighbors, and family members residing in other households. Own-household provided transportation includes driving, receiving rides from one's spouse or other household members, walking, or riding a bicycle.

Table 4.1 shows the usual modes of travel to selected activities outside of older individuals' homes. As can be seen in the bottom row, almost all respondents shop, bank, receive medical care, and visit friends and relatives outside of their homes, and about 80 percent attend religious activities. By contrast, less than half engage in volunteer activities, only about 30 percent participate in senior center activities, and just under 15 percent still work. Hence, when we indicate that 87 percent of respondents report driving to work, we are referring to 87 percent of the 15 percent of the sample who work, and similarly for the other activities.

Primarily, Table 4.1 shows that two thirds or more of nonmetropolitan older individuals drive themselves to activities outside of their homes as their usual means of transportation. They are most likely to drive themselves to work or to volunteer and are somewhat less likely to drive themselves when engaging in social activities or visiting friends and family. Almost no older people in these nonmetropolitan counties rely on formal arrangements, such as public buses, as their usual means of transportation. Cortland County's public bus and dial-a-ride services had been in operation only three years at the time of the survey, and low usage may reflect unfamiliarity with the county's public transportation. Only a limited number of bus routes (four) were in operation, and only one of those routes ran between the city of Cortland and a few smaller communities in the county a few days per week. Seneca County does not have a public bus system, but van transportation from a senior citizens' center is available to take individuals to and from the center, to doctor's appointments, and to grocery stores. Both demand and supply factors may have affected the choice of transportation mode among these nonmetropolitan older persons. Only between 6.5 and 26.6 percent of respondents reported using a combination of two or more transportation modes as their usual arrangement to various activities, which usually included driving and getting rides from members of networks. This finding further underlines respondents' dependence on their own household transportation modes, particularly driving.

Nonmetropolitan older women were somewhat less likely than men to drive themselves to different activities, but they were more likely to rely on other household members and family, friends, and neighbors from outside the household for rides. (Data not shown.)

Table 4.1. Usual Modes of Transportation or Travel to Selected Activities among Nonmetropolitan Older Persons, 1995

Travel Mode	Activity (%)								
	Shopping	Banking	Medical Care	Work	Volunteer	Religious Activity	Senior Citizen's Activity	Other Social and Recreational Activities	Visit Family and Friends
Informal Arrangement									
Own Household									
Drive self	69.9	70.6	70.6	86.9	77.3	68.4	66.7	61.3	64.1
Spouse/other hh member drives	5.2	4.8	5.1	1.1	3.0	5.8	3.1	5.4	5.7
Walk or bicycle	0.9	3.6	0.7	1.1	3.7	6.0	6.3	0.9	0.9
Not Own Household									
Ride from family, friend, neighbor, or paid helper	6.1	4.8	7.5	2.2	2.0	5.4	5.7	5.6	6.1
Formal Arrangement									
Bus, taxi, senior citizens' van, or other common carrier	0.9	0.3	1.4	2.2	1.3	0.5	3.6	0.2	0.9
Combination (2 or more modes)	17.0	15.9	14.7	6.5	12.7	13.9	14.6	26.6	22.3
Engaged in each activity outside of home (%)	98.0	96.3	98.5	14.8	42.9	79.5	28.4	89.9	96.7

Gender differences were statistically significant, except for transportation to work; the majority of both older men and women who work drive themselves. Regardless of gender, the dominant mode of transportation was driving one's personal vehicle.

We further examine nonmetropolitan older individuals' transportation arrangements by investigating whether rural older people *ever* use infrequently used modes of transportation. Findings from a set of questions that asked respondents how often they get rides from family, friends, neighbors, and paid helpers indicated that almost two thirds get rides from family and friends at least yearly. (Data not shown.) But more than 80 percent never get rides from their neighbors, and almost no one ever pays anyone in their informal network to give them a ride. Apparently, rural older people are only likely to get rides from informal network members with whom they have an affective tie.

Respondents were asked whether or not they ever use public buses or senior citizens' van transportation; only 4 percent and 7 percent, respectively, ever do so. (Data not shown.) Thus, not only are formal modes not the usual means of transportation; the vast majority of the older rural respondents *never* use them. Both supply and demand factors probably play a role in this pattern of usage. The findings may also suggest a greater preference among rural older people for reliance on informal networks rather than formal transportation services, when unable to drive.

Using data from national level surveys collected in 1983 and 1990, Rosenbloom (1995) found a small increase among rural older persons in the proportion of all trips made on public transit. But in 1983 the percentage was zero, and the proportion of all trips made on public transit was still minuscule by 1990 (fewer than 1% of trips, except among the aged 85 and older group, among whom 3.4 percent of trips were by public transit). Rosenbloom speculated that the existence of rural public transit systems had increased between 1983 and 1990. In fact, the public bus system in Cortland County had been in operation only three years at the time of this study's survey. As the county's older residents become more familiar with the system, their use of public buses may increase over time. Rosenbloom's (1995) national-level study, however, found low public transit usage among both rural and urban older residents. Such findings suggest that public transit usage will remain low over time among Cortland's older population.

Cumulative Advantage and Disadvantage

In the 1995 survey, 85 percent (or 621) of the respondents were current drivers, and 15 percent (116 respondents) were non-drivers. Because the majority of nonmetropolitan older people drive as their usual mode of transportation, the decision was made to analyze factors associated with being a driver versus a non-driver. In Table 4.2, driving status is defined as current drivers and current nondrivers, with the non-driver category comprising former drivers and those who never drove.

Table 4.2 compares the sociodemographic characteristics of drivers

Table 4.2. Selected Characteristics of Older Nonmetropolitan Drivers and Nondrivers, 1995

Characteristic	Driving Status (%)		Chi Square	
	Driver (N = 621)	Nondriver (N = 116)		
Age				
65–74	90	10	26.5	P<.001
75 and older	76	24		
Gender				
Male	94	6	35.9	P<.001
Female	77	23		
Marital Status				
Married	92	8	52.1	P<.00
Unmarried	72	28		
Household Income				
Under $10,000	62	38	71.8	P<.000
$10,000–$19,999	82	18		
$20,000–$39,999	95	5		
$40,000 and over	99	1		
Health Status				
Excellent	94	6	41.8	P<.000
Very good	87	13		
Good	87	13		
Fair or poor	68	32		
Residence				
Open country rural	91	9	13.3	P<.05
Village or small town	84	16		
City	78	22		

versus non-drivers. Non-drivers are more likely to be older, female, unmarried, low income, and to report poorer health. These findings are similar to past research, which found women, frail, and low-income rural older persons to be those most likely to be non-drivers and to experience transportation difficulties (Patton, 1975; Revis & Revis, 1978; Richardson, 1987). Older nonmetropolitan drivers, on the other hand, show a set of characteristics suggesting cumulative advantage. Not only do they have the autonomy and independence of being a driver, they are also better situated in society, as indicated by health status, marital status, and income.

Presumably, rural countryside residents have a greater need to remain drivers during old age than do in-town residents, and the analysis of driver/non-driver status by type of residence supports that hypothesis (Table 4.2). Compared to those living in town, older rural countryside residents are more likely to be drivers. Demographic analysis has shown a tendency among older rural countryside residents to move into town as they advance in age (Glasgow & Beale, 1985), probably because of declines in health status and the need to be closer to goods, services, and possibly social acquaintances. Some of this study's respondents who experienced declining health may have moved into town and subsequently relinquished driving. Or it may be simply that a higher proportion of open-country than in-town older residents continues to drive because options for doing otherwise are very limited. *These findings confirm that context does make a difference in whether or not one drives.* All differences between drivers and non-drivers are significant, using chi-square tests of significance (Table 4.2).

Life Stage and the Cessation of Driving

A consideration of life stage and driving status allows us to explore the issue of the timing of the transition from driver to former driver status, as well as something about rural older people's driving history. Moen (1995) conceptualizes social roles, relationships, and statuses as shaped by whether one is female or male and gender as key in establishing the *context* of an individual's life course. Age and gender shape "driving careers" as well. Table 4.3 displays the proportions of older men and women by age group who were current drivers, former drivers, or who never drove. Consistent with past research, older men are more likely than older women to be current drivers, regardless of

Table 4.3. Nonmetropolitan Men and Women Driving, by Age Group, 1995 (in %)

	Aged 65–69		Aged 70–74		Aged 75–79		Aged 80–84		Aged 85 and over	
	Male	Female	Male	Female	Male	Female	Male	Female	Male	Female
Current driver	97.1	85.3	94.2	86.1	96.6	78.7	88.2	63.8	78.6	41.7
Former driver	2.9	4.4	4.7	6.5	3.4	13.5	8.8	22.4	21.4	38.9
Never driven	0	10.3	1.2	7.4	0	7.9	2.9	13.8	0	19.4

age group. But the proportions of current drivers diminish among both men and women of more advanced age. The "current driver" status among older men ranged from approximately 97 percent in the 65–69 age group to almost 79 percent in the aged 85 and older group. Among older women, more than 85 percent of the 65–69 age group but only about 42 percent of women aged 85 or older were current drivers. The proportions currently driving did not decline precipitously among men or women until age 80 and older, and then the decline was sharper among women than men.

Driving at some time during their lives was almost universal among older men in this study (only four of the 305 males in the sample never drove), but there were distinct cohort differences in "never driver" status among older women. Over nineteen percent of the women aged 85 or older reported that they had never driven, compared to only about 10 percent of women aged 65–69 (Table 4.3). Rosenbloom (1995) estimates that among future cohorts of older people, having been a driver for a large part of adult life will be almost universal among both males and females, but being a driver or former driver is not universal among current cohorts of older women.

By age 85 and older, women are almost twice as likely as men to be former drivers (39% versus 21%), and thus driving is a status that older women are more likely to relinquish than men (Table 4.3). Burkhardt and colleagues (1996) examined a different question than this study, namely, the proportion licensed to drive rather than the proportion driving. Their national-level study found that 55 percent of men and 25 percent of women aged 85 and older were licensed to drive, whereas this study found that 79 percent of men and 42 percent of women aged 85 and older were still driving. Even though the questions posed in the two studies differ slightly, and some people drive without a license while others with a license do not drive, a comparison of the two studies suggests the rate of driving is higher among older rural New Yorkers than older people nationally.

Gender and Marital Status Context of Driving

Gender and marital status are among the personal characteristics that set the *context* of individuals' lives. Further, marital status is one area in which the lives of older men and women differ. Older men are more likely married, whereas the majority of older women are widowed (see Chapter 1). Women's greater longevity and their tendency to marry men somewhat older than themselves largely account for observed marital status differences. A common stereotype regarding gender differences associated with driving is that older married women stop driving or never start and rely on husbands as the household's driver. In Table 4.2 we saw that married older people are more likely than are unmarried older people to drive. But is that more the case for older men or women? What is the association of gender, marital status, and driving status among rural older people? Can driving be viewed as a household rather than an individual characteristic?

Table 4.4 shows that, among both males and females, married older people are more likely than their unmarried counterparts to drive currently. Ninety-five percent of older married men and 89 percent of older married women were driving, compared to 91 percent of unmarried males and only 67 percent of unmarried older women. Being married thus is more strongly associated with driving among older women than it is among men. This analysis suggests that older married women do not stop driving to rely on husbands as household drivers. The large majority of people falling into the "unmarried" category are widowed, however, and those who are widowed are older on average than the married older people. Because of the confounding effect of age and marital status, one might also speculate that there are cohort differences in life-course propensities to drive among the younger married versus the older unmarried women in the sample.

In a multivariate analysis, which controlled several independent variables simultaneously, marital status was not significantly related to the driving status of older women (Glasgow & Brown, 1997). Among older rural residents, both men and women may view driving as a necessity, and thus the tendency may not be as strong among rural older women to rely on husbands to drive, as may be the case among urban

Table 4.4. Driving Status, by Marital Status and Gender of Nonmetropolitan Older Persons, 1995

Driving Status	Married (%)		Unmarried (%)	
	Male (N = 231)	Female (N = 207)	Male (N = 65)	Female (N = 220)
Current driver	95.3	88.9	90.8	66.8
Former driver	4.3	7.2	7.7	16.8
Never driven	0.4	3.9	1.5	16.4

older women. That is an issue for research of a more comparative nature to explore, however.

Transportation and Indicators of Social Integration

Also important is the effect of transportation arrangements on nonmetropolitan older persons' social integration. Moen and colleagues (1989; 1992) emphasize participation in *social roles* as important indicators of social integration. Thus, to assess the consequences of different transportation arrangements for the social integration of older rural people, we examine whether drivers versus non-drivers show higher levels of participation in different social roles.

We expected more effective transportation arrangements (in this case driving) to be associated with higher levels of participation in social roles. The findings displayed in Figure 4.1 confirm this hypothesis. Older nonmetropolitan drivers are significantly more likely than non-drivers to be club members or volunteers, to attend religious services, and to be caregivers. Participation in the first three roles almost certainly would take one outside of one's home. While caregiving may be provided in the caregiver's home, caregivers are likely to be called upon to provide emergency or other necessary transportation for care recipients, or they may travel to the care recipient's home to provide the care. Accordingly, we hypothesized that caregiving would be affected by an individual's transportation arrangements, and that appears to be the case.

Participation as club members or volunteers and in church has been shown in past research to be positively associated with health and longevity (see, e.g., Chapter 2 of this volume; Berkman & Syme, 1979; Moen et al., 1989; Seeman et al., 1987; Sugisawa et al., 1994; Young & Glasgow, 1998). This study does not assess the health outcomes of

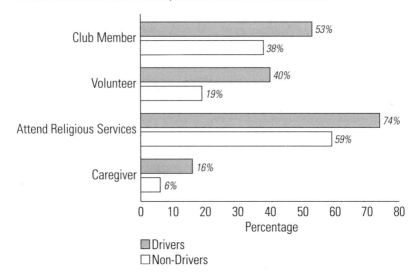

Figure 4.1   Percent Participation in Social Roles among Older Nonmetropolitan Drivers and Non-drivers, 1995. Using chi-square tests, drivers were significantly more likely than non-drivers (at the .01 level or better) to participate in these social roles.

social role participation, but it is worth noting that effective transportation arrangements and, hence, social participation may positively affect the health and well-being of older people.

Frequency of interaction with social networks, often defined by researchers as *social support*, provides another set of indicators of social integration (see, e.g., Chapter 2; and Thoits, 1986). Findings on the frequency of social interaction through visiting with relatives, friends, and neighbors are displayed in Figure 4.2. Drivers and non-drivers are *not* significantly different in the frequency with which they visit relatives. Questions on the frequency of visiting were worded on the survey questionnaire to specify face-to-face visits as that being inquired about (not telephone calls, letters, or e-mail, for example), but there was no specification of where visits take place. Relatives of non-drivers may feel enough obligation and affection to visit non-drivers in their homes, rather than expecting older non-drivers to visit in the homes of relatives who drive. This interpretation of the nonsignificant finding, however, is speculative. Drivers do visit friends and neighbors significantly more frequently than do the non-drivers (Fig-

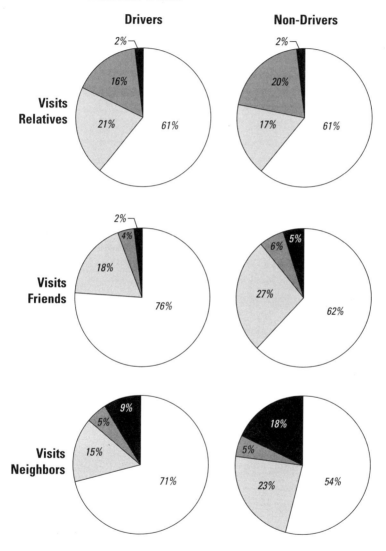

Figure 4.2   Social Network Interaction of Older Nonmetropolitan Drivers and Non-drivers, 1995.

ure 4.2). Social integration thus appears to be enhanced among rural older people who still drive. In summary, the findings in Figures 4.1 and 4.2 show that drivers participate in a greater number of social roles, and they visit with friends and neighbors more frequently than non-drivers.

Comparing former drivers with persons who never drove, former drivers were found to be significantly less likely than those who never drove to participate in social activities. (Data not shown.) Those who never drove have had a lifetime in which to adapt to getting around by means of transportation other than driving, and they may have an advantage over former drivers. The former drivers may still be adapting to disruptions in their social participation. We cannot draw firm conclusions about an adaptive process while using cross-sectional data, but findings on social participation differences between older former drivers and those who never drove suggest an adaptive process.

Transportation and Quality of Life

Inadequate transportation has a negative effect on the satisfaction and morale of rural older people (Fengler & Jensen, 1981; McGhee, 1984). Such findings raise questions about the quality of life of rural older people who cannot drive and who may not have formal transportation available. The drivers in this study were significantly more satisfied than non-drivers with their transportation. (Data not shown.) But satisfaction was relatively high among both drivers and non-drivers, perhaps suggesting that adaptation occurs in conjunction with changes in transportation. Carp (1971) found that the anticipation of stopping driving was perceived quite negatively. For those who had stopped driving, however, retrospective assessments of the meaning of stopping driving were not as negative. This study's finding on satisfaction with transportation arrangements and Carp's earlier research suggest a psychological and emotional adaptation to the cessation of driving.

A question that asked whether respondents are able to get out as often as they want was also used to examine perceived quality of life among drivers versus non-drivers. Drivers and non-drivers assessed their situations differently, with 85 percent of older rural drivers compared to only 56 percent of non-drivers reporting being able to go out as often as they want. (Data not shown.) The risk of social isolation thus is greater among non-drivers than drivers.

Figure 4.3 displays findings on whether being able to get out as

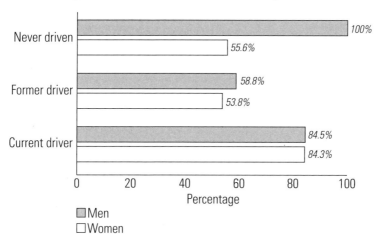

Figure 4.3   Percent of Older Nonmetropolitan Males and Females Who Report That They Are Able to Go Places as Often as They Like, by Driving Status, 1995.

often as one likes varies by gender and driver status. Among current drivers, males and females are equally likely to report being able to get out as often as they want (more than 80% of each group). Older men, however, are advantaged in getting out as often as they want over older women who were former drivers and those who never drove. This finding may be due to the higher marriage rate of older men and, consequently, their greater likelihood of having a spouse available to drive. It is striking that 100 percent of the older men who never drove reported getting out as often as they want, but only four older men in the sample never drove. Thus, we must interpret that finding with extreme caution. Interestingly, the proposition that persons who never drove will be better adapted than former drivers does not seem to apply to older women. Approximately equal percentages of older women who never drove versus former drivers reported going places as often as they wanted (fewer than 60% in each group).

CONCLUSION

This analysis has shown the utility of using a life-course framework to understand the association between older individuals' transportation transitions and trajectories and their social integration.

Driving oneself is the dominant mode of transportation for nonmetro-politan older persons in upstate New York to participate in daily ac-tivities. Dependence on the automobile was strong among both men and women, but older men were especially likely to continue driving in old age. Just as gender roles affect other areas of the lives of men and women, gender roles also affect critical life-course transitions in the reduction and cessation of driving. Gender differences in driving place older women at greater risk of social isolation than their male coun-terparts. Several indicators of cumulative advantage—being male, younger-old, married, and in better health—are associated with con-tinued driving during old age. And older drivers were shown to be more socially integrated than their non-driving counterparts and to have a higher perceived quality of life. To adapt Carp's (1988) terminology, the *person-environment fit is better among rural older persons who drive.*

Driving is a normative activity among the majority of older resi-dents of nonmetropolitan New York. Why are people so reluctant to give up driving in old age? The explanation seems to be both structural and attitudinal. Attitudinally, rural older individuals, like older Ameri-cans in general, associate driving with independence and self-reliance. Hence, their reluctance to cease driving is partly explained by self-concept.

From a structural standpoint, transportation alternatives are lim-ited in rural areas, and consequently driving facilitates social integra-tion. Older people, especially older rural residents, continue driving to facilitate participation in social networks, community activities and social roles, and to maintain access to goods, services, and facilities. Our finding that rural countryside residents were more likely than those living in town to drive currently shows the usefulness of exam-ining variation within nonmetropolitan areas. Given the deficit of for-mal services and the greater economic vulnerability of older rural residents, it was important to gain a better understanding of how trans-portation transitions and trajectories affect the social integration of older rural residents. Future research comparing across metropolitan and nonmetropolitan areas could lend additional insights into how transportation affects older individuals' social integration.

REFERENCES

Berkman, L. F., & Syme, S. L. (1979). Social networks, host resistance, and mortality: A nine-year follow-up study of Alameda County residents. *American Journal of Epidemiology, 109*, 186–204.

Burkhardt, J. E., & Berger, A. M. (1997). *The mobility consequences of the cessation of driving.* Paper presented to the Transportation Research Board Annual Meeting, Washington, DC.

Burkhardt, J. E., Berger, A. M., & McGavok, A. T. (1996). *The mobility consequences of the reduction or cessation of driving by older women.* Paper presented to the Second National Conference on Women's Travel Issues, Baltimore.

Bylund, R. A., & Crawford, C. O. (1987). An examination of selected dimensions of independent living among a sample of 900 older persons. *Agricultural Experiment Station, Bulletin 864.* University Park, PA: Pennsylvania State University, College of Agriculture.

Carp, F. (1971). On becoming an ex-driver: Prospect and retrospect. *The Gerontologist, 11*, 101–103.

Carp, F. (1972). Retired people as automobile passengers. *The Gerontologist, 12*, 67–71.

Carp, F. (1980). Environmental effects upon the mobility of older people. *Environment and Behavior, 12*, 139–156.

Carp, F. (1988). Significance of mobility for the well-being of the elderly. In *Transportation in an aging society: Improving mobility and safety for older persons, Vol. 2* (1–20). Washington, DC: National Research Council.

Cordes, S. M. (1985). Biopsychological imperatives from the rural perspective. *Social Science and Medicine, 21*, 1373–1379.

Coward, R. T. (1987). Factors associated with the configuration of the helping network of noninstitutionalized elders. *Journal of Gerontological Social Work, 10*, 113–132.

Coward, R. T., Bull, C. N., Kukulka, G., & Galliher, G. M. (1994). *Health services for rural elders.* New York: Springer.

Coward, R. T., & Cutler, S. (1989). Informal and formal health care systems for the rural elderly. *Health Services Research, 23*, 785–806.

Eisenhandler, S. A. (1990). The asphalt identikit: Old age and the driver's license. *International Journal of Aging and Human Development, 30*, 1–14.

Fengler, A. P., & Jensen, L. (1981). Perceived and objective conditions and predictors of life satisfaction of urban and non urban elderly. *Journal of Gerontology, 36*, 750–752.

Glasgow, N. (1988). *The nonmetro elderly: Economic and demographic status.* Washington, DC: U.S. Department of Agriculture Economic Research Service. Rural Development Research Report, No. 70.

Glasgow, N., & Beale, C. L. (1985). Rural elderly in demographic perspective. *Rural Development Perspectives, 21,* 22–26.

Glasgow, N., & Blakely, R. (2000). Older nonmetropolitan residents' evaluations of their transportation arrangements. *Journal of Applied Gerontology, 19,* 95–116.

Glasgow, N., & Brown, D. L. (1997). *Gender differences in driving behavior among nonmetropolitan older residents: Problems and prospects.* Paper presented to the Gerontological Society of America Annual Meeting, Cincinnati.

Glasgow, N., & Brown, D. L. (1998). Older, rural, and poor. In R. T. Coward and J. A. Krout (Eds.), *Aging in rural settings: Life circumstances and distinctive features* (187–207). New York: Springer.

Holden, C. (1987). Why do women live longer than men? *Science, 238,* 158–160.

Iutcovich, J. M., & Iutcovich, M. (1988). Assessment of the transportation needs of Pennsylvania's rural elderly. *Journal of Gerontology, 7,* 515–529.

Lee, G. R., & Cassidy, M. L. (1985). Family and kin relations of the rural elderly. In R. T. Coward and G. R. Lee (Eds.), *The elderly in rural society* (151–169). New York: Springer.

Lee, G. R., & Whitbeck, L. B. (1987). Residential location and social relations among older persons. *Rural Sociology, 52,* 89–97.

Marottoli, R. A., Ostfeld, A. M., Merril, S. S., Perlman, G. D., Foley, D. J., & Cooney, L. M., Jr. (1993). Driving cessation and changes in mileage driven among elderly individuals. *Journal of Gerontology: Social Sciences, 48,* S255–S260.

McGhee, J. L. (1984). The influence of qualitative assessment of the social and physical environment on the morale of the rural elderly. *American Journal of Community Psychology, 12,* 709–723.

Moen, P. (1995). Gender, age, and the life course. In R. H. Binstock and L. George (Eds.), *Handbook of aging and the social sciences,* 4th ed. (171–187). San Diego: Academic Press.

Moen, P., Dempster-McClain, D., & Williams, R. M., Jr. (1989). Social integration and longevity: An event history analysis of women's roles and resilience. *American Sociological Review, 54,* 635–647.

Moen, P., Dempster-McClain, D., & Williams, R. M., Jr. (1992). Successful aging: A life course perspective on women's multiple roles and health. *American Journal of Sociology, 97,* 1612–1638.

National Eldercare Institute on Transportation. (1994). *Meeting the challenge: Mobility for elders.* Washington, DC: National Eldercare Institute on Transportation.

Patton, C. V. (1975). Age groupings and travel in rural areas. *Rural Sociology, 40,* 55–63.

Revis, J. A., & Revis, B. D. (1978). Transportation and disability: An overview of problems and prospects. *Rehabilitation Literature, 39,* 170–179.

Richardson, H. (1987). The health plight of women. *Women and Health, 12,* 41–54.

Rosenbloom, S. (1988). The mobility needs of the elderly. In *Transportation in an aging society: Improving mobility and safety for older persons, Vol. 2* (21–71). Transportation Research Board, Special Report 218. Washington, DC: National Research Council.

Rosenbloom, S. (1995). Travel by the elderly. *Demographic Special Reports: 1990.* Nationwide Personal Transportation Survey Report Series (3–1 through 3–49). Washington, DC: U.S. Department of Transportation, Federal Highway Administration.

Scheidt, R. J., & Norris-Baker, C. (1990). A transactional approach to stress among older residents of rural communities: Introduction to a special issue. *Journal of Rural Community Psychology, 11,* 5–30.

Seeman, T., Kaplan, G. A., Knudsen, L., Cohen, R., & Guralnik, J. (1987). Social network ties and mortality among the elderly in the Alameda County study. *American Journal of Epidemiology, 126,* 714–723.

Sugisawa, H., Liang, J., & Lu, X. (1994). Social networks, social support, and mortality among older people in Japan. *Journal of Gerontology, Social Sciences, 49,* S3–S13.

Taietz, P., & Milton, S. (1979). Rural-urban differences in the structure of services for the elderly in Upstate New York counties. *Journal of Gerontology, 34,* 429–437.

Talbot, D. M. (1985). Assessing the needs of the rural elderly. *Journal of Gerontological Nursing, 11,* 39–43.

Thoits, P. A. (1986). Social support as coping assistance. *Journal of Consulting and Clinical Psychology, 54,* 416–423.

Youmans, E. G. (1977). The rural aged. *Annals of the American Academy of Political Science, 429,* 81–90.

Young, F., & Glasgow, N. (1998). Voluntary social participation and health. *Research on Aging, 20,* 339–362.

CHAPTER FIVE

Social Integration and Family Support

Caregivers to Persons with Alzheimer's Disease

Karl Pillemer and J. Jill Suitor

The present volume, like others in the field that have recently appeared, highlights the positive aspects of "successful" aging. As has been noted in preceding chapters, social integration contributes substantially to productive well-being in later life. However, the unfortunate fact remains that many people spend the final chapter of their lives suffering from disability or chronic illness. And contrary to the popular view of family breakdown and abandonment of older persons, in such situations care for the impaired individual is usually assumed by relatives.

Over the past three decades, scholarly interest in the problems of these "family caregivers" has grown dramatically. Research reports have established the incidence and prevalence of family care provision. A host of studies has examined the negative consequences of becoming a primary caregiver to an impaired elder, focusing in particular on the experience of "burden" from helping responsibilities and resultant psychological distress. Further, a literature on intervention programs designed to improve the lives of family caregivers has developed (Pillemer, 1996; Pillemer & Suitor, 1994).

Given the plethora of studies on this topic, a surprising number of questions regarding the role of social integration in the caregiving experience remain unanswered. We believe that family caregiving situations provide an excellent "laboratory" for examining the effects of social integration in situations of prolonged and unremitting stress.

In this chapter, we explore several issues related to the social integration of caregivers to persons with Alzheimer's disease (AD). We begin by addressing the question, Are AD caregivers at risk of social isolation? Next, we propose an innovative theoretical model for understanding family caregiving, based on the concept of caregiving as a life-course transition. We discuss the major implication of this theoretical model—the critically important role of similar others in promoting social integration. We then provide several illustrative findings from our research.

ALZHEIMER'S DISEASE CAREGIVING: A THREAT TO SOCIAL INTEGRATION?

It has been amply documented that most families do not abandon their frail elderly members but instead perform almost heroically in their attempts to assist them. Research has also shown the emotional toll that such assistance takes on family members. Schulz and colleagues (1995) conducted a comprehensive review of the literature on family caregiving and found overwhelming evidence for increased psychological distress among caregivers, compared to persons not providing care.

Physical health may also be affected. Some studies have found that caregivers report themselves to be in poorer health than comparison groups, although the evidence is somewhat mixed (Haley, 1997; Schulz et al., 1995). There is even evidence suggesting that the stress of caregiving has a negative impact on the functioning of the immune system, which may in turn lead to increased physical morbidity (Kiecolt-Glaser & Glaser, 1994).

Nowhere are such problems so great as among family caregivers to persons suffering from Alzheimer's disease (AD) and other related types of dementia. The symptoms of AD are by now well known. The hallmark is memory loss, especially for recent events. This is not, however, what is sometimes stereotyped as the "benign forgetfulness" of old age. Even in the early stages of AD, victims forget important events entirely and can never recall them. Over time, the memory loss is so profound that the patient cannot recall the previous sentence in a conversation, follow a television story line, or identify familiar places or objects. Finally, the victim becomes unable even to recognize the names or faces of loved ones.

Just as difficult for many family members are the striking behavioral changes AD patients undergo. They often exhibit a wide range of troubling and bizarre behaviors, including agitation, wandering, sleeplessness, delusions, obsessive behavior, and even violence. Research has demonstrated the burden and stress experienced by family caregivers in dealing with both the mental deterioration and the problematic behaviors of AD patients (Haley, 1997).

AD is definitely a family affair. Family members encounter many costs in caring for a dementia patient, including:

— The things they most loved about the patient in his or her healthy years—intellect, wit, thoughtfulness—may be gone.
— Families lose the loved one as a source of closeness and support, as their activities become almost entirely devoted to caregiving.
— Families have to come to terms with an intense sense of loss— the living death of a person they once loved. They feel grief, anger, and anxiety as part of an anticipatory grieving process.
— For some families, severe economic costs result from caring for a relative with AD.

Because of these experiences, family caregiving to dementia patients provides an appropriate focus for studies of the effects of social support and social relationships on persons undergoing chronic stress. The devastating nature of the disease and the responsibilities placed on family members are likely to compromise their social relationships. Further, the deterioration of potentially supportive relationships may have negative effects on caregivers' physical and psychological well-being.

Impact on Social Relationships

A common finding from the past two decades of research is that individuals' involvement with friends and family often declines after they become primary caregivers (Archbold, 1982; Brody & Lang, 1982; Cantor, 1983; Chenoweth & Spencer, 1986; Fengler & Goodrich, 1979; Grafstroem & Winblad, 1995; Mace, 1984; Moritz et al., 1989). However, the question arises of whether this effect is due simply to caregiving, or to special characteristics of AD that cause greater disruptions in social relationships than occur in situations where the care recipient is not demented. Birkel and Jones (1989) contrasted aspects of the social networks of caregivers to demented and non-demented elders. They argued that the presence of dementia can actually *decrease* the amount of help others provide to the care recipient.

Birkel and Jones suggested that such a decrease can occur for several reasons. First, the mood swings and disruptive behaviors that often accompany dementia may discourage others from providing assistance. Second, the shame associated with mental illness may cause caregivers to isolate themselves. Third, non-demented elders can help maintain relationships with persons outside the household, whereas demented persons generally cannot. They hypothesize that families caring for demented persons will rely on resources within the household and that the primary caregiver will be less likely to receive help from persons outside the household.

The authors compared elderly physically disabled persons without dementia with individuals who had both physical disability and dementia. As hypothesized, the dementia group had smaller overall networks and fewer helpers from outside the household. Household members provided a greater number of hours of care for dementia patients; fewer hours were provided by non-household members. Overall, dementia caregivers identified fewer out-of-household supporters. Thus, Birkel and Jones's study indicates that responsibility for caring for non-demented individuals is shared to a greater extent than the care of demented persons. When the care recipient had dementia, responsibility fell on a smaller number of household members.

Other research concurs with these findings. Shaw et al. (1991) compared the support received by caregivers to Alzheimer's patients and caregivers to frail, non-demented elders. Alzheimer's caregivers were more likely to identify unmet needs for social support. They also reported having fewer non-kin supporters. Similarly, Clipp and George (1990) compared caregivers to dementia patients with persons caring for cancer patients. Overall satisfaction with social activities was substantially lower for dementia caregivers. They also were more likely to report feeling alone and to need more help from friends and family. Thus, becoming an AD caregiver appears to reduce social interaction, and caregivers cannot assume that they will be provided with adequate support. (However, for an exception, see Catternach & Tebes, 1991.)

Another critical question is, Do patterns of support and interaction change throughout the course of the illness? George and Gwyther (1986) used data on 376 AD caregivers to test whether six sets of caregiver characteristics and needs predicted levels of support over time. In general, patterns of support remained stable over the course of one year, with only about 15 percent of the respondents reporting decreases in either instrumental support or perceived support over that period.

When changes occurred, however, caregivers in greatest need of support were paradoxically those who were least likely to receive it. Persons who either had high support at both time points, or who received increasing support over the year, were likely to be better educated and have higher incomes, to have frequent contact with friends and family, and to be caregivers to a person who was institutionalized. Those persons who were either low in support at both times, or whose support decreased, were disproportionately older and had lower incomes. They reported higher stress and were mostly caring for relatives in their homes.

Effects of Social Relationships on AD Caregivers

The preceding discussion suggests that social integration is compromised for AD caregivers. We now turn our attention to the *impact* of social relationships on caregivers. It is important to note that inconsistencies exist among studies in terms of sampling strategy, definitions of key concepts, and selection of independent and dependent variables. Therefore, generalizations about the relationship between social support and psychological well-being among caregivers must be made with caution. However, the more methodologically sound studies provide at least preliminary support for two points. First, satisfaction with social support leads to psychological well-being in caregivers. Second, interpersonal stress has a negative effect on psychological well-being among caregivers. We provide supporting evidence for these points here.

Satisfaction with Social Support. Several studies support the first assertion. Fiore and colleagues (1986) studied caregivers to spouses with Alzheimer's disease and found that satisfaction with support was the best predictor of depression and negative psychological symptoms. Similarly, George and Gwyther (1986) examined the impact of a measure of perceived need for more social support on several well-being measures. This item was strongly predictive of both self-rated physical health and several measures of psychological well-being. Zarit et al. (1986) and Stuckey and Smyth (1997) found that caregivers' subjective rating of the adequacy of support received predicted caregiver burden. Finally, Creasey et al. (1990) examined the impact of the spousal relationship on caregiver burden. Again, perception of support from the spouse was negatively associated with burden.

Interestingly, it does not appear that mere contact or the *potential* provision of support results in better psychological outcomes for caregivers. For example, in the study by Fiore and colleagues (1986) mentioned above, frequency of contact with network members, frequency with which the respondent called on network members for support, and extent to which the network members were perceived as available for support were *not* found to predict caregiver well-being.

Several other studies confirm this finding. Chiriboga et al. (1990) found that measures of the simple presence of *possible* supporters— such as the number of friends living nearby, number of siblings, marital status, and involvement in self-help groups—were not consistently related to caregivers' psychological well-being. Moritz et al. (1989) found no relationship between social isolation—measured as having no monthly "visual contacts" with friends or relatives other than children—and depression. Cohen et al. (1994) found measures of network structure and social contact to have very little impact on caregiver well-being, as did Stuckey and Smyth (1997).

Interpersonal Stress. It appears, then, that perceptions of social support have some potential for explaining caregiver well-being, while measures of contact, network structure, and instrumental support have a less clear effect. However, although most researchers have emphasized the positive effects of social support on psychological well-being, there are both theoretical and empirical bases upon which to suggest that *negative* interactions with network members may have more pronounced and detrimental effects (Rook, 1984). In the past decade, investigators have paid increasing attention to what has been variously described as "negative support," or "interpersonal stress."

Interestingly, one of the earliest studies of AD caregivers provided evidence that negative interactions were particularly predictive of distress. Fiore and colleagues (1983) found that the experience of upset within the social network owing to unmet expectations of support or to negative interactions with others was by far the best predictor of depression among AD caregivers. Upset in the area of "cognitive guidance" was most strongly predictive of depression; this area includes interactions that are designed to increase the caregiver's understanding of problems like the illness course and that help to put the situation into perspective. Social network helpfulness was not related to depression in this study.

Further supporting evidence is available for the importance of interpersonal stress in explaining caregiving outcomes. For example,

Creasey et al. (1990) found that for adult daughters caring for elderly parents with AD, negative interactions with their spouses were strongly positively associated with burden. Semple (1992) also found that conflict over family members' attitudes and actions toward the caregiver were related to depression.

Spouses' negative behaviors relating to caregiving also appear to affect the quality of marital relationships. Suitor and Pillemer (1996) used quantitative and qualitative data to examine the factors explaining marital satisfaction among women who recently began caring for an elderly parent with Alzheimer's disease or a related dementia. The findings indicated that husbands' hindrances of their wives' caregiving, as well as failure to provide them with support, had a negative effect on marital satisfaction.

Franks and Stephens' (1992) research is also worth noting in this context. Franks and Stephens interviewed women primary caregivers to elderly family members who were living in the community. In addition to the caregiving role, they examined stress in two other roles: those of wife and mother. Most of the stress items relating to the wife and mother role measured various types of negative interactions (e.g., in the wife role, conflicts over children, insufficient emotional support, not enough appreciation). Stress in both roles was negatively related to psychological well-being, with stress in the mother role a particularly strong predictor. In a related study, Stephens et al. (1994) examined not only the stressful aspects of roles but also the rewards received. Again, stress in the maternal role most strongly predicted the measures of distress. Interpersonal stress with intimates appears to be a potentially powerful predictor of caregiver distress.

Summary

In this discussion, several points become clear. First, AD caregivers experience deficits and problems in their social relationships. Second, the degree of perceived support from others has a beneficial impact on caregivers' well-being. And third, negative interactions with network members cause distress for care providers. Our review of the literature indicates a paradox: although social integration is of great importance to AD caregivers, social support and relationships are in fact threatened by taking on this role, with potential detrimental effects on caregivers.

NEW DIRECTIONS: CONCEPTUALIZING FAMILY
CAREGIVING AS A LIFE-COURSE TRANSITION

Where should we go from here? We believe that it is possible to move beyond such descriptive findings and to advance our knowledge of caregiving and social support in major new directions. In particular, it is important to study the issue of social support and caregiving in the context of broader sociological theory regarding interpersonal relationships. Consistent with the theme of the present volume, we hold that conceptual frameworks for research and intervention on family caregiving should be based on a life-course approach (see Chapter 2).

The life-course approach suggests that researchers should examine issues of support and caregiving from a dynamic perspective. Caregiving has typically been viewed as a specific *activity*, rather than as a status that individuals move into and out of at various points in the life course (Moen et al., 1994). In contrast, we hold that "family caregiver" meets the sociological definition of a social status—particularly when individuals assume primary responsibility for the care of an elderly relative (Suitor & Pillemer, 1990).

This conceptualization allows investigators to view becoming an AD caregiver as a *status transition*, similar to other transitions in the life course, such as becoming a new parent, a widow, or a retiree. As we demonstrate below, reconceptualizing caregiving as a life-course transition allows us to develop a theoretical framework for understanding social relations and caregiving, as well as to provide suggestions for planning interventions.

Further, the life-course approach suggests that social networks will change in response to critical transitions and that different people in a lifetime "convoy" of support (Antonucci, 1990) will be activated as needed. This point is related to House's classic question regarding social support: *"Who* gives *what* to *whom* regarding *which* problems?" (1981: 22). A great deal of work has been directed toward answering this question in the intervening years, with considerable attention focused on identifying associates who are most likely to be sources of support for persons who have experienced negative life events. Our goal has been to extend this line of research to the study of AD caregivers.

Finally, an expanded perspective on caregiving leads us to examine more systematically the role of interpersonal stress in AD caregiving relationships. The preliminary evidence discussed above suggests that negative interactions with network members are as or more strongly related to caregiving outcomes than emotional and instrumental support. It is therefore important to identify both the sources of interpersonal stress, as well as its consequences.

Over the past several years, we have been involved in a program of research designed to address these issues. In this section, we summarize the conceptual framework we have developed to guide this research and briefly note several examples of empirical research we have conducted to test components of the theoretical framework. We then turn to the application of this framework in an intervention for AD caregivers.

Family Caregiving as a Status Transition

Why should we consider the position of family caregiver as a social status? One basis for this argument is that "family caregiver" is a position in society that has specific behavioral and attitudinal expectations attached to it (Suitor & Pillemer, 1990). Individuals who assume the care of an elderly relative are expected to provide both physical and emotional support for the care recipient, and to do so with a minimum of resentment (Cicirelli, 1981; George, 1986; Gubrium, 1988; Zarit & Knight, 1996).

Research on attitudes regarding filial responsibility illustrates the persistence of these norms. Friends and relatives expect adult children and spouses to provide elderly parents with assistance for activities of daily living and expenses, even when doing so requires that the caregiver alter family plans and work responsibilities (Jarrett, 1985; George, 1986; Gubrium, 1988; Lawton, 1996; Zarit et al., 1998). These informal prescriptions to provide assistance are reinforced by laws in most states regarding elder neglect that provide formal standards for adequate performance of caregiving responsibilities (cf. Crystal, 1986; Wolf & Pillemer, 1989).

Based on this argument, we suggest that becoming a caregiver involves a status acquisition that is similar in many ways to those experienced when individuals acquire other new social statuses in adulthood, such as becoming a parent, becoming divorced, retiring, or entering the labor force or college. The event that triggers the status transition to family caregiver is usually the onset of the relative's illness or injury, or the relative's discharge from the hospital following serious illness or injury.

In the case of AD, however, there may not always be an abrupt change in well-being that initiates caregiving. However, there are two bases upon which to argue that caregiving responsibilities are likely to become most clearly defined at the time that a *formal diagnosis* of dementia is made. First, prior to diagnosis, the individual may have given nonmedical interpretations to the older person's condition. After the illness has been identified and labeled, the caregiver must recognize that the patient is seriously ill and begin to plan for his or her long-term care. Second, once the patient's condition has been brought to the attention of medical personnel, they will expect the relative who has been listed as the primary contact/responsible person to begin enacting the role of caregiver, thus creating social pressure on the individual to perform that role. Therefore, we would argue that in most cases, there is a point that marks the transition to the status of caregiver, even in the case of victims of dementia.

Status Transitions and the Benefits of Similar Others

If becoming a family caregiver is viewed as a status transition, a great deal of research literature becomes applicable. This research shows that acquiring a new social status generally produces changes in individuals' social networks that affect both the provision of social support and psychological well-being. Most important, when people acquire new statuses, they often reduce contact with associates to whom they have become less similar and intensify existing relationships (or develop new ones) with others to whom they have become more similar (see Bell, 1981; Belsky & Rovine, 1984; Gouldner & Strong, 1987; Hetherington et al., 1976; Suitor et al., 1995).

This pattern of increased status similarity appears to augment the positive effect of social support on psychological well-being. Lin and colleagues (Lin et al., 1985, 1986) found that support from individuals who were similar to the respondents (e.g., in terms of similarity of age or occupational prestige) was associated with lower levels of depression following undesirable life events, while support from dissimilar sources was not.

More important than structural types of similarity, such as age, occupation, and gender, is what we term *experiential similarity*. Thoits

(1986) has cogently argued that particularly important is similarity of *situational experience:* empathic understanding, which is critical to the support process, is more likely to come from similar others. Based on Thoits's model, we suggest that the benefits occur for several reasons.

First, distressed persons frequently fear that something is seriously wrong with them. Others who have been through the same experience can help the stressed individual to view his or her feelings as acceptable, to be expected, and within the range of normality. Similar others may be less likely to reject persons because of their distress or strong emotions. This greater sense of acceptance may allow stressed individuals more freedom to discuss their feelings than they experience with non-similar associates.

Thus, a distressed person must perceive empathic understanding from potential helpers in order to receive maximum benefit from their assistance. Situationally similar persons will provide the most helpful support because they can offer the stressed individual precisely this: understanding based on shared experience (Pillemer & Suitor, 1996; Thoits, 1986). The positive effects also occur because similarity decreases the likelihood that social interactions will have detrimental consequences on well-being. That is, experiential similarity can reduce the amount of interpersonal stress that occurs in a relationship. We suggest that the potentially negative consequences of social support are less likely when support is offered by network members to whom the individual is more similar.

The basis for this expectation is that individuals who share social statuses may be more accepting of one another's temporary inability to reciprocate support. This may occur in part because status similarity is associated with greater closeness, and there is more tolerance of a short-term violation of the norm of reciprocity among intimates. But it is also likely that individuals who are status similar have a greater understanding of one another's resources and ability to reciprocate, and are therefore more tolerant of temporary periods of non-reciprocity (see Suitor & Pillemer, 1990, for a more complete discussion of this issue).

Another potential source of stress associated with network contact has been alluded to earlier: unmet expectations of support and negative input from network members are possibly more important in explaining psychological well-being than is perceived helpfulness. The greater value similarity associated with status similarity is likely to reduce criticism (cf. Suitor 1987a; 1987b). Research on ineffective and miscarried support further bolsters the importance of similar others. Advice and intervention is more likely to be perceived as stressful when it comes from associates who are not similar.

RESEARCH EXAMPLES

Based on the discussion above, conceiving of family caregiving as a life-course transition leads us to the following hypothesis: experiential similarity will be particularly important in explaining which associates will be sources of support and stress, and in predicting psychological well-being. In the remainder of this section, we summarize several findings from our own research that illustrate this approach. In accordance with the perspective we presented in Chapter 2, we pay attention to both subgroup variations (with gender as an example) and to longitudinal findings. The examples are drawn from two independent but conceptually related studies we have conducted over the past several years.

Study 1

This research project involved a longitudinal study of caregivers to relatives with AD called "Caregivers across Time." It is beyond the scope of this chapter to describe the methods of this study in detail (see Pillemer & Suitor, 1996; Suitor & Pillemer, 1996). To summarize, the first wave of data was collected between January 1989 and March 1992 during two-hour interviews with 256 individuals who were identified as the primary caregivers to elderly relatives with some form of irreversible dementia. The participants were referred to the study by physicians at major medical centers in the northeastern United States that have dementia screening programs. The Wave 1 sample included 118 daughters, 14 sons, 30 daughters-in-law, 53 wives, 25 husbands, 7 siblings, 6 other relatives, and 3 nonrelatives who were viewed by the respondents as equivalent to kin. Interviews were conducted one year and two years following the original interview.

Respondents were also asked for detailed information about members of their social networks. For each of the more than two thousand network members named, we collected data on the individual's demographic characteristics (age, educational attainment, gender, marital status, employment status, etc.), and whether the associate had experience caring for an elderly relative. Respondents were also asked about ways the associates had been supportive and the extent to which they were sources of interpersonal stress.

Study 2

The second study uses data collected for the Peer Support Project study. Because this study is described in detail in Chapter 11, we will not provide extensive information here. In brief, the data for the Peer Support Project were collected between March 1994 and April 1997 on 145 individuals, using essentially the same measures and procedures as those employed in the Caregivers Across Time study. There were only two differences in the procedures. First, all respondents were recruited through one major medical center, located in Syracuse, New York. Second, all potential respondents were informed that if they participated in the study, they might be asked to spend one hour a week for eight weeks with a "friendly visitor" discussing caregiving, in addition to completing three interviews across a period of one year. The friendly visitor was an experienced caregiver who had been trained to provide support and information to the respondent. It is important to note that only Wave 1 data were used in the analysis discussed below, and thus all of the interviews took place prior to the "friendly visitor" intervention.

Using these data sets (either individually or linked), we have conducted a series of analyses that shed light on the theoretical framework outlined above. Here, we summarize several of the most relevant and interesting findings.

Explaining Support and Interpersonal Stress

Using only the Caregivers Across Time data set, we conducted a multivariate analysis of factors affecting support and stress. This analysis clearly demonstrates the importance of status similarity in explaining whether individual network members were a source of support or interpersonal stress. We found that associates who had themselves provided care to an elderly relative were more likely to have been a source of support. Further, network members with caregiving experience were less likely to have been a source of interpersonal stress,

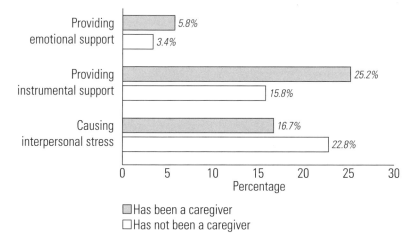

Figure 5.1   Comparison of Associates with and without Caregiving Experience.

such as criticism, direct interference, or unmet expectations for support (see Figure 5.1).

The respondents were often aware of the importance of caregiving similarity in explaining which associates were most likely to be sources of support or stress. Caregivers' responses to open-ended questions indicated that relatives and friends who were sources of stress had little sense of the responsibilities and emotions involved in caring for a parent suffering from dementia, owing to their inexperience as caregivers. For example:

> Everyone will put their two cents in on how they think it should be. . . . If you don't live with an Alzheimer's patient, you have no idea. It's like you're in a world unto yourself because [my mother] will go out and do absolutely nothing in front of somebody else and be as normal as normal can be and [my relatives and friends] think that [I'm] exaggerating. Walk in my shoes kind of thing. . . .

> [I told my brother that mother] is just really terrible. She wets all over the place, she couldn't remember anything or anyone. [He] just didn't want to believe me . . . he thought I was just being ridiculous and crazy and all that. . . . I think that not being involved in giving care made it [hard] for him to [understand] what was going on.

People don't really [understand]. . . . [A friend] annoyed me because I always felt, you're not walking in my shoes and I said [to myself] you don't know what you're talking about. I never told her but it made me feel, you know, bad.

The Role of Gender

These findings demonstrate the importance of experiential similarity. Another question is also relevant, however: To what extent does gender affect patterns of similarity and support from network members? We conducted analyses to shed light on this question. (A full report of this study can be found in Suitor & Pillemer, in press.)

We believed that there were grounds to argue that experiential similarity may be even more important for men than women in explaining the circumstances under which individuals seek and accept emotional support. The literature is very consistent about gender differences between men's and women's patterns of support. Although men are generally more likely than women to receive high levels of support from their spouses (cf. Lynch, 1998; Okun & Keith, 1998), they are far less likely than women to receive support from all other sources throughout the life course (cf. Harrison et al., 1995; Okun & Keith, 1998; Rossi & Rossi, 1990). It has been suggested that these gender differences exist because men's socialization leads them to be (1) less willing than women to admit needing or desiring support, (2) less willing than women to accept support when offered, (3) less proficient than women at soliciting support, and (4) less willing and able than women to reciprocate support (cf. Barbee et al., 1993; Dunkel-Schetter & Slokum, 1990; Riggio & Zimmerman, 1991).

In the face of such obstacles to receiving support, the greater empathy and understanding between associates with shared experiences may be even more necessary for men than women to both ask for and accept support. Further, experiential similarity may be especially important when men experience focal events that are generally experienced by women, such as becoming a caregiver. Women who become caregivers step into a more familiar "kinkeeping/caring" role (cf. Gerstel & Gallagher, 1993). In contrast, men are unlikely to have been socialized to these roles, and therefore they may feel less competent and comfortable. As a result, men may particularly benefit from the support from similar others. In addition, men's greater difficulty in reciprocating emotional support may be less of a problem with associates who have had similar experiences, because these individuals have greater understanding of the way in which stressful events diminish the ability to reciprocate (cf. Pillemer & Suitor, 1996).

To explore this issue, we conducted analyses to investigate whether experiential similarity affects how men and women obtain social support. To do so, we used a combined data set that included the Time 1 data for both the Caregivers Across Time study and the Peer Support Project study. When the two studies were combined, the sample contained 401 caregivers, including 169 daughters, 34 sons, 35 daughters-in-law, 98 wives, 46 husbands, 8 siblings, 8 other relatives, and 3 nonrelatives who were viewed by the respondents as equivalent to kin. Sixty-six percent were women; 34 percent were men.

To investigate whether experiential similarity was equally important in explaining men's and women's pattern of support, we conducted a series of logistic regression analyses using the associate as the unit of analysis. In these analyses, we examined whether associates with caregiving experience were more likely named as sources of support by both men and women.

Throughout these analyses, the following variables were controlled: (a) the associate's age; (b) the respondent's age; (c) the respondent's marital status; and (d) the number of miles that the associate lived from the respondent.

The findings demonstrated clear differences in the importance of experiential similarity in explaining men's and women's patterns of support. Multivariate analyses revealed that caregiving similarity was a consistent predictor of which associates were named as sources of support to women respondents. In fact, this variable was important across all of the dimensions of support on which we collected data. In contrast, for men, caregiving similarity was important only in explaining which associates provided instrumental support specific to caregiving.

Perhaps the higher significance of experiential similarity for women than men can be explained by the greater importance and demands of the caregiving role for women, often resulting in decreases in women's time and energy for social interaction. If interaction must be limited, perhaps restricting contact to those associates who have the greatest understanding of the difficulties and constraints of caregiving reduces stressful interactions for women caregivers (Pillemer & Suitor, 1996, Suitor & Pillemer, 1993, 1996; Suitor et al., 1995).

Our qualitative data suggest that, in fact, the women chose to spend time with others who had been caregivers specifically because of the increased empathy associated with experiential similarity. For example, two women reported:

> [When you talk to others who have been caregivers] you're able to verbalize your feelings, what you're going through, what's happening . . . You get the support of each other . . . They have the full understanding of what you're going through. . . . That's a big help in itself.

> [My friend Laura and I] are a sounding board for one another. She's here with me every day. She went through [caring for her mother] last year. Her mother [was in a nursing home] and I was very supportive of her too.

In contrast, none of the men mentioned the issue of caregiving similarity when discussing their relationships with network members. For men, such discrimination among associates in terms of caregiving similarity may be less important, since their caregiving activities are a less central focus of their day-to-day lives. It appears that gender differences emerge in the role that similar others play in the lives of people undergoing stress. For women, such associates play a critical role in providing support; for men, this effect is much less evident.

Changes across Time

The findings discussed above demonstrate the importance of experiential similarity, particularly for women, during the early period following the transition to family caregiver. But they do not tell us about the long-term effects of similarity on patterns of support and interpersonal stress. It is possible that experiential similarity continues to affect support and stress long after an individual becomes a caregiver. However, it is also possible that similarity becomes less important in explaining support and stress as the caregiver moves further from the status transition.

Why might the importance of experiential similarity diminish over time? First, as caregiving continues, friends and relatives can observe the time and effort involved, and thereby become more understanding, even if they have not been caregivers themselves. In addition, caregivers may become more proficient at explaining their situation to others. This would place them in a better position to directly ask for support from associates who do not have caregiving experience. Over time, they may also learn how to deflect criticism from these individuals. Caregivers may also become more confident in their roles and therefore may need to rely less on others who have provided care to elderly relatives as they spend more time caregiving. In sum, the need for similar others may be especially acute for the novice caregiver and diminish as he or she becomes more confident and experienced (a pattern that has been anecdotally noted about new parents).

To examine this hypothesis, we used data on the fifty-seven married daughters from the Caregivers Across Time study who were still providing care to their mothers after two years (Suitor et al., 1995). As noted earlier, the caregivers completed a total of three interviews at one-year intervals, beginning shortly after the relative's diagnosis. Since we were concerned with changes across a longer period, we chose to use only the data from the Time 1 and the Time 3 interviews for this analysis.

The logistic regression analysis we conducted using these data revealed that experiential similarity became less important in explaining patterns of emotional support across the first two years of caregiving, as we anticipated. Associates who had been caregivers themselves at Time 1 were much more likely to provide emotional support than were associates without caregiving experience. However, this effect had almost disappeared by Time 3.

In contrast, experiential similarity continued to be important in explaining which associates provided instrumental support (that is, concrete help with caregiving tasks or related assistance). In fact, experiential similarity was the only factor (besides relationship to the caregiver) that helped to explain patterns of instrumental support at both Time 1 and Time 3. Thus, even though caregivers became less reliant on others with similar caregiving experience for emotional support, they maintained their reliance on fellow caregivers for instrumental support.

What might these differences in the long-term effects of experiential similarity on patterns of emotional and instrumental support result from? We believe that the explanation may lie in differences in the obstacles to providing caregivers with these two types of support. Providing emotional support requires only that a friend or relative become more sensitive to the concerns expressed by the caregivers. In contrast, providing the sorts of instrumental support that the caregivers reported most frequently (e.g., respite, personal care of the parent, etc.) requires skills that most associates would not have developed if they did not have direct prior experience assisting frail or impaired elderly.

Interestingly, changes in the effects of experiential similarity on interpersonal stress paralleled those found in the analysis of emotional support. While associates without caregiving experience were more likely to have been sources of interpersonal stress at Time 1, they were no more likely than previous caregivers to have been named by Time 3. The decrease in the importance of experiential similarity in explaining emotional support and interpersonal stress was also reflected in the qualitative data. Indeed, at Time 3, the issue of caregiving experience was not raised when the women discussed either associates' emotional supportiveness or their negative attitudes and behaviors.

In sum, these findings show that experiential similarity becomes less important as the caregiving career progresses. As discussed earlier, it is possible that as an individual moves further from a transition, he or she becomes better at informing others about his or her needs and difficulties. This increased ability might reduce differences between how caregivers are treated by associates with and without caregiving experience. Further, as individuals become more confident in their caregiving role, they may feel less need to ask for emotional support primarily from associates with caregiving experience, because they can increasingly rely on their own experience and knowledge. This may be particularly true for our sample, in which relatives were recently diagnosed, because a major function of associates is probably cognitive guidance—that is, helping the new caregivers to interpret their situation in this novel and unsettling early stage. This type of cognitive guidance is more important in early stages of the caregiving career, because the individual can draw on his or her own resources at later stages.

The qualitative data support these explanations. At Time 1, the women's statements indicated that they greatly relied on other caregivers because these were the only individuals who "truly understood" their situation and could guide them in their decisions regarding care. However, by Time 3, the women increasingly referred to their own experiences when trying to solve problems and no longer appeared to feel that only other caregivers understood their situation.

One alternative explanation is possible: perhaps the effect of experiential similarity also diminished because the respondents experienced less caregiving stress or reduced their actual caregiving responsibilities. However, neither of these explanations can account for the reduced effect of experiential similarity. We conducted several analyses to examine whether experiential similarity was important for some subgroups but not for others. We divided the sample on the basis of subjective stress, number of caregiving tasks performed, hours spent providing care, and nursing home placement. Analyses across all of these subgroups revealed the same pattern shown in the full sample.

Effects of Status-Similar Others on the Well-Being of Caregivers

This set of findings shows that status similarity is a powerful predictor of the provision of support and interpersonal stress by network members. The theoretical framework outlined above also proposed that the presence of status-similar others in social networks would reduce psychological distress among caregivers. In another analysis, we investigated this second question by examining the effect of experiential and structural similarity on caregivers' well-being. We anticipated that the presence of a larger proportion of other caregivers in the respondents' social networks would be positively related to psychological well-being (for a complete discussion of this study, see Pillemer & Suitor, 1996).

A multivariate analysis confirmed our hypotheses. The number of other caregivers in the respondents' social networks significantly predicted lower levels of depression. Further, the effect of similar others was even stronger in the portion of the sample where caregiving stress was greatest. Specifically, among persons whose relatives exhibited serious disruptive behaviors, the number of other caregivers in the network emerged as more strongly related to depression than self-reported health, amount of help provided, or living arrangement.

Summary

In sum, the findings presented here contribute to a growing literature showing that associating with others who have experienced the same status transition leads to greater support and less interpersonal stress. Specifically, similar associates are more likely to provide support and less likely to be sources of interpersonal stress. The studies also suggest that this pattern is more likely to occur among women than men and becomes less important for some dimensions of interpersonal relations as individuals acquire more experience enacting their new roles. Further, respondents who named a larger proportion of other caregivers in their networks had lower depression scores, especially in situations of greater stress. Taken together, these findings support our conceptual framework, in which we argued that persons undergoing a stressful life course transition—in this case to the status of AD care-giver—are benefited by networks with heavier concentrations of associates who have experienced the same transition.

CONCLUSION

In this chapter we have attempted to identify both consistent findings as well as major gaps in the literature on the social relationships of AD caregivers. In addition, we provided a conceptual framework and described several empirical analyses to demonstrate a new and, we believe, promising approach to the study of caregiving and social support. From a research perspective, we believe that it is important for investigators to avoid methodological problems that limit the utility of many of the research findings. Most important, many studies have been largely atheoretical, examining questions that emerged from clinical practice rather than grounding the hypotheses firmly on a theoretical basis. Researchers should frame their studies in light of sociological and psychological theory. We believe that the research program described in this chapter, which used theory related to life-course transitions and status similarity, provides a compelling example of the benefits of such theoretical grounding.

Ultimately, the beneficiaries of these refinements will be not only the scientific community but also persons professionally and personally concerned with assisting family caregivers to AD patients. Little is known as yet about social support interventions for dementia caregivers. Demonstration projects are needed that examine the mechanisms through which support is effective. The fruits of such targeted intervention studies will be improvements in practice. Examining changes in social support, interpersonal stress, and psychological distress across the caregiving career will increase our ability to target interventions to persons who need them most, at the points when they will have the greatest benefit. Theoretically grounded and empirically sound research on this topic will enhance our ability to successfully provide support to caregivers and, in turn, ease the strain and distress they experience. The Peer Support Project intervention, described in Chapter 11, provides one example of work that moves in this direction.

REFERENCES

Archbold, P. G. (1982). All-consuming activity: The family as caregiver. *Generations, 7,* 12–13, 40.

Antonucci, T. C. (1990). Social supports and relationships. In R. H. Binstock & L. K. George (Eds.), *Handbook of Aging and the Social Sciences,* 3d ed. (205–226). New York: Academic Press.

Barbee, A. P., Cunningham, M. R., Winstead, B. A., Derlega, V. J., Gulley, M. R., Yankeelov, P. A., & Druen, P. B. (1993). Effects of gender role expectations on the social support process. *Journal of Social Issues, 49,* 175–190.

Bell, R. R. (1981). *Worlds of friendship.* Beverly Hills: Sage.

Belsky, J., & Rovine, M. (1984). Social-network contact, family support, and the transition to parenthood. *Journal of Marriage and the Family, 46,* 455–462.

Birkel, R. C., & Jones, C. J. (1989). A comparison of the caregiving networks of dependent elderly individuals who are lucid and those who are demented. *The Gerontologist, 29,* 14–119.

Brody, E. M., & Lang, A. (1982). They can't do it all: Aging daughters with aged mothers. *Generations, 7,* 18–20, 37.

Cantor, M. (1983). Strain among caregivers: A study of experience in the United States. *The Gerontologist, 23,* 597–604.

Catternach, L., & Tebes, J. K. (1991). The nature of elder impairment and its impact on family caregivers' health and psychosocial functioning. *The Gerontologist, 31,* 246–255.

Chenoweth, B., & Spencer, R. (1986). Dementia: The experience of family caregivers. *The Gerontologist 26,* 267–272.

Chiriboga, D. A., Weiler, P. G., & Nielsen, K. (1990). The stress of caregivers. In D. Biegel & A. Blum (Eds.), *Aging and caregiving: Theory, research, and policy* (1221–137). Newbury Park, CA: Sage.

Cicirelli, V. (1981). *Helping elderly parents: Role of adult children.* Boston: Auburn House.

Clipp, E. C., & George, L. K. (1990). Caregiver needs and patterns of social support. *Journal of Gerontology: Social Sciences, 45,* S102–111.

Clipp, E. C., & George, L. K. (1993). Dementia and cancer: A comparison of spousal caregivers. *The Gerontologist, 33,* 534–541.

Cohen, C., Teresi, J., & Blum, C. (1994). The role of caregiver social networks in Alzheimer's disease. *Social Science and Medicine, 38,* 1483–1490.

Creasey, G. L., Myers, B. J., Epperson, M. J., & Taylor, J. (1990). Couples with an elderly parent with Alzheimer's disease: Perceptions of family relationships. *Psychiatry, 53,* 44–51.

Crystal, S. (1986). Social policy and elder abuse. In K. Pillemer & R. S. Wolf (Eds.), *Elder abuse: Conflict in the family* (331–40). Dover, MA: Auburn House.

Dunkel-Schetter, C., & Slokum, L. (1990). Determinants of social support provisions in personal relationships. *Journal of Social and Personal Relationships, 7,* 435–450.

Fengler, A. P., & Goodrich, N. (1979). Wives of elderly disabled men: The hidden patients. *The Gerontologist, 19,* 175–183.

Fiore, J., Becker, J., & Coppel, D. B. (1983). Social network interactions: A buffer or a stress? *American Journal of Community Psychology, 11,* 423–439.

Fiore, J., Coppel, D. B., Becker, J., & Cox, G. B. (1986). Social support as a multifaceted concept: Examination of important dimensions for adjustment. *American Journal of Community Psychology, 14,* 93–111.

Franks, M. M., & Stephens, M. A. P. (1992). Multiple roles of middle-generation caregivers: Contextual effects and psychological mechanisms. *Journal of Gerontology: Psychological Sciences, 47,* S123–S129.

George, L. K. (1986). Caregiver burden: Conflict between norms of reciprocity and solidarity. In K. Pillemer & R. S. Wolf (Eds.), *Elder abuse: Conflict in the family* (67–92). Dover, MA: Auburn House.

George, L. K., & Gwyther, L. P. (1986). Caregiver well-being: A multidimensional examination of family caregivers of demented adults. *The Gerontologist, 26,* 253–259.

Gerstel, N., & Gallagher, S. K. (1993). Kinkeeping and distress: Gender, recipients of care, and work-family conflict. *Journal of Marriage and the Family, 55,* 598–607.

Gouldner, H., & Strong, M. S. (1987). *Speaking of friendship: Middle-class women and their friends.* New York: Greenwood Press.

Grafstroem, M., & Winblad, B. (1995). Family burden in the care of the demented and nondemented elderly: A longitudinal study. *Alzheimer's Disease and Associated Disorders, 9,* 78–86.

Gubrium, J. F. (1988). Family responsibility and caregiving in the qualitative analysis of the Alzheimer's disease experience. *Journal of Marriage and the Family, 50,* 197–207.

Haley, William E. (1997). The family caregiver's role in Alzheimer's disease. *Neurology, 48,* S25–S29.

Harrison, J., Maguire, P., & Pitceathly, C. (1995). Confiding in crisis: Gender differences in patterns of confiding among cancer patients. *Social Science and Medicine, 41,* 1255–1260.

Hetherington, E. M., Cox, M., & Cox, R. (1976). Divorced fathers. *Family Coordinator, 25,* 417–428.

House, J. (1981). *Work stress and family support.* Reading, MA: Addison-Wesley.

Jarrett, W. H. (1985). Caregiving within kinship systems: Is affection really necessary? *The Gerontologist, 25,* 5–10.

Kiecolt-Glaser, J. K., & Glaser, R. (1994). Caregivers, mental health, and immune function. In E. Light, G. Niederehe, & B. D. Lebowitz (Eds.), *Stress effects on family caregivers of Alzheimer's patients* (64–75). New York: Springer.

Lawton, M. P. (1996). The aging family in a multigenerational perspective. In G. H. S. Singer, L. E. Powers, & A. L. Olson (Eds.), *Redefining family support: Innovations in public-private partnerships* (135–149). Baltimore: Paul H. Brookes.

Lin, N. (1986). Conceptualizing social support. In N. Lin, A. Dean, & W. Ensel (Eds.), *Social support, life events, and depression* (1730). New York: Academic Press.

Lin, N., Woelfel, M. W., & Light, S. C. (1985). The buffering effect of social support subsequent to an important life event. *Journal of Health and Social Behavior, 26,* 247–263.

Lynch, Susan A. (1998). Who supports whom? How age and gender affect the perceived quality of support from family and friends. *The Gerontologist, 38,* 231–238.

Mace, N. (1984). Self-help for the family. In W. E. Kelly (Ed.), *Alzheimer's disease and related disorders* (185–202). Springfield, IL: Charles Thomas.

Moen, P. E., Robison, J., & Fields, V. (1994). Women's work and caregiving roles: A life course perspective. *Journal of Gerontology, 49,* S146–S186.

Moritz, D. J., Kasl, S. V., & Berkman, L. F. (1989). The health impact of living with a cognitively impaired elderly spouse: Depressive symptoms and social functioning. *Journal of Gerontology: Social Sciences, 44,* S17–S27.

Okun, M. A., & Keith, V. M. (1998). Effects of positive and negative social exchange with various sources on depressive symptoms in younger and older adults. *Journals of Gerontology: Psychological Sciences, 53*, P4–P20.

Pillemer, K. (1996). Family caregiving: What would a Martian say? *The Gerontologist, 36*, 269–271.

Pillemer, K. A., & Suitor, J. J. (1994). Violence in caregiving relationships: Risk factors and interventions. In E. Light, G. Niederehe, and B. D. Lebowitz (Eds.), *Stress effects of family caregivers of Alzheimer's patients: Research and Interventions* (205–221). New York: Springer.

Pillemer, K., & Suitor, J. J. (1996). It takes one to help one: Status similarity and well-being of family caregivers to relatives with dementia. *Journal of Gerontology: Social Sciences, 51*, S250–S257.

Riggio, R. E, & Zimmerman, J. (1991). Social skills and interpersonal relationships: Influences on social support and support seeking. In W. H. Jones & D. Perlman (Eds.), *Advances in Personal Relationships: A research annual, 2*, 133–155.

Rook, K. (1984). The negative side of social interactions: Impact on psychological well-being. *Journal of Personality and Social Psychology, 46*, 1097–1108.

Rossi, A. S., & Rossi, P. H. (1990). *Of human bonding: Parent-child relationships throughout the life course.* Hawthorne, NY: Aldine de Gruyter.

Schulz, R., O'Brien, A. T., Bookwala, J., & Fleissner, K. (1995). Psychiatric and physical morbidity effects of dementia caregiving: Prevalence, correlates, and causes. *The Gerontologist, 35*, 771–791.

Semple, S. J. (1992). Conflict in Alzheimer's caregiving families: Its dimensions and consequences. *The Gerontologist, 32*, 648–655.

Shaw, L. B., O'Bryant, S. L., & Meddaugh, D. L. (1991). Support system participation in spousal caregiving: Alzheimer's disease versus other illness. *Journal of Applied Gerontology, 10*, 359–371.

Stephens, M. A. P., Franks, M. M., & Townsend, A. L. (1994). Stress and rewards in women's multiple roles: The case of women in the middle. *Psychology and Aging, 9*, 43–52.

Stuckey, J. C., & Smyth, K. A. (1997). The impact of social resources on the Alzheimer's disease caregiving experience. *Research on Aging, 19*, 423–441.

Suitor, J. J. (1987a). Mother-daughter relations when married daughters return to school: Effects of status similarity. *Journal of Marriage and the Family, 49*, 435–444.

Suitor, J. J. (1987b). Social networks in transition: Married mothers return to school. *Journal of Social and Personal Relationships 4*, 445–461.

Suitor, J. J., & Pillemer, K. (in press). Gender, social support, and experiential similarity during chronic stress: The case of family caregivers. In B. Pescosolido & J. Levy (Eds.), *Advances in Medical Sociology: Social Networks*. New York: JAI Press.

Suitor, J. J., & Pillemer, K. (1990). Family caregiver as a social status: A new conceptual framework for studying social support and well-being. In S. Stahl (Ed.), *The legacy of longevity: Health, illness, and long-term care in later life*. Newbury Park, CA: Sage.

Suitor, J. J., & Pillemer, K. (1993). Support and interpersonal stress in the social networks of married daughters caring for parents with dementia. *Journal of Gerontology: Social Sciences, 48,* S1–S8.

Suitor, J. J., & Pillemer, K. (1996). Sources of support and interpersonal stress in the networks of married, caregiving daughters: Findings from a 2-year longitudinal study. *Journals of Gerontology, 51B,* S297–S306.

Suitor, J. J., Pillemer, K., & Keeton, S. (1995). When experience counts: The effects of experiential and structural similarity on patterns of support and interpersonal stress. *Social Forces, 73,* 1573–1588.

Thoits, P. A. (1986). Social support as coping assistance. *Journal of Consulting and Clinical Psychology, 54,* 416–423.

Wolf, R. S., & Pillemer, K. (1989). *Helping elderly victims*. New York: Columbia University Press.

Zarit, S. H., Johansson, L., & Jarrott, S. E. (1998). Family caregiving: Stresses, social programs, and clinical interventions. In I. H. Nordhus, G. R. Vandenbos, S. Berg, & P. Fromholt (Eds.), *Clinical Gerontology* (345–360). Washington DC: American Psychological Association.

Zarit, S. H., & Knight, B. G. (1996). *A guide to psychotherapy and aging: Effective clinical interventions in a life stage context*. Washington, DC: American Psychological Association.

Zarit, S. H., Todd, P. A., & Zarit, J. M. (1986). Subjective burden of husbands and wives as caregivers: A longitudinal study. *The Gerontologist, 26,* 260–266.

CHAPTER SIX

Future Housing Expectations in Late Midlife

The Role of Retirement, Gender, and Social Integration

Julie T. Robison and Phyllis Moen

Along with food and clothing, adequate and appropriate housing is one of humankind's basic survival needs. However, the relative importance of living arrangements can shift at different stages of the life course. Housing location and design features take on increasing significance in later adulthood in the face of illness or disability, a changing or shrinking social network, or major changes in social roles.

Various types of supportive housing can facilitate individuals' independent functioning and delay institutionalization, thus preventing a significant break in contact with family and friends. Of course, many older people maintain excellent health and functioning but see dramatic changes in their social networks as some of their friends and family members move away, become ill, or die. A supportive living arrangement embodying a strong network of neighbors (see Chapter 7), whether in a traditional neighborhood or a retirement community, can be vital in this situation as well. Moreover, later life transitions (such as retirement) often lead to an increase in the sheer number of hours spent at home, increasing the relative importance of an appropriate and acceptable living environment.

Growing demand for various levels of supportive housing is occurring in tandem with the growing population of older Americans. Most people over age 65 are healthy and live independently in their own homes, but along with longevity they face an increasing likelihood of chronic disease, frailty, and widowhood, making their current housing arrangements no longer viable. We are witnessing an expanding diversity of older individuals' housing needs and preferences, from independent living to retirement communities with various services, and informal home sharing, in addition to assisted living and long-term-care facilities.

As individuals age, they assess the probability of a move for a variety of reasons, from amenities to assisted living. But do their current social ties lessen their future expectations of moving? It is not clear how social integration shapes housing choices and expectations or, conversely, how housing choices and experiences shape social integration. Research to date examining the links between later life living arrangements and social integration primarily falls into two categories. The first examines later life migration patterns, focusing on how social relationships influence migration probabilities and types of moves. The second type of research looks at the level of social connectedness of older adults in various housing arrangements, along with how social relationships influence residential decisions and expectations.

In this chapter we first present our life-course approach to housing experiences and expectations in the later years of adulthood, reviewing research on housing for older people and later life residential patterns as they relate to issues of social integration. We then draw on data from the *Cornell Retirement and Well-Being Study* to explore links between older workers' and recent retirees' later life housing expectations and dispositions and various measures of their social integration. Our model of expectations related to residential arrangements draws on a life-course perspective, retirement migration theory, and economic theories of expectations and intentions.

A LIFE-COURSE PERSPECTIVE

As previous chapters have noted, a life-course perspective underscores the importance of continuity and change over the life span, emphasizing cumulative role trajectories and patterns (Elder, 1995; Giele & Elder, 1998; Moen, 1995; 1996). Later-life transitions are influenced and shaped by earlier experiences; they, in turn, shape the life course as it progresses. Residential expectations and choices in later adulthood can thus be seen as the outcome of past experiences and relationships in addition to current influences (cf. Atchley, 1989).

A life-course formulation also emphasizes the significance of human agency. Individuals' subjective assessments and expectations frequently reflect strategies of adaptive response, affecting both current and subsequent life choices. For example, Elder (1995) describes *control cycles*, whereby individuals modify their expectations and behavior in response to changes in either needs or resources (see also Moen & Wethington, 1992).

A final focus of the life-course perspective concerns the importance of *context*, the situational exigencies and circumstances shaping perceptions and choices. Decisions such as those related to housing are not made in a vacuum; rather, ongoing role involvements and situational factors influence actions and expectations. For example, one's past history of mobility, community and family involvements, and personal and family health, in combination with current economic, social, and health situations, may well shape housing plans and expectations. Such a life-course approach has at least implicitly guided research and theoretical development in the study of retirement migration (see also Krout et al., 1998; Robison & Moen, in press).

RETIREMENT MIGRATION

Shifts in residence mirror other life-course transitions and trajectories. In general, more families want to move than actually intend to do so; however, the *desire* to move generally decreases with age (McHugh et al., 1990; Rossi, 1980; Yee & Van Arsdol, 1977). Life stage changes can be a key impetus for moving (Rossi, 1980). For example, the addition or subtraction of children from the household or the aging of couples can create pressures to change housing. Indeed, as children leave the home (as well as with widowhood), housing needs contract. Nevertheless, mobility remains low for adults in late midlife and beyond. Rossi (1980) refers to this type of household as "overfilled," proposing that it is much easier to adjust to too much living space than to too little without moving.

Litwak and Longino (1987) draw on the family life-cycle framework in their approach to migration after age 60. They describe three distinct types of moves during later life: a *primary retirement move for amenities*, a move to *adapt to moderate disability levels*, and a move in the face of major, *chronic disability* that usually results in institutionalization. Each type of move is affected differently by retirement lifestyle, family ties, and health. About 5 percent of the U.S. population aged 65 and over undertakes an "amenities move" shortly after retirement, which frequently involves relocating a significant distance away from children and other family members. These migrants are typically in their late sixties, married, college-educated homeowners with a relatively high income. They commonly have preexisting ties to their new communities (Glasgow, 1980).

Litwak and Longino (1987) argue that modern technology, such as the telephone and affordable air travel, allows these migrants to maintain adequate ties to their children and other relatives. However, when older people experience the onset of health problems or moderate disability, they may need to move again, this time to relocate closer to caregiving family members. The third type of move occurs when older people require a great deal of health care, frequently a combination of family and formal care. Although many individuals may go through three (or more) post-retirement life stages involving changes in health, few people actually make all three types of moves.

A few researchers have made useful minor adjustments or additions to this three-stage model. In a study of 814 older migrants (aged 40 to 90s) to western North Carolina, Serow and Haas (1992) found that people seriously considered relocating for an average of 5.75 years before they actually moved. Respondents had thought about moving for an average of 3.4 years before retiring and 2.1 years after retiring before their eventual move. These findings prompted these scholars to suggest an additional stage, preceding the first retirement move, called "remote thoughts" (Serow & Haas, 1992). Although Litwak and Longino's theory has typically been used to describe long-distance migration, Jackson et al. (1991) argue that local moves, modifications to current homes, and changes in living arrangements that do not involve residence changes should also be conceptualized in terms of this framework. They refer to this broader concept as "environmental adjustment." Their analysis of data from the Longitudinal Study on Aging (LSOA) found that change in instrumental activities of daily living from 1984 to 1986 predicted the probability of making such environmental adjustments, as predicted by Litwak and Longino's original model.

This model has framed much of the research on later life migration. For example, Reshovsky and Newman (1990), in an analysis of the 1979 Survey of Housing Adjustment, found that both frail and non-frail older people tend to move at the same rate, but that moves by frail persons are more concentrated among renters. They speculate that moving from one's own home is more difficult for a frail person than moving from a rental unit. Of the frail respondents, those most likely to move are younger and with a higher income.

Speare et al. (1991) studied moves or changes in living arrangements accompanying changes in health (using the 1984 and 1986 waves of the LSOA). They found that disability in 1984 predicted institutionalization or living with others two years later (1986). A *change* in disability between 1984 and 1986 predicted changes in living arrangements. Using the same sample, Longino and colleagues (1991) found that higher levels of disability and especially change in functional level are related to the second type of move, that is, to be closer to relatives.

Frequently this second type of move is seen as a *return* migration, that is, a return to one's state of birth. One study (using 1980 census data) found that migrants returning to their native states are older and more dependent than non-return migrants, characteristics that accompany the second type of later life move. However, return migrations more likely represent a return from a Sunbelt retirement destination to an earlier place of residence, rather than to one's birth state. Rogers (1990) supports this conclusion with his finding that older people are no more likely to return to their place of birth than the general population. In a study of African Americans (1980 census respondents), Longino and Smith (1991) found that those people who moved to the South were younger, healthier, and more likely to be married than older African Americans moving North. Thus, a return to the region of birth for African Americans actually characterizes an amenities (type 1) move, whereas a migration to the North, where children and a previous place of residence may be, represents an assistance (type 2) move. These findings indicate that return migration destinations are primarily based on where you have lived in the past and where your relatives live; for people who formerly lived in an area of the Sunbelt, a move to this area may be both an amenities *and* a return move.

Social Networks and Housing Types

A few studies have focused on the relationship between housing arrangements and social connectedness. The strength of these relationships varies widely both across outcomes and in the operationalization of social integration (or social support). Studies of the relationship between different kinds of housing arrangements for older adults and social integration have focused principally on the benefits of age-segregated versus age-integrated living arrangements. For example, Rosow (1967) emphasized the importance of continuity of past patterns of behavior in later adulthood, including social interactions and roles. He argued that segregating older people into separate housing complexes interfered with their connectedness and was thus detrimental to their health and well-being. Others have suggested that residents of planned "senior citizen" housing are surrounded by a network of similar peers and friends, and therefore will actually experience higher levels of social integration. Overall, high age-concentrated settings appear to facilitate social interaction, yet the relationship to morale or life satisfaction is mixed.

Another study looked for variations in the social networks among three types of community-based housing for older people and any concomitant differences in psychological health and functioning (Robison et al., 1996). Specifically, it examined differences among residents of public elderly housing, private elderly housing, and older residents in the community in their social, physical, and emotional functioning (using the first three years of the New Haven EPESE [Established Population for Epidemiologic Studies of the Elderly] data). Analyses show that, net of basic demographic and socioeconomic indicators, residents of both private and public housing facilities tend to have weaker social networks than do those living on their own in the community. In addition, the effects of changes in disability over three years on depression vary depending on housing type. Residents of public senior housing show fewer depressive symptoms when they recover from some disability, as well as a higher level of depression in the face of a new disability, than do residents of community housing. However, the strength of social networks does not explain changes or differences in psychological health across housing types.

EXPECTATIONS AND INTENTIONS
FOR FUTURE HOUSING ARRANGEMENTS

In past decades, aging adults either had to function completely independently, rely on relatives for care, or face institutionalization. But the options for later life housing and long-term care have expanded exponentially in recent years. A wide continuum of living arrangements now exists, giving older people and their families a broad range of choices for the best residential setting in which to spend their post-retirement years. As yet, however, it is unclear which of these options current and future generations of older people are most likely to choose.

Because we are in the midst of this transformation in lifestyle options, it is important to investigate the intentions of those in late midlife to move at all as they age, as well as their expectations regarding choosing particular types of housing or living arrangements. Numerous characteristics and circumstances may influence such expectations, including health, socioeconomic factors, and social integration in their current setting (in terms of social relationships and multiple role involvements). For example, one study examining correlates of older people's plans or intentions to move focused on the importance of health, psychological and social factors, and life events among 3,097 residents of two rural Iowa counties (Colsher & Wallace, 1990). They found factors representing level of social integration—specifically living alone, change in work duties, and someone else moving in (i.e., early caregiving)—predicted an intention to move.

Drawing on data from the *Cornell Retirement and Well-Being Study*, the remainder of this chapter focuses on a group of recent retirees and older workers' expectations about eight later life housing arrangements (for details about the sample, see Chapter 3, this volume). We use a life-course perspective, retirement migration theory, and economic theories regarding decision making and intentions to develop a model of later life housing expectations. In addition, we examine four dispositions about future housing that relate to issues of social integration.

Prospect Theory

Choices about specific housing arrangements for the retirement years can be examined in light of two streams of research: decision-making behavior and expectations or intentions about future activities. There is an ongoing dialogue in the fields of economics and psychology addressing choice, judgment, and decision-making behavior (e.g., Tallman & Gray, 1990). Kahneman and Tversky argue that actual choices do not always follow what might be seen as rational decision making (Kahneman & Tversky, 1983; Tversky & Kahneman, 1981, 1991; Tversky et al., 1988). They offer an alternative model of decision-making behavior, called *prospect theory*, which applies particularly to risky or uncertain choices. "Risky" choices are defined as de-

cisions that are made "without advance knowledge of their consequences," for example, whether or not to take an umbrella or whether
or not to go to war (Kahneman & Tversky, 1983: 341). In their experiments, Kahneman and Tversky ask how likely people are to make
particular choices under various circumstances and what rules of decision making can be discerned from these observations.

They find that people primarily conceptualize outcomes in terms
of *gains* or *losses* relative to a given reference point, rather than as
final assets. Losses usually loom larger than gains; an individual is
more distressed at the prospect of a loss than pleased by a potential
gain. This concept is termed "loss aversion." Therefore, people are
unlikely to plan a later life move when a choice involves simply a
potential gain over their current residential arrangement. People tend
to be risk *averse.* But when they perceive that staying in their current
arrangement might mean a possible loss, risk *seeking* is observed
(Thaler, 1980). Clearly, moving from their current homes is a risky
choice for older people. Some might see it as a potential gain over
staying in what is already an acceptable situation. Others will view
remaining in their current homes as a potential loss (especially given
the specter of poor health) compared to moving to a more supportive
or amenity-oriented environment. Those who feel satisfied with their
current arrangements will avoid the risks involved in moving, while
those who feel they cannot (now or at some future point) manage in
their current homes will take on the risks associated with moving.

The difficulty is that decisions about moves in one's later years
are made without advance knowledge of the consequences or of future
circumstances, particularly in regard to individual and family members' health. Healthy people may have different expectations about
their future health status, as they face their seventies and eighties,
which can also affect their housing plans. Those in late midlife already in poor health or with an ill spouse may foresee a necessary
move; those who are currently healthy may not. Decisions regarding
later life living arrangements are thus contingent upon expectations,
aspirations, social comparisons, and norms (Thaler, 1980; Tversky &
Kahneman, 1991), which in turn are influenced by various social structural characteristics, including age, health status, family composition,
educational and occupational background, gender, and nonmetropolitan
or metropolitan residence. What is not clear is whether and when these
factors tip the balance away from maintaining the status quo (not
moving) toward choosing an alternative housing arrangement.

Expectations and Intentions

Until the mid-1970s, social psychologists described intentions in terms of traditional "expectancy multiplied by value" models, where people acted on behaviors with the highest combination of expectation of achieving the goal and the personal value of the goal (Kuhl & Beckman, 1985). Ajzen and Fishbein have since improved on this model with significant empirical support (Yordy & Lent, 1993). In its most recent formulation, the *theory of planned behavior* states that intention combined with perceived behavioral control (defined as one's *perceived ability* to perform some behavior) most accurately predicts actual performance. Furthermore, intentions are determined by one's personal attitude toward the behavior, subjective norms, and perceived behavioral control reflecting past experiences, second-hand information, and anticipated obstacles (Ajzen, 1988, 1991; Ajzen & Fishbein, 1980; Fishbein & Ajzen, 1975). When a certain behavior does not require a high level of personal control or ability (such as going to work in the morning), intention alone is an adequate predictor. However, in situations where acting in a certain way depends on one's abilities or situational factors, like losing weight or "aging in place," perceived behavioral control, in addition to measures of intention, significantly improves predictions of actual behavior (Ajzen, 1991).

Both prospect theory and the theory of planned behavior can be extended to individuals' predictions about post-retirement housing. According to prospect theory, those people who view moving simply as a potential (but not certain) *gain* over their currently acceptable living arrangements will be risk averse and will predict a lower probability of moving in the future. However, those people who view staying in their current homes as a potential *loss* compared to the more likely gains involved in moving to a more supportive environment will be willing to take on the risks of moving and will predict a higher probability of moving. The way this choice is framed (i.e., as a gain or loss) depends on other characteristics like age, health, and mobility history.

Similarly, phrased in terms of the theory of planned behavior, the expectation to "age in place" will be affected both by intention (reflecting desire) and perceived behavioral control—whether individuals actually believe they will be able to live independently in their current housing for the rest of their lives. Again, health, family composition, and other factors will influence one's perceived behavioral control. For example, current health, the availability of informal family caregivers, income, and other resources will affect confidence in one's ability to live independently and maintain one's current home.

Examining retirement housing expectations from the vantage point of a life-course perspective, retirement migration theory, and theories of expectation and intention raises the following research questions: Who is more likely to see "aging in place" as a viable option? What groups will feel that the risks associated with staying in their current housing outweigh the risks associated with moving? Are particular housing arrangements perceived as greater or smaller risks? Are there clear patterns of expectations based on gender, area of residence, or retirement status? How do life-course events and trajectories, such as health problems, social integration, productive activity, or previous mobility affect housing expectations?

To address these questions, we propose a model with four categories of explanatory factors affecting older peoples' expectations about their future mobility and living arrangements: background characteristics, housing history, social integration, and health (see Figure 6.1). In addition to examining the direct effects of these factors on expectations to move (as well as on specific arrangements), we also study potential interactions between particular factors. For example, do expectations differ for men versus women, for nonmetropolitan versus metropolitan residents, or for the retired versus pre-retired older workers?

Specifically, we examine individuals' expectations about eight housing or long-term care options, arrayed as relatively low, medium, or high risk. Extending Kahneman and Tversky's (1979, 1983) prospect theory and Elder's (1995) conception of control cycles, we define risk categories based on each option's implied level of *dependence.* Independence is a primary American norm; our society expects adults of all ages to take care of themselves, both in terms of physical functioning and financially. Older people vastly prefer to remain in their own homes and live independently for as long as possible. Thus, those housing arrangements that indicate higher potential levels of dependence are categorized as higher risk. We hypothesize that individuals' expectations about housing options within the same risk categories will relate to similar sets of personal characteristics.

We anticipate that those respondents more likely to experience physical or financial dependence—specifically older individuals, the retired, women, metropolitan residents, lower income, or non-white—will have greater expectation probabilities of ever living in a setting

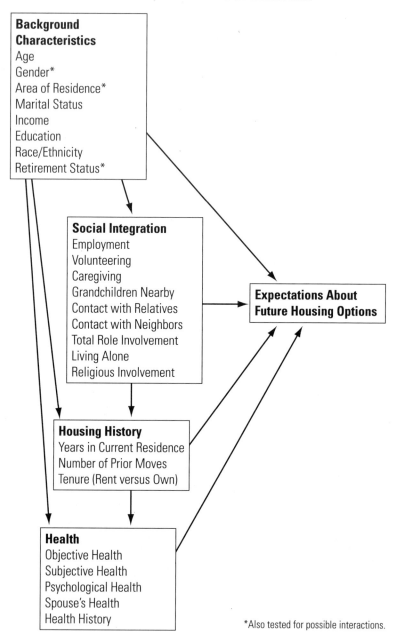

Figure 6.1   A Conceptual Model of Older Adults' Expectations about
Future Housing Options.

with a high level of implied dependence (that is, in our terms, a setting of high risk). This is because they have (or expect they will have) fewer of the resources needed to maintain an independent household. Renters (versus homeowners) and mortgage holders (versus those who own their homes outright) should also anticipate a greater likelihood of living arrangements implying a high level of dependence, because they have fewer ties to their current residence and, in the case of renters, less control over their housing in general. Individuals who have lived in their homes for fewer years or have made more moves over their life courses should have weaker ties to their current homes and be more open to other options. Therefore, they are more likely to expect to live in the more supportive housing types.

Ties to one's neighborhood or community can influence expectations of mobility. Measures of social integration (conceptualized both as multiple role occupancy and as contact with social network members) also reflect ties to individuals' current homes and neighborhoods. We expect that those respondents who are less socially integrated will have higher expectations of "riskier" (that is, more dependent) living arrangements, as will those in worse health or with less healthy spouses.

Measures

Respondents' expectations, plans, and dispositions about their current and future housing arrangements were assessed using modified questions from the 1989 version of the American Association of Retired Persons' (AARP) *Understanding Senior Housing for the 1990s* survey (1992), a random telephone survey of 1,514 Americans aged 55 and over. The AARP study asked three "yes" or "no" questions about each type of living arrangement: whether the respondent had already made the arrangement, if they were currently seriously considering the arrangement, and whether they would consider it in the future. These questions are modified in the current study as Juster (1964, 1966, 1997) suggests, by wording them in terms of the likelihood of ever having each particular arrangement at some time in the future, on a scale of 0 to 100. If the respondent is already living in one of the options, they receive 100 on the scale, and the date of the change to this option is recorded.

Respondents' expectations of ever making each of eight different housing or long-term care arrangements are arrayed on a scale from 0 to 100. The eight options (clustered by risk/dependency level) include always living in one's current home or modifying one's home for special needs (low risk of dependency); living in a retirement community, purchasing long-term care insurance, or getting a reverse mortgage (medium risk of dependency); living with a family member, sharing a household with unrelated people, or living in a separate housing unit located on a relative's property (ECHO cottage) (high risk of dependency). This method measures the strength of the respondents' expectations of living in each housing option rather than simply asking whether or not they will move at some point in the future. This approach elicits much finer information and more accurately reflects future behavior.

We investigate the housing-related characteristics of the sample of late midlife workers and retirees as well as the factors predicting their expectations of moving or of living in particular arrangements. The amount of planning for future housing ranges from a lot, some/ a little, to not at all. Whether people rent or own their homes, and (among the homeowners) whether they have mortgages or own their homes outright, determines housing tenure. The number of moves is counted since age 30, as well as the duration, in years, of living in the current residence. Four variables assess dispositions about housing in later life on a "yes," "no," or "don't know" basis: whether respondents want to live in a community with people of all different ages, whether they are counting on their children to help take care of them when they get older, whether they want to live only with people their own age, and whether they would like to live alone.

RESULTS

Housing Characteristics and Dispositions

On average, the people in this study see their odds as about 57 (on a scale of 1 to 100) that they will never move—only a little over 50/50. In fact, there is no "sure thing" in terms of housing futures. The odds of moving to a retirement community are seen as about one in five (23 out of 100).

Our sample falls fairly evenly into three categories in terms of the amount of planning for future housing needs: a lot, some or a little, or not at all. Those with the highest income are most likely to report a lot of planning, while the lowest income group more frequently reports no planning. Similar proportions of retirees and pre-retirees have done a lot of planning, but two out of five pre-retired workers report having done no planning for future housing at all, compared to one fifth of retirees. The amount of planning does not differ across gender, area of residence, or age cohort.

There are subgroup differences in wanting to live with people of different ages, with more men, people with higher incomes, those in their fifties, and pre-retired workers preferring to have age diversity. Eighty percent of the sample as a whole disagree with (and 9% do not know how they feel about) the statement that they are counting on their children for help; none of the individual characteristics relate significantly to this disposition. Few people say they want to live with people of the same age, but those with the lowest incomes are slightly more apt to do so. Although most of those in the study do not want to live alone, women, those with less income, those in their sixties and early seventies, and retirees tend to agree with this statement more often than do their counterparts.

Degree of Expectations

Overall, respondents uniformly perceive living with a family member, sharing a home with unrelated people, or living in an ECHO cottage on a relative's property as *very* unlikely future housing arrangements. (Mean expectation probabilities, on a scale of 0 to 100, for these three options are 12%, 9%, and 7%, respectively.) Expectations about other housing and long-term-care options show a high degree of variability. We collapse each of these five measures into three categories of expectancy: almost certain *not* to have the particular arrangement (less than 30% expectancy rate on the 0–100 scale), *uncertain* about whether or not they will have the arrangement (30%–70% expectancy rate), and reasonably certain in *expecting* to have the arrangement (over 70% expectancy rate). Each of these expectancy categories is then compared across five demographic indicators (gender, area of residence, income, age cohort, and retirement status) using the chi-square statistic.

Moving or not?

Just under half (45%) of the people in our study are quite certain about expecting that they will always live in their current house; the rest of the sample splits evenly between being certain they will move (28%) and uncertain about their expectations (27%). Note that men feel more certain that they will move from their current home; women are more certain that they will stay. Those from metropolitan areas, with the highest incomes, in their fifties, and not yet retired from their career jobs all feel more certain they will move in the future. Conversely, other groups—those from nonmetropolitan areas, with low incomes, in their sixties to early seventies, and retired—tend to expect with a strong degree of certainty that they will stay in their current homes. Most uncertain about this possibility are metropolitan residents, those with middle incomes, and those in their early fifties.

Modifying one's home?

Just over one third (36%) of the people we interviewed are sure they will make (or already have made) some adjustments to their home in order to stay there, while 39 percent are certain they will not. A fourth do not know what to expect about this option. Women are more likely to feel sure they will make some modifications; men are more certain they will *not* make adjustments but are also more uncertain about their expectations than are women. Those with low incomes are the most certain they will make some modifications, followed by middle and then upper income groups. Those in the middle income bracket express the most uncertainty about making modifications. Workers not yet retired from their career jobs are more certain that they will not modify their homes, whereas retirees feel more sure they will make adjustments for special needs.

Long-term-care communities or insurance?

Only 9 percent of those in our study feel certain about expecting to move to a retirement/continuing care community, another 19 percent are uncertain, and 72 percent are fairly sure they will *not* move to such a community. The likelihood of expecting to move to a retirement community does not differ by gender, age, income, retirement status, or area of residence.

By contrast, the degree of expectancy of purchasing long-term-care (LTC) insurance shows significant relationships with three individual characteristics—income, age, and retirement status. Almost one in five (18%) either already have or feel certain they will buy this insurance, one fourth are unsure, and three out of five (57%) feel fairly certain they will not buy it. Those who have lower incomes, who are in their sixties and seventies, and who are retired feel sure they will *not* buy LTC insurance; those with higher incomes, in their fifties, and who are not yet retired tend to be either undecided or certain about expecting to purchase long-term care insurance.

Reverse mortgage?

More than three fourths of the people in our study express certainty that they will not obtain a reverse mortgage, 15 percent are unsure, and 8 percent are certain they will. Those with the lowest incomes (who would potentially benefit most from such an arrangement) feel the most certain that they will *not* get a reverse mortgage in the future, while those in the middle and upper income brackets feel more sure they might. While few anticipate getting a reverse mortgage, individuals in their fifties and those not yet retired from their career jobs are somewhat more likely to expect to do so, compared to older, retired respondents.

MULTIVARIATE ANALYSES

We now turn to a more complex analysis, to see how expectations about future housing options relate to background characteristics, previous housing history, social integration, and health. Table 6.1 provides a summary overview of our findings.

Who expects to remain in their current home?

First, expectations about always staying in one's current home relate significantly to gender, income, years in the current home, number of moves, tenure, volunteering, and depression (see column 1, Table 6.1). Women's likelihood of expecting to remain in their current homes is five percentage points higher than that of men's. Lower income relates to an increased expectation to age in place. Number of years in the home increases the expectation of remaining there, but a history of more moves over the life course, and especially status as a renter (as

Table 6.1. The Effects of Background Characteristics, Housing History, Social Integration, and Health on Expectations about Future Housing Arrangements

	Never Move	Modify Home	Retirement Community	LTC Insurance	Reverse Mortgage	Family Member	Shared Housing	ECHO Cottage
Background Variables								
Age	.45	−.19	−.06	−.31	−.25	−.14	−.40[b]	.19
Women	5.19[c]	.70[b]	−1.59	−2.76	−1.68	1.80	−2.45[b]	−.54
Income	−3.19[a]	.58	1.60[a]	1.89[a]	.08	−.53	.07	−.46
Married	6.05	4.45	−8.17[a]	−6.59[c]	.63	−5.77[a]	−5.70[a]	−1.26
Non-white	−4.27	12.98[b]	−2.60	3.68	6.88	−.01	−5.11[c]	4.53
Housing History								
Years in residence	.25[c]	.20	−.31[a]	−.03	−.27[b]	−.06	−.13[c]	−.03
Number of moves	−1.55[c]	−.11	−.30	−.79	−.66	−.54	.37	.20
Rent home	−19.06[a]	−10.90[c]	−.72	−6.58	−12.60[b]	4.90	4.00	−.61
Own home outright	1.31	4.99	7.12[a]	.03	1.30	−.71	5.84[a]	.29
Social Integration								
Volunteering	5.21[c]	−2.04	3.84[c]	7.05[b]	2.42	.54	1.90	.43
Caregiving	−3.18	−.36	7.61[a]	7.00[b]	.11	1.23	−.85	−1.67
See relatives often	−1.80	−6.04[c]	−3.62	−7.34[b]	−.83	.56	−.13	.34
See neighbors often	.77	4.99[c]	1.84	1.50	−.04	2.50	−.65	1.23
Grandchildren near	4.24	5.94[c]	2.69	−3.24	1.12	2.57	−.22	1.27
Religious involvement	4.24	−4.37	−.10	−5.10[c]	4.16[c]	−1.04	.30	−.75

Health

Self-esteem	−.70	6.63	−4.67	7.69	−9.08[b]	−5.76[c]	−3.53	.67
Depression	−.61[b]	−.05	.23	.39	.32	.08	.20	.40[a]
Health history	−.67	.88	−.56	.19	−.06	−.14	−.05	−.30
F	6.08[b]	2.39[b]	2.09[b]	2.73[b]	1.45[a]	1.75[a]	2.52[b]	1.06
R^2	.21	.10	.08	.11	.06	.07	.10	.04
N	586	565	584	559	568	571	579	580

Note: Not related to any housing arrangement expectation are urban *vs.* metropolitan residence, retirement status, objective health (being ill in past year), subjective health, spouse's health, health history of self or spouse. These coefficients are therefore omitted from the table.

[a] $p < .01$

[b] $.01 < p < .05$

[c] $.05 < p < .10$

opposed to a homeowner) decreases the expectation of remaining in the current home. Respondents who volunteer in the community have an expectation rate of aging in place that is five points higher than those who are not currently volunteering, but no other measure of social integration relates significantly to this expectation. Finally, the more depressive symptoms respondents report, the stronger their anticipation of moving at some future time. Surprisingly, none of the measures of current or past physical health or of spouse's health are related to expectations about moving.

Who expects to modify their current home?

Gender and ethnicity both relate to expectations about modifying one's home to adjust for special needs (see column 2, Table 6.1), with women's expectancy rate seven points higher than men's and nonwhite individuals' rate thirteen points higher than whites. Not surprisingly, renters are less likely than homeowners to expect to modify their homes. The expectation rates of modifying one's current home of those who see their neighbors often and those with grandchildren nearby are five and six percentage points higher than those who do not interact frequently with their neighbors or live near grandchildren. However, individuals who see their relatives often have a lower expectation rate of modifying their homes than those who do not keep in close contact with relatives. Neither physical nor psychological health relates to anticipating modifying one's current home environment.

Who expects to move to a retirement community or buy long-term-care insurance?

Both moving to a retirement community and purchasing long-term-care insurance (see columns 3 and 4, Table 6.1) are positively associated with income but negatively associated with being married; those who are single, divorced, or widowed have higher expectancies for these two options than their married counterparts. Owning one's home outright increases the level of expectation to live in a retirement community by seven percentage points over homeowners with a mortgage. Both current volunteering and caregiving increase respondents' degree of expectation of moving to a retirement community and of buying long-term-care insurance significantly as well. But those who see their relatives often and those more religiously involved are less likely to expect to buy long-term-care insurance. Surprisingly, one's own or one's spouse's health is again unrelated to expectations of a retirement community move or of purchasing long-term-care insurance.

Who expects to get a reverse mortgage?

The expectation of obtaining a reverse mortgage is related to time in one's current home. Individuals who have spent more years in their current homes are *less likely* to expect to get a reverse mortgage, even though they would stand to gain the most from such an arrangement. Not surprisingly, renters are much less likely than homeowners to expect to get a reverse mortgage. While none of the social integration indicators are related to this expectation, people with low self-esteem have a higher likelihood of expecting to obtain a reverse mortgage.

Who expects to live with (or very near) others?

People in this late midlife sample have a higher likelihood of expecting to move in with a family member if they are single and have lower self-esteem. Several demographic factors relate to anticipating sharing one's home with a non-relative. Those in their fifties, male, unmarried, and white all have a higher expectancy of sharing a residence with a non-relative. Those who have spent fewer years in their current home, as well as individuals who own their homes outright (versus holding a mortgage), also perceive home-sharing as a more likely option. Only depressive symptoms increase the expectation of living in an ECHO cottage.

Differences by Gender, Retirement Status, and Residential Location

Studies that examine the retirement transition and concomitant plans and expectations have focused almost exclusively on men; however, women are disproportionately likely to live to be old and to need supportive housing. One third of the people in this study lives in nonmetropolitan counties, a group who likely have unique housing needs and expectations. We also expect that people in late midlife who are retired might be more likely to think about and plan for future housing needs than those in this same age group who are not yet

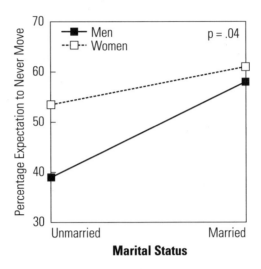

Figure 6.2   Moderating Effect of Gender on Marital Status
for the Expectation to Never Move.

retired.[1] We find a link between marriage, gender, and expectations about moving versus remaining in one's own home. Specifically, unmarried men report a much lower expectation of staying in their current house than do unmarried women, while married men and women have similar expectations (see Figure 6.2).

Gender also is linked to age, retirement status, and objective health in predicting expectations of moving to a retirement community (Figure 6.3). Age makes a larger difference for women, with older women more apt to expect to eventually live in a retirement community. Men show the opposite trend, with less difference across age groups. Retirement and health status also affect women's expectations more than men's. Retired women and women who have been sick in the past year have higher expectations of moving to a retirement community.

---

[1] We examine the interaction effects between gender, area of residence, and retirement status and a subset of individual characteristics on the likelihood of expecting four of the more policy-relevant options: remaining in one's current home, moving to a retirement community, purchasing long-term-care insurance, and obtaining a reverse mortgage. The subset of characteristics includes age, marital status, retirement status, volunteering, and objective health. The interactions are tested in individual regression models, each of which controls for age, income, race, and gender.

For men, being pre-retired and healthy relate to a higher expected likelihood of retirement community living at some point in the future. Retirement status also moderates the effects of volunteering on the expectations of moving to a retirement community; those who are already retired have higher levels of expectation about living in such a community if they currently volunteer, while the pre-retired show the opposite tendency (Figure 6.3).

Gender and retirement status are both related to the expectation of buying long-term-care insurance. Pre-retired men have stronger

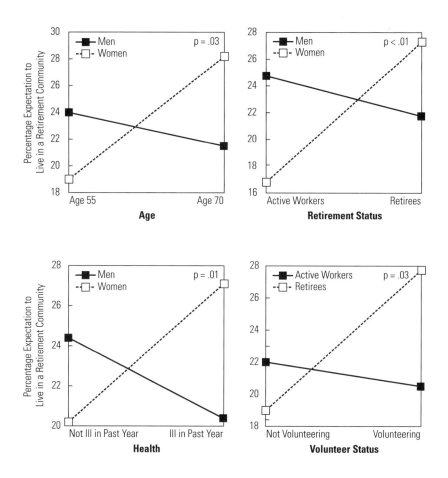

Figure 6.3   Moderating Effects of Gender and Retirement Status for the Expectation to Live in a Retirement Community.

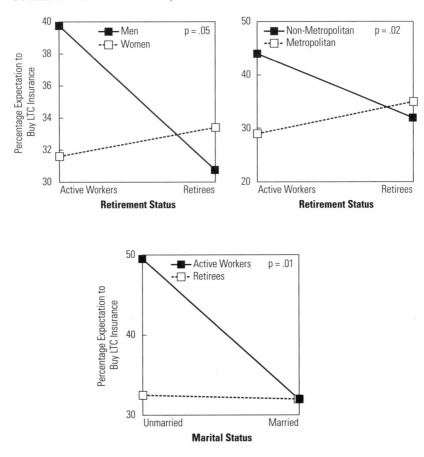

Figure 6.4   Moderating Effects of Gender, Area of Residence, and Retirement
Status for the Expectation to Buy LTC Insurance.

expectations of buying long-term care insurance than retired men, but
women show the opposite pattern (Figure 6.4). And retirement status is
linked to area of residence regarding expectations of buying long-term-
care insurance. Retirement status does not greatly affect metropolitan
dwellers' expectations about this option, but pre-retired nonmetropolitan residents have a higher rate of expecting to buy LTC insurance
than retired nonmetropolitan dwellers (Figure 6.4). Single, pre-retired
individuals have higher expectations about buying LTC insurance than
married pre-retired workers.

Gender and volunteer participation, as well as area of residence and age, shape expectations of obtaining a reverse mortgage (see Figure 6.5). Women who volunteer in the community having higher expectations of getting a reverse mortgage than those who do not volunteer. Metropolitan residents in their fifties have higher expectations

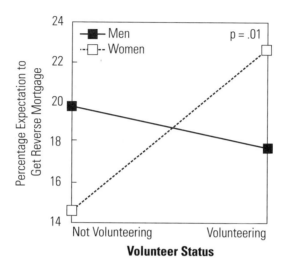

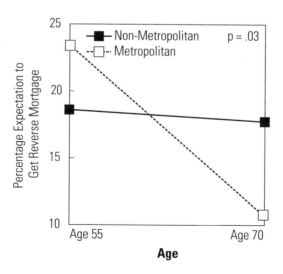

Figure 6.5   Moderating Effect of Gender and Area of Residence
for the Expectation to get a Reverse Mortgage.

of obtaining a reverse mortgage than do metropolitan residents in their sixties and early seventies.

Discussion

A life-course perspective on housing emphasizes the importance of resources, past experiences, and contextual considerations in shaping subjective choices and expectations. In this chapter we have shown that individuals vary in their housing expectations, depending on a range of factors. In particular, women, members of ethnic minorities, and those integrated in their communities (through neighboring and volunteering) are more likely to expect to "age in place" by modifying their current homes.

Arraying the range of housing options in terms of the risk of increasing dependency (and reduced independence) reveals a pattern of greater certainty about *not* using options with a high risk of dependency.[2] Nine out of ten rate their chances of someday living with a family member or sharing housing as less than 30 percent. And three out of ten respondents believe there is less than a 30 percent chance they will move into a retirement community, for example (which could be viewed as having a more moderate risk of dependency). By contrast, almost half believe there is a greater than 70 percent chance they will age in place, staying in their own homes. The general trend—cutting across gender, area of residence, income level, age cohort, and retirement status—is away from counting on one's children for help, reflecting an underlying desire for independence and avoidance of "becoming a burden." This finding points to the growing need to plan for alternate housing and community-based, long-term-care arrangements that will enable people in later adulthood to function as independently as possible.

---

[2] The findings from this study also underscore the utility of drawing on several theoretical paradigms in developing a model of housing expectations. The literature on decision making and intentions (Ajzen & Fishbein, 1980; Fishbein & Ajzen, 1975; Kahneman & Tversky, 1979, 1983; Tversky & Kahneman, 1981, 1991) would suggest that expectations about future courses of action, such as housing choices, are grounded in degree of risk.

Housing Expectation Patterns by Income and Gender

As anticipated, people with higher incomes are more likely than those with lower incomes to expect to move from their current homes, to live in a retirement community, and to purchase long-term-care insurance. Women, compared to men, have higher expectation rates of never moving or of modifying their current homes. They also have lower rates (than men) for shared housing. Despite the reality that women and those with less income disproportionately use alternative housing arrangements as they age, they are the least likely to expect to do so.

Housing Expectation Patterns by Current Housing Circumstance and History

Those who own their homes outright anticipate a higher likelihood of sharing housing in the future, an unexpected finding. Additional analysis shows that those who hold a mortgage have significantly higher incomes than homeowners without a mortgage; those owning their own homes may see shared housing as an option that would allow them to retain their independence and remain in their homes while generating some income. As hypothesized, renters do not expect to remain in their current homes or modify their homes for special needs, yet they are not any more likely than homeowners to expect any of the high-risk options.

Housing Expectation Patterns by Social Integration

Individual measures of social integration have some unique relationships with expected housing options. Both volunteering and caregiving are associated with the expectation of moving into a retirement community and of purchasing long-term-care insurance. Volunteering and caregiving experiences may well increase awareness of the frailties that often accompany aging and may reinforce a desire to take control over one's housing future in order to optimize both care and independence.

In contrast, seeing relatives is related to a lower likelihood of expecting to modify one's home or to purchase long-term-care insurance (as is religious involvement). Respondents with active kin networks may feel that they can rely on their family members for care (although they do not foresee actually moving in with family members).

Housing Expectation Patterns by Current Health Circumstances and History

Unexpectedly, neither current nor prior physical health problems are linked to the expectations of those in late midlife about their future living arrangements. However, individuals with poorer psychological health (as measured by depressive symptoms and low self-esteem) are more apt to anticipate a future dependency than are those with more psychological resources. Specifically, those with symptoms of depression or low self-esteem have higher expectations of having a reverse mortgage, living with a family member, or living in an ECHO cottage and lower expectations of remaining in their current home. This illustrates a key proposition of the theory of planned behavior related to perceived behavioral control. Individuals with low self-esteem and depressive symptoms may doubt they will be able to remain in their current homes.

The Importance of Context

As a life-course formulation would suggest, we find that expectations and the processes shaping them may well differ across subgroups of the population. For example, older or retired women have higher expectations of living in a retirement community than do men in these same circumstances. And the marital status and age of pre-retirees have a noticeable effect on their expectations about long-term-care insurance or reverse mortgages. By contrast, retirees appear to be more similar than different in risk aversion as they contemplate the housing choices in their future. Retirees are, in fact, more risk averse in terms of dependency than are pre-retirees, possibly because they are closer to the reality of these options than are those older workers who are not yet retired.

POLICY IMPLICATIONS

From a policy perspective, our findings show that expectations about specific housing options vary widely. Policy makers recognize the diversity in preferences and degree of planning among those in late midlife confronting their housing futures. This suggests the necessity of providing a wide range of residential and long-term-care options for those individuals approaching old age.

Only 28 percent of this sample expresses a high degree of certainty that they will move from their current homes at some point in the future, whereas almost half—45 percent—feel quite certain that they will not do so. Clearly, a large proportion of older workers and retirees plans to age in place. This group of "stayers" will require access to a wide variety of community-based services. These services could well include skilled "retro-fitting" of homes to make adjustment for special needs; 60 percent of this sample appears open to such a possibility.

About a fourth of the people in this study believe there is at least a 30 percent chance they will move into a retirement community that provides meals, housekeeping, transportation, and other services. Many types of assisted living environments exist, from high-rise apartment buildings with a single service coordinator to continuing care retirement communities with all-inclusive health care, but a large proportion are not affordable for the average person. Since this type of residence promotes maximum independence, it is likely that it will increase in popularity in the future.

Corporations and other employers considering including long-term-care insurance in their benefits packages (as well as insurance companies that sell these policies) should know that 43 percent of employees in their fifties and sixties in this study express interest in this option, especially those who are more educated or in upper-level occupations. This finding may reflect an emerging shift in employee preference, as younger cohorts of individuals begin to confront the reality of long lives in retirement. Employers and organizations that offer retirement planning and counseling, or sponsor retirement clubs, could include information about retirement housing options, educating their audience as to the range of and tradeoffs among options.

It is instructive that none of the three high dependency risk options assessed in this study are popular among our respondents. Sharing a home with a nonrelative did appeal slightly more to some groups than to others (specifically men, those not married, those who are white, individuals in their fifties, and individuals who have lived in their homes for fewer years but own them outright), but the rate of expectation remains low. Moving in with a family member or living in an ECHO cottage are *not* expected. Informal family solutions to the long-term-care needs of older Americans appear not to be popular options; practically no one in this sample desires or anticipates living with a family member. The resistance expressed by our respondents toward moving in with a relative reflects current reality; while up to 15 percent of adult daughters may live with an older parent at some point (Weinick, 1995), roughly only 3 percent of older people move in with a family member because they need care (Pillemer & Suitor, 1991). The majority of two- or three-generation households that include older people either have always had that arrangement (i.e., the children never moved out) or else involve adult children moving in due to their own financial or health needs (Crimmins & Ingeneri, 1990).

The fact that poor physical health is *not* related to expectations about housing options suggests that individuals in their fifties, sixties, and early seventies do not translate poor health into perceptions of future physical dependency. However, physical health problems may become more salient in shaping housing expectations as these individuals move into their mid-seventies and eighties. A key policy challenge is how to assist individuals in learning about and assessing housing options and requirements as they age, so that their housing expectations and choices conform more closely to the reality of their future needs, resources, and possibilities.

REFERENCES

Ajzen, I. (1988). *Attitudes, personality, and behavior.* Chicago: Dorsey Press.
Ajzen, I. (1991). The theory of planned behavior. *Organizational Behavior and Human Development Processes, 50,* 179–211.
Ajzen, I., & Fishbein, M. (1980). *Understanding attitudes and predicting social behavior.* Englewood Cliffs, NJ: Prentice-Hall.
Ajzen, I., & Madden, T. J. (1986). Prediction of goal-directed behavior: Attitudes, intentions, and perceived behavioral control. *Journal of Experimental Social Psychology, 22,* 453–474.
American Association of Retired Persons. (1992). *Understanding senior housing for the 1990s.* Washington, DC: AARP.
Atchley, R. C. (1989). A continuity theory of normal aging. *The Gerontologist 29,* 183–190.
Beale, D. A., & Manstead, A. S. R. (1991). Predicting mothers' intentions to limit frequency of infants' sugar intake: Testing the theory of planned behavior. *Journal of Applied Social Psychology, 21,* 409–431.

Colsher, P. L., & Wallace, R. B. (1990). Health and social antecedents of relocation in rural elderly persons. *Journal of Gerontology: Social Sciences, 45*, S32–S38.

Crimmins, E. M., & Ingeneri, D. G. (1990). Interaction and living arrangements of older parents and their children: Past trends, present determinants, future implications. *Research on Aging, 12*, 3–35.

Doll, J., & Ajzen, I. (1992). Accessibility and stability of predictors in the theory of planned behavior. *Journal of Personality and Social Psychology, 63*, 754–765.

Elder, G. H., Jr. (1995). The life course paradigm: Social change and individual development. In P. Moen, G. H. Elder, Jr., & K. Lüscher (Eds.), *Examining lives in context: Perspectives on the ecology of human development* (101–139). Washington, DC: American Psychological Association.

Fishbein, M., & Ajzen, I. (1975). *Belief, attitude, intention, and behavior: An introduction to theory and research.* Reading, MA: Addison-Wesley.

Giele, J., & Elder, G. H., Jr. (1998). *Methods of life course research: Qualitative and quantitative approaches.* Thousand Oaks, CA: Sage.

Glasgow, N. (1980). The older metropolitan migrant as a factor in rural population growth. In A. J. Sofranko & J. D. Williams (Eds.), *Rebirth of rural America: Rural migration in the Midwest* (87–104). Ames, IA: North Central Regional Center for Rural Development.

Jackson, D. J., Longino, C. F., Jr., Zimmerman, R. S., & Bradsher, J. E. (1991). Environmental adjustments to declining functional ability: Residential mobility and living arrangements. *Research on Aging, 13*, 289–309.

Juster, F. T. (1964). *Anticipations and purchases: An analysis of consumer behavior.* Princeton: Princeton University Press.

Juster, F. T. (1966). *Consumer buying intentions and purchase probability: An experiment in survey design.* New York: National Bureau of Economic Research.

Juster, F. T. (1997). On the measurement of expectations, uncertainty, and preferences. *Journal of Gerontology: Social Sciences, 52B*, S237–S239.

Kahneman, D., & Tversky, A. (1979). Prospect theory: An analysis of decision under risk. *Econometricia, 47*, 263–350.

Kahneman, D., & Tversky, A. (1983). Choices, values, and frames. *American Psychologist, 39*, 341–350.

Krout, J. A., Moen, P., Oggins, J., & Bowen, N. (1998). Reasons for relocation to a continuing care retirement community. Pathways Working Paper No. 2. Ithaca: Bronfenbrenner Life Course Center, Cornell University.

Kuhl, J., & Beckman, J. (1985). *Action control: From cognition to behavior.* Berlin: Springer-Verlag.

Litwak, E., & Longino, C. F., Jr. (1987). Migration patterns among the elderly: A developmental perspective. *The Gerontologist, 27,* 266–272.

Longino, C. F., Jr., Jackson, D. J., Zimmerman, R. S., & Bradsher, J. E. (1991). The second move: Health and geographic mobility. *Journal of Gerontology: Social Sciences, 46,* S218–S224.

Longino, C. F., Jr., & Smith, K. J. (1991). Black retirement migration in the United States. *Journal of Gerontology: Social Sciences, 46,* S125–S132.

Madden, T. J., Ellen, P. S., & Ajzen, I. (1992). A comparison of the theory of planned behavior and the theory of reasoned action. *Personality and Social Psychology Bulletin, 18,* 3–9.

McHugh, K. E., Gober, P., & Reid, N. (1990). Determinants of short- and long-term mobility: Expectations for home owners and renters. *Demography, 27,* 81–95.

Moen, P. (1995). A life-course approach to post retirement roles and well-being. In L. A. Bond, S. J. Cutler, & A. Grams, *Promoting successful and productive aging* (230–257). Thousand Oaks, CA: Sage.

Moen, P. (1996). Gender, age and the life course. In R. H. Binstock & L. George (Eds.), *Handbook of aging and the social sciences,* 4th ed. (171–187). San Diego: Academic Press.

Moen, P., & Wethington, E. (1992). The concept of family adaptive strategies. *American Sociological Review, 18,* 233–251.

Pillemer, K., & Suitor, J. J. (1991). Relationships with children and distress in the elderly. In K. Pillemer & K. McCartney (Eds.), *Parent-child relations throughout life* (163–178). Hillsdale, NJ: Erlbaum.

Radloff, L. S. (1977). The CES-D scale: A self-report depression scale for research in the general population. *Applied Psychological Measurement, 1,* 385–401.

Reshovsky, J. D., & Newman, S. J. (1990). Adaptations for independent living by older frail households. *The Gerontologist, 30,* 543–552.

Robison, J. T., Kasl, S. V., Mendes de Leon, C., & Glass, T. (1996). *Housing type and social networks: Effects on disability and depression.* Paper presented to the annual meeting of the Gerontological Society of America, Washington, DC, November 1996.

Robison, J., & Moen, P. (in press). A life course perspective on later life housing expectations and realities. *Research on Aging.*

Rogers, A. (1990). Return migration to region of birth among retirement-age persons in the United States. *Journal of Gerontology: Social Sciences, 45,* S128–S134.

Rosenberg, M. (1986). *Conceiving the self.* Melbourne, FL: Academic Press.

Rosow, I. (1967). *Social integration of the aged.* New York: The Free Press.

Rossi, P. H. (1980). *Why families move,* 2d ed. Beverly Hills: Sage.

Serow, W. J., & Haas, W. H., III. (1992). Measuring the economic impact of retirement migration: The case of western North Carolina. *Journal of Applied Gerontology, 11,* 200–215.

Speare, A., Jr., Avery, R., & Lawton, L. (1991). Disability, residential mobility, and changes in living arrangements. *Journal of Gerontology: Social Sciences, 46,* S133–S142.

Tallman, I., & Gray, L. N. (1990). Choices, decisions, and problem-solving. *Annual Review of Sociology, 16,* 405–433.

Thaler, R. H. (1980). Toward a positive theory of consumer choice. *Journal of Economic Behavior and Organization, 1,* 39–60.

Thaler, R. H., & Johnson, E. J. (1990). Gambling with the house money and trying to break even: The effects of prior outcomes on risky choice. *Management Science, 36,* 643–660.

Tversky, A., & Kahneman, D. (1981). The framing of decisions and the psychology of choice. *Science, 211,* 453–458.

Tversky, A., & Kahneman, D. (1991). Loss aversion in riskless choice: A reference-dependent model. *Quarterly Journal of Economics, 106,* 1039–1061.

Tversky, A., Sattath, S., & Slovic, P. (1988). Contingent weighting in judgment and choice. *Psychological Review, 95,* 371–384.

U.S. Bureau of the Census. (1990). *Census of population, summary population and housing characteristics.* Washington, DC: U.S. Government Printing Office.

U.S. Bureau of the Census. (1994). *Housing in metropolitan areas—Movers and stayers.* Washington, DC: U.S. Government Printing Office.

U.S. Bureau of the Census. (1995). *Housing of the elderly.* Washington, DC: U.S. Government Printing Office.

Weinick, R. M. (1995). Sharing a home: The experience of American women and their parents over the twentieth century. *Demography, 32,* 281–297.

Yee, W., & Van Arsdol, M. D., Jr. (1977). Residential mobility, age and the life cycle. *Journal of Gerontology, 2,* 211–221.

Yordy, G. A., & Lent, R. W. (1993). Predicting aerobic exercise participation: Social cognitive, reasoned action, and planned behavior models. *Journal of Sport and Exercise Psychology, 15,* 363–374.

CHAPTER SEVEN

Neighboring as a Form of Social Integration and Support

Elaine Wethington and Allison Kavey

A key informal source of social support is neighboring: regular social interaction with those living in close proximity. Yet research on social relationships, social support, and health has neglected the role of neighboring in several domains: the maintenance of independent living situations for older adults, the nature and development of neighboring relationships, and the association of these relationships with mental and physical health and positive health maintenance behaviors. Research on the demographic correlates of neighboring, moreover, has been informed by a traditional community-level perspective rather than by research on social support (Logan & Spitze, 1994). This chapter proposes a theoretical model of neighboring as an aspect of *social support* and the dependence of neighboring on other social support resources. It presents data from two pilot studies on neighboring and health. Factors underlying this association are explored, including availability of support from family, personality characteristics believed to promote sociability, physical characteristics of different neighborhoods, and pre-existing levels of health.

We define neighboring social support as the characteristics of congeniality, amicability, respect, and availability for help that characterize friendly but not necessarily close or intimate relationships between people who live in the same neighborhood. The seeking of help from neighbors while in need may in itself be considered a naturally occurring, self-motivated "intervention," in that people seek help from neigh-

I am grateful to Alexis Krulish, Nina Delligati, and Melissa Trepiccione for their expert research assistance.

bors to substitute for support gaps in the more intimately connected network (Cantor, 1979).

WHY FOCUS ON NEIGHBORING?

The current lack of attention to the role of neighboring in social support, personal relationships, and health research seems curious given the focus of early research (predating 1975) on social support. Most recent social support research focuses on close relationships (such as family and friends) and personality factors underlying relationship functioning. This focus has directed attention away from provocative research findings in the 1960s and 1970s, which suggested that support from neighbors was critical to the health and well-being of older people who did not live with their children (e.g., Rosow, 1967; Cantor, 1979). Interventions to promote health through neighboring (e.g., Ross, 1983) have been relatively rare.

The early research indicated that neighboring may be an important complement to family support systems, especially for older adults with no or limited family support (Rosow, 1967; Cantor, 1979). Neighboring can enhance the safety of older people through a monitoring or "watching" function, improve their access to critical goods and services, such as grocery shopping, medical care, and household maintenance, promote their independence and positive feelings about themselves, and enhance their general psychological well-being and social involvement. Although neighboring can provide an important protection against isolation and neglect, it is undermined by privacy concerns, fear of others, time constraints, declining health, and a lack of community facilities that promote social interaction.

There are pressing reasons to pursue a study of the potential health effects of social support derived from less close relationships, such as neighboring. First, there is evidence that non-family members frequently serve as caregivers and other types of essential helpers for frail older people. Recent demographic trend studies show that 12 percent of all reported caregivers in the United States are non-related adults (see Pearlin et al., 1990). Many of these caregivers are likely to be neighbors.

Second, it is likely that the importance of non-related others, including neighbors, in providing social support to older people will increase. As discussed in Chapter 1, the members of the baby-boom cohort are at somewhat greater risk for lacking close family ties in old age than are the members of their parents' generation (Butler, 1984). It is expected that a substantial number of women born during the baby boom will reach old age without living children. Beginning in the 1960s, the fertility rate of married women began to decline (McLanahan & Casper, 1995). The lifetime divorce rate among baby boomers, moreover, is estimated to be in excess of 50 percent (Norton & Moorman, 1987). Lack of support from one's children may be particularly critical for divorced fathers, many of whom permanently lose contact with their children after divorce (Cherlin, 1999). Therefore, non-family relationships, such as neighbors, may be crucial to baby boomers' well-being in later life.

The neglect by researchers of neighboring as a form of social support seems to have occurred for three reasons. Research has tended to focus on the relationship between support from intimate others and physical and psychological health, since in community health studies, these correlations tend to be much larger than those seen between health and support from non-intimate others (House et al., 1988). In addition, many researchers have reported virtually no relationship between measures of network size and well-being (e.g., Kahn et al., 1987), implying that a few close relationships are adequate for maintaining well-being. Current research, particularly in the field of psychology, also strongly emphasizes the relationship between personality factors and reports of social interaction (e.g., Cohen et al., 1986), which could be taken to imply that the broader social setting is irrelevant to health.

For the purposes of this chapter, we have identified five important strands of research on neighboring and its potential relationship to health. Although general research on social support and health is germane to this project, this review of findings will concentrate on studies of neighboring behavior, its relationship to other forms of social support, and its hypothesized positive relationship to good physical and psychological health, primarily through enhancement of good health behavior. The five strands of research are organized by six research questions.

RESEARCH QUESTIONS

Does neighboring enhance the quality of life and the physical and psychological health of older adults?

Researchers (e.g., Cantor, 1979; Fischer, 1982; Hochschild, 1973) have identified five important functions of support potentially available from neighbors: (1) watching and monitoring; (2) the provision of instrumental aid, primarily through the exchange of goods and services; (3) crisis assistance; (4) everyday socializing and peer interaction; (5) the opportunity for intimate exchange, confiding, and reassurance, as well as a source of replacement for relationship loss through illness or death. In general, the availability or presence of these types of support appears to be related to good psychological and physical health (House et al., 1988). The research of Wentowski (1981), moreover, suggests that the equal exchange of such support functions among older people and their neighbors promote psychological morale by maintaining older people's independence and feelings of competence and self-worth.

Is neighboring promoted by participation in voluntary and religious organizations?

Church and voluntary group membership has been shown to promote neighboring behaviors through two mechanisms: providing a context for positive social interaction with others (e.g., Chatters et al., 1986; Fischer, 1982; Van Willigen, 1989); and the development of values favoring social interaction with acquaintances (Fiske, 1991; Rosow, 1967). These are among the most well researched and consistent findings in the literature on neighboring.

Is neighboring associated with the stability, physical type, socioeconomic status, and propensity for crime in the neighborhood?

The associations of neighborhood stability, physical type, and socioeconomic status with neighboring behavior are also well established. More stable neighborhoods—and longer residence in them—are associated with more neighboring activity (e.g., Fischer, 1982). Interaction between neighbors is less frequent among people of lower socioeconomic status (Chatters et al., 1986). It has been suggested that this is due to the burdens of interacting with others undergoing economic stress (Belle, 1983); inadequate access to financial resources that promote equal exchanges and reciprocity among neighbors (Wentowski, 1981); and more frequent reliance on kin when economic resources are scarce (Stack, 1974). It may also be due to a fear of crime (Sampson, 1988).

Does neighboring provide an important complement and, in some cases, a substitute for the family support system?

Cantor (1979), in an important study of older people in New York City, proposed that support from friends, neighbors, and formal social organizations becomes important to health only when kin, particularly children, are not available as supporters. Cantor's study documents that the older people report seeking help from children and other close family members for all sorts of tasks and believe that seeking support from kin is more appropriate than seeking support from less-close others, when close others are available. This is referred to as *hierarchical-compensatory* substitution (see also Rook & Schuster, 1996). In contrast, Litwak (1985) has argued that older adults seek support from different sorts of network members—including neighbors—according to the tasks that need to be addressed. This is referred to as *task-specific* substitution (see also Litwak & Szelenyi, 1969). Both models make assumptions about the efficacy of different sorts of support received in promoting health. Cantor's theory assumes that support from normatively inappropriate others is less efficacious. Litwak's hypothesis assumes that support from task-inappropriate others is less efficacious. In contrast, other possible models of support substitution (each supporter performs random tasks, or no efficacious substitution is possible) imply that neither task specificity nor normative expectations affect the support process.

The task-specific hypothesis is distinguished from other models of support substitution in assuming that efficacy is determined by the helping/support task to be performed. From this perspective, different supporters are more appropriate for different sorts of support tasks: kin provide intimacy; friends provide peer group interaction and the opportunity to have a good time without pressing obligations; and neighbors provide crisis assistance and support tasks that require being in geographic proximity.

Cantor's perspective assumes that there is a culturally determined order of preference for support. Americans rate kin first, followed by other significant relationships, then acquaintances and formal organizations. The hierarchical-compensatory model assumes that when a "preferred" supporter is absent, another supporter can compensate. However, when a preferred supporter is available, substitution is less efficacious. Cantor's (1979) research has been interpreted to mean that supporters can be substituted for helping/support tasks only if a supporter from a more primary relationship is not available (cf. Peters & Kaiser, 1985).

Reviews of the literature on neighboring (Peters & Kaiser, 1985; Rook & Schuster, 1996) suggest that efficacy of support substitution is related to both task-specific and hierarchical compensatory factors. For example, support from intimates does appear to be especially efficacious; indeed, the presence of a spouse is associated with lower risk of mortality (House et al., 1988) and the presence of children with better health behaviors (Umberson, 1987). More specifically, Litwak and Messeri (1989) presented macro-level data on mortality consistent with the task-specific model, while Hochschild (1973) observed specific instances of the substitution of neighbor support for daily social interaction needs. As well, Cantor (1979) demonstrated that "norms" for seeking support reported by the older people follow a hierarchical-compensatory pattern; and Lieberman (1986) argued that only close family members could provide efficacious support in times of deep bereavement.

Relatively little has been done, however, to test explicitly the underlying assumptions about support efficacy from different sources. Neither the task-specific or hierarchical-compensatory hypothesis has been tested against data on support substitution behavior and levels of reported physical and psychological health. Some important questions need to be addressed: Are there aspects of life that neighboring can enhance for everybody (as Cantor's research implies)? Under what specific circumstances can neighboring substitute for family support and still promote good psychological morale and maintain positive health behaviors? Does the efficacy of the substitution for maintaining health differ by type of problem, severity of problem, availability of related others, and internalized norms about what type and source of support is appropriate?

Such hypotheses have been developed (e.g., Cantor, 1979; Chatters et al., 1986; Litwak, 1985; Litwak & Messeri, 1989) but not tested against relative levels of physical or psychological health, as measured by standardized reliable instruments. For example, Cantor presents data suggesting that people have "norms" about whether family or less-close connections should be called on for help in crisis or stressful situations, but she shows no data suggesting that people who consult the normatively appropriate supporters report better outcomes after a crisis. Hochschild (1973) argues that support from neighbors cannot substitute effectively for the sort of support that maintains high self-worth and esteem, but she did not directly assess the psychological or physical health of those who had support versus those who did not. Chatters and her colleagues (1986) present data that are consistent with objective substitution of less close relationships for close ones in the networks of older African Americans but do not demonstrate the relationship of such substitution to health.

> Can the good effects of neighboring on psychological and physical health and general quality of life be undermined by (1) privacy concerns; (2) fear of others; (3) real and perceived time constraints; (4) aging and physical decline?

It is well known that people vary a great deal in their preferences for and habits of affiliation and socializing. Rosow (1967) identified types of older people whose preferences for affiliation and typical interaction styles made it more or less likely for them to engage in affiliative behavior with neighbors. Their interaction and personality styles sometimes prevented the development of new relationships or made it less likely for them to experience satisfaction in their relationships with others. Rosow's research is significant in that it suggests that individual preference for affiliation, norms about privacy, and interaction styles mediate the relationship between giving and receiving social support and health. The existence of these factors partly determines the efficacy of any specific supportive transaction (Eckenrode & Wethington, 1990). These factors also have relevance to the substitution hypothesis, in that the specification of these attitudes, personality traits, interaction styles, and cognitions could represent a more specific elaboration of the phenomenon of support substitution.

Privacy concerns. Preferences for privacy and the ways in which people guard their privacy make intervention and giving formal help difficult. This relatively informal clinical observation has been used to inform the more social psychologically based research relevant to privacy concerns in personal relationships (e.g., Derlega & Chaikin, 1975). These preferences for privacy are undoubtedly related to the propensity for seeking help.

Concomitant with the desire for privacy are social practices in regard to personal *disclosure* of thoughts and feelings and help-offering and help-seeking in various types of relationships (Jourard, 1971). These social practices in regard to disclosure correlate, in the ideal-typical sense, with the distinction between intimate and non-intimate relationships (Derlega & Chaikin, 1975).

Rules for self-disclosure and help exist in non-intimate as well as intimate relationships. In voluntarily formed intimate relationships, there is generally a long history of successful needs fulfillment that relates to emotional and physical well-being. Once trust is established, there are strong expectations that affect disclosure, protecting the privacy of the person who discloses and the ways in which help is offered and sought. These interrelated expectations are (1) availability when help is asked for or sought (Lieberman, 1986; Veroff et al., 1981); (2) appropriateness when giving help (Coyne et al., 1988); (3) knowing ways to offer help so that the potential for insult is minimized, such as avoiding the implication that the subject is dependent, incompetent, or unable to solve the problem (Fisher et al., 1982); (4) readiness to help even when aid is not explicitly sought by the subject (Wethington & Kessler, 1986); (5) willingness to wait for reciprocation, that is, not expecting an immediate payback (Clark et al., 1979). Failures, or lack of sensitivity to the "rules," are apt to lead to an erosion of trust in relationships.

These observations are relevant for a study of neighboring and its efficacy as a social support. Forced or inappropriate ways of neighboring complicate the cross-sectional associations that we observe. (Some obvious examples of rule violations would be intrusiveness and attempts to establish unwanted intimacy.) An understanding of how "rules" apply to neighboring relationships is necessary for recommending interventions that promote neighboring (see also Ross, 1983).

Fear of others. Personality research suggests that stable personal characteristics affect relationship functioning. Neuroticism, lack of trust in others, deficits in social skills, and shyness are all associated with less ease and competence in relationships (e.g., Cohen et al., 1986). Extraversion and friendliness are associated with maintaining more relationships (Eysenck & Eysenck, 1976). Research on isolated older people (e.g., Eckert, 1982), moreover, suggests that a history of social isolation may reflect this sort of personality style (see also Takahashi, 1990).

Time constraints. Demands on time from family and other obligations may also undermine neighboring relationships. If one's time is absorbed by other responsibilities (caregiving in the household, kin keeping, voluntary associations outside the household), less time is left for maintaining neighborly ties. This is a reasonably simple extension of role conflict models of human interaction (Goode, 1960).

There is a problem, though, with assuming that objective time constraints are related to less neighboring. For example, outgoing and extraverted people may keep many relationships going at once (cf. Sieber, 1974). Excellent social skills attract others, and the rewards of good associations with others reinforce friendly, neighborly behavior. A more sophisticated model of this process would take account of perceptions of time constraints, as well as objective demands (cf. Schorr, 1991). A sophisticated model among older people would also try to account for the observed contraction of the social network as people age (Carstensen, 1992).

METHODS

Sample

To address some of these questions, we conducted two pilot studies on neighboring. The two pilot studies were conducted in the cities of Elmira and Ithaca, New York.

The Ithaca pilot study examined neighboring behavior and its relationship to physical and psychological health, network structure, personality, and network characteristics. The respondents for the Ithaca study (n = 70) were selected from eight physically distinct "neighborhoods" selected randomly from a street and topographical map of the city. The respondents were aged 55 and over. The respondents for the pilot study in Elmira (n = 25) were selected from a public housing project. This study was a focus group, especially constructed to discuss the role of crime in affecting the propensity to neighbor. The site was selected in order to see how reports of neighboring behavior would be related to fear of crime. Use of this site also produced racial diversity for our pilot work. Response rates for both of these studies were very good (78% for the Ithaca study, and 70% focus group participation in Elmira).

Respondents in Ithaca completed a fifty-minute face-to-face interview. The interview contained demographic assessments, a standard set of items measuring perceived health, disability, and chronic conditions (House, 1997); depression and anxiety (Derogatis, 1977); memory impairment (House, 1997); organizational membership, religious participation, social interaction, and support (Mattlin et al., 1990); neuroticism and extraversion (Eysenck & Eysenck, 1976); and roles, tasks, and burdens that might produce time constraints on neighboring, such as work, household duties, and giving care to dependent others. The interview also contained measures assessing attitudes toward interacting with others, including concerns about privacy and the reliance on people outside of family, derived from Fischer (1982). The two trained interviewers (both mature women) also filled out a neighborhood and respondent observation form, which included assessments of health, disability, and mood (Fischer, 1982). In addition, we developed a series of measures on satisfaction with neighboring, level of neighboring activity, and the types of help sometimes sought from neighbors.

The major dependent variable in this chapter is "neighboring activity," an index of nine items. Respondents were asked if they had "done any of these things with any of your neighbors in the past 12 months": have long conversations, visit in each other's home, borrow things from one another, help fix something or work on a project together, provide transportation for each other, provide child care, give favors such as mowing the lawn or running errands, help out in a health or other type of crisis, and confide about personal problems or troubles. Responses were either yes or no; all yes responses were summed to form the index. The mean of neighboring activity reported was 4.34 (s.d. = 2.52), with a range from 0 to 9.

The Ithaca sample is fairly small, consistent with its pilot status. Thus we lack statistical power to examine more complex research questions involving substitution of support because they require multivariate specification. The sample is 61 percent female, and its mean age is 61.1 years.

RESULTS

Neighboring and Demographic Factors

Neighboring activities are significantly related to income ($r = .228$; $p < .05$) and education ($r = .196$; $p < .05$). Predicted relationships to female gender and age did not hold, probably because of small sample size (see Table 7.1).

NEIGHBORING AND HEALTH

As expected, neighboring activities are significantly related to re-ported physical health, as well as to interviewer observation of re-spondent health (see Table 7.1). Neighboring activities are positively related to self-reported health (r = .423; p < .01), and negatively re-lated to the number of self-reported health problems (−.423; p < .01) and to self-reported level of physical disability (−.280, p < .05). Neigh-boring activities are not significantly related to self-reported depres-sion (r = −.165; n.s.), self-reported anxiety (r = −.045, n.s.), or memory problems (r = .003; n.s.).

Table 7.1.   The Relationship of Neighboring Activity to Demographic Factors, Health, and Group Membership (Correlations)

Demographic Factors	
Gender (Female = 1)	−.035
Age (in years)	.104
Years of education	.196[a]
Income (in $1,000 units)	.288[b]
Health	
Perceived health	.423[b]
Number of health problems	−.423[b]
Level of disability	−.280[a]
Depression	−.165
Anxiety	−.045
Memory problems	.003
Interviewer rating—R has difficulty moving	−.426[a]
Interviewer rating—R health	.449[a]
Group Membership	
Organization membership	.105
Religious participation	.015
Volunteer status	.103
Enjoy volunteering	−.034
Number of organizations	.099
Any organizational participation	.031

[a] p < .05 (one-tailed test).
[b] p < .01 (one-tailed test).

Neighboring and Organization Membership

Perhaps the more surprising finding was that neighboring activity was not related to organizational membership, religious participation, or volunteer status (see Table 7.1). A summary measure of group participation (a sum of the number of organizations the respondent belonged to, religious participation, and volunteer status) was similarly not related to neighboring activities.

Neighboring and Neighborhood Factors

The focus group study in Elmira was designed to measure perceptions of neighboring and neighboring activity in a setting assumed to be hostile toward social activity and cohesion—a housing project. Participants were unanimously nostalgic for neighborhoods that encouraged or permitted neighboring. But they were also of one voice about the paucity of spontaneous neighbor contact near their own dwellings. Neighbors were assumed to be the major source of threat and crime in their neighborhood, since turnover in the project was high and residents had no say over who could move into the project. As a consequence, few interactions were spontaneous. Few believed that they could trust next-door neighbors, and even if they did, they did not feel they could trust the relatives and visitors of the neighbors.

The random selection of Ithaca neighborhoods did not include any congregate, low-income housing. (Most of the units sampled were single-family homes, followed by multi-unit houses.) However, assessments of safety varied a great deal across neighborhoods. Consistent with the Elmira focus group findings, neighboring activities are strongly related to perceptions of neighborhood safety ($r = .326$; $p < .01$), as shown in Table 7.2.

Does Neighboring Substitute for Social Support?

One key assertion of the simple substitution hypothesis is that people would seek to fill a deficit in social relationships by forming relationships in the wider social network. An alternative to the substitution hypothesis is that those who seek and engage in neighboring are in fact just more gregarious and friendly.

Table 7.2 summarizes a number of simple analyses done to test for simple versions of the substitution hypothesis. Married people are no

Table 7.2.   The Relationship of Neighboring Activity to Neighborhood Factors and Social Support (Correlations)

Neighborhood Factors	
Neighborhood safe	.326[b]
Years in neighorhood	.035
Has speaking relations with neighbors	.415[c]
Owns home	.138
Interviewer rating—neighborhood cleanliness	.196
Social Support	
Married	.157
Children live in area	−.149
Has confidant	.236[a]
Perceived support from marital partner	.068
Marital conflict	−.210
Perceived support from children	.142
Perceived support from friends	.139
Good friends live in neighborhood	.437[b]
Prefers to keep problems to self	−.118
Prefers to talk out problems	.242[a]
Family preferred source of support	−.074
Enjoy helping others	.376[b]
No contact with children	−.120

[a] p < .05 (one-tailed test).
[b] p < .01 (one-tailed test).
[c] p < .001 (one-tailed test).

more likely than the currently unmarried to engage in neighboring activities (r = .157; n.s.), which suggests that neighboring is not a simple substitute for the lack of a primary confiding relationship. Neighboring activity is also not related to marital conflict (r = −.210; n.s.), implying that the sort of social contact involved in neighboring is not likely to compensate for difficulties in primary relationships. (As well, perceived support from one's marital partner [r = .068] does not predict neighboring.) Neighboring activity is strongly related to having good friends in the neighborhood (r = .437; p < .01, one-tailed), a finding that needs a more detailed context to constitute evidence for support substitution. (People who have neighbored more in the past will have more close friends in the neighborhood; moreover, people more inclined to neighbor may have based their previous housing decision on having friends in the neighborhood.)

A key component of the more complicated substitution hypotheses, however, is that attitudes toward receiving support underlie the seeking of support from less close others. Preferring to keep problems to oneself is not related to neighboring activity. However, preferring to talk out problems with others is related to neighboring activity ($r = .242$; $p < .05$), implying that gregariousness or openness may be important. A major component of the hierarchical-substitution hypothesis, though, is not related to neighboring: the belief that the family should be the preferred source of support is not significantly negatively related to neighboring activity. Consistent with the gregariousness interpretation of neighboring, those who enjoy helping others are more likely to engage in more neighboring activities ($r = .376$; $p < .01$).

Another way to approach the substitution hypothesis is to assess the degree to which people seek help from their neighbors. What functions of support do people get from their neighbors, and how many people engage in this type of activity? Table 7.3 analyzes the nine types of help and interaction included in the neighboring activities measure. Data are presented separately for men and women. In addition,

Table 7.3. Seeking and Getting Support from Neighbors, by Type of Support or Interaction (in %)

Support or Interaction	Men	Women
Have long conversations	93	84
Visit in each other's homes	63	79
Borrow things	59	58
Help fix something	44	35
Provide transportation	41	56
Provide child care	7	12
Give favors	48	44
Help out in health or other crisis	37	37
Confide in	26	40
Has neighbor who		
watches house	70	84
notices activities	89	77
monitors strangers	59	40
calls family if help needed	85	79

we present reports of receiving help from neighbors in monitoring the safety of the neighborhood.

There are no significant gender differences in the nine different types of help people seek from or give to neighbors, or in the four types of neighborhood monitoring. However, the propensity to do these activities seems to increase when the activity involves less intimate contact (e.g., "long conversations") in comparison to interactions that involve a longer-term commitment or personal involvement (e.g., giving help during a crisis, confiding, and childcare). Of the thirteen support items presented, only one is significantly related to length of time residing in the neighborhood and to age of respondent. That item is whether the respondent has a neighbor who would call family if he or she needed help.

Personality and Neighboring

Neighboring does not relate, as hypothesized, to neuroticism. It does relate to extraversion, in the predicted direction ($r = .258$; $p < .05$). Reported neighboring activities also correlate with the interviewer's judgment of the respondent's skill in handling people ($r = .305$; $p < .01$), but not with interviewer observation of respondent self-confidence.

Table 7.4.   Neighboring Activity in Relationship to Personality Traits and Time Constraints (Correlations)

Personality Traits	
Neuroticism	−.006
Extraversion	.258[a]
Interviewer rating—R's skill at handling people	.305[b]
Interviewer rating—R's self-confidence	.114
Time Constraints	
R is caregiver	.095
Currently working	−.026
Worked in past year	−.078
Number of household tasks	.243[a]
Number of household members	.098

[a] $p < .05$ (one-tailed test)
[b] $p < .01$ (one-tailed test)

Time Constraints and Neighboring

Neighboring activity is not related to most of the various measures of time constraints, not to working in the past year, present work status, giving care to others (inside or outside the household), or number of household members. However, the number of household activities and chores that the respondent performs is positively related to neighboring ($r = .243$; $p < .05$). The number of household activities is related to reported physical health and to disability, and that may explain the association.

DISCUSSION

The pilot data analyses presented here confirm several early analyses of neighboring as a source of social support. People with more education and income engage in more neighboring activities. People in poorer health or who are physically disabled report fewer contacts with neighbors. Neighborhood safety, which correlates with education and income, is associated with more neighboring activity. Neighboring activity is associated with having speaking relationships with people in the neighborhood, but in cross-sectional data the direction of this effect is not clear. Given other findings, it is likely that personal gregariousness is at work: those who report that very good friends live in the neighborhood, who prefer talking out their problems with others, who enjoy helping others, and who are extraverted report more neighboring activity.

Several factors hypothesized to be related to neighboring activity were not found to be significantly correlated in the pilot data. Level of depression, anxiety, and memory problems are not associated with neighboring activity. Religious and group participation did not predict neighboring activity. Length of time living in the neighborhood (in years) was not related to neighboring activity.

As noted above, the small size of the sample makes it impossible to test more the complicated hypotheses relating to the substitution of support from neighbors for support from family. In general, there is no support from the pilot data that neighbors can "substitute" for lack of support from spouse or children. Being married or not, having children living in the area, or perceived support from partner, children, and friends were not related to neighboring activities. The data more strongly indicate that those who seek or have support—that is, those who have good friends in the neighborhood or who have confidants— engage in more neighboring activity, not the reverse.

The data suggest that substitution is not easy to effect across relationships, because the support that people give and receive from neighbors is not the sort of support they may typically exchange within more intimate relationships. Neighboring activity is very prevalent in this sample. But the help most likely to be exchanged involved passive help ("monitoring"), short-term exchange, or problem-focused exchange in an emergency.

We have also been able to confirm, in a general way, that many older people view their neighbors as a potential source of emergency assistance. Particular neighbors are viewed as reliable and trustworthy helpers.

Can neighboring *per se* significantly promote better health among socially isolated persons who are "at risk"? Several research studies have established the association of social integration with better health behaviors (e.g., Umberson, 1987). In addition, a few interventions have been conducted to promote neighboring assistance for frail older people (Pynoos et al., Hade-Kaplan, & Fleisher, 1984) or to encourage use of health services (Ross, 1983). The relative success of these interventions suggest that informal neighborhood information and assistance networks can be promoted to encourage better preventive health care among older people, at least among those who are comfortable interacting with neighbors.

These pilot data, however, argue for caution and conservatism when promoting interventions to increase neighboring activities among older people. Naturally occurring neighboring activity is more likely among the gregarious and the extraverted. This implies that norms relating to the appropriateness of seeking help from others will limit what can be gained from interventions to increase neighboring activities. Perhaps the most efficient way to promote neighboring activity is to provide settings where more people who wish to meet others can safely meet new and different people. It is unclear whether even these relatively superficial activities can be transformed into a source of support critical to well-being. Clearly, the conservative answer is, "it depends." Neighboring is dependent on context, and whether or not a particular person seeks support is dependent on personal, historical, and situational factors.

REFERENCES

Antonucci, T. A., & Akiyama, H. (1987). Social networks in adult life and a preliminary examination of the convoy model. *Journal of Gerontology, 42,* 519–527.

Belle, D. (1983). The impact of poverty on social networks and social supports. *Women and Health, 1,* 89–103.

Butler, R. N. (1984). *A generation at risk: When the babyboomers reach Golden Pond.* Austin, TX: Hogg Foundation.

Cantor, M. (1979). Neighbors and friends: An overlooked resource in the informal support system. *Research on Aging, 1,* 434–463.

Carstensen, L. (1992). Social and emotional patterns in adulthood: Support for socioemotional selectivity theory. *Psychology and Aging, 7,* 331–338.

Chatters, L., Taylor, R. J., & Jackson, J. S. (1986). Aged blacks' choices for an informal helper network. *Journal of Gerontology, 41,* 94–100.

Cherlin, A. (1999). *Public and private families,* 2d ed. New York: McGraw-Hill.

Clark, M. S., Gotay, C. C., & Mills, J. (1979). Acceptance of help as a function of similarity of the potential helper and opportunity to repay. *Journal of Applied Social Psychology 3,* 224–229.

Cohen, S., Sherrod, D., & Clark, M. S. (1986). Social skills and the stress-protective role of social support. *Journal of Personality and Social Psychology, 50,* 963–973.

Coyne, J. C., Wortman, C. B., & Lehman, D. R. (1988). The other side of support: Emotional overinvolvement and miscarried helping. In Gottlieb, B. H. (Ed.), *Marshalling social support* (305–330). Beverly Hills: Sage.

Derlega, V., & Chaikin, A. (1975). *Sharing intimacy.* Englewood Cliffs, NJ: Prentice-Hall.

Derogatis, L. (1977). *SCL–90: Administration, scoring, and procedures manual for the revised edition.* Baltimore: Clinical Psychometrics Research Unit, Johns Hopkins School of Medicine.

Eckenrode, J., & Wethington, E. (1990). The process of mobilizing social support. In S. Duck (Ed.), *Personal relationships and social support* (83–103). Beverly Hills: Sage.

Eckert, J. K. (1982). *The unseen older people: A study of marginally subsistent hotel dwellers.* San Diego: Campanile Press.

Eysenck, H. B., & Eysenck, S. B. G. (1976). *Psychoticism as a dimension of personality.* London: Hodder and Stoughton.

Fischer, C. (1982). *To dwell among friends.* Chicago: University of Chicago.

Fisher, J. D., Nadler, A., & Witchner-Alagna, S. (1982). Recipients' reactions to aid. *Psychological Bulletin, 91,* 27–54.

Fiske, A. P. (1991). *Structures of social life: The four elementary forms of human relations.* New York: Free Press.

Goode, W. (1960). A theory of role strain. *American Sociological Review, 45,* 483–496.

Hochschild, A. R. (1973). *The unexpected community.* Englewood Cliffs, NJ: Prentice-Hall.

House, J. S. (1997) Americans changing lives: Wave I and II, 1986 and 1989. Ann Arbor: Survey Research Center, University of Michigan.

House, J. S., Umberson, D., & Landis, K. L. (1988). Structures and processes of social support. *Annual Review of Sociology, 14,* 293–318.

Jourard, S. (1971). *Self-disclosure.* New York: Wiley.

Kahn, R. L., & Antonucci, T. C. (1981). Convoys of social support: A life course approach. In S. B. Kiesler, J. N. Morgan, & V. C. Dopenheimer (Eds.), *Aging: Social change.* New York: Academic Press.

Kahn, R. L., Wethington, E., & Ingersoll-Dayton, B. (1987). Social support and social networks: Determinants, effects, and interactions. In R. Abeles (Ed.), *Life-span perspectives and social psychology* (139–163). Hillsdale, NJ: Erlbaum.

Lieberman, M. (1986). Social supports—the consequences of psychologizing: A commentary. *Journal of Consulting and Clinical Psychology, 4,* 461–465.

Litwak, E. (1985). *Helping older people.* London: Guilford Press.

Litwak, E., & Messeri, P. (1989). Organizational theory, social supports, and mortality: A theoretical convergence. *American Sociological Review, 54,* 49–66.

Litwak, E., & Szelenyi, I. (1969). Primary group structures and their functions: Kin, neighbors, and friends. *American Sociological Review, 34,* 465–481.

Logan, J., & Spitze, G. (1994). Family neighbors. *American Journal of Sociology, 100,* 453–476.

Mattlin, J., Wethington, E., & Kessler, R. C. (1990). Situational determinants of coping and coping effectiveness. *Journal of Health and Social Behavior, 31,* 103–122.

McLanahan, S. A., & Casper, L. (1995). Growing diversity and inequality in the American family. In R. Farley (Ed.), *State of the union: America in the 1990s, Vol. 2* (1–46). New York: Russell Sage.

Norton, A. J., & Moorman, J. E. (1987). Current trends in marriage and divorce among American women. *Journal of Marriage and the Family, 49,* 3–14.

Pearlin, L. I., Mullan, J. T., Semple, S. J., & Skaff, M. N. (1990). Caregiving and the stress process: An overview of concepts and measures. *The Gerontologist, 30,* 583–594.

Peters, G. R., & Kaiser, M. A. (1985). The role of friends and neighbors in providing social support. In W. J. Sauer & R. T. Coward (Eds.), *Social support networks and the care of the older people* (123–158). New York: Springer.

Pynoos, J., Hade-Kaplan, B., & Fleisher, D. (1984). Intergenerational neighborhood networks: A basis for aiding the frail older people. *The Gerontologist, 24,* 233–237.

Rook, K., & Schuster, S. (1996). Compensatory processes in the social networks of older adults. In G. R. Pierce, B. R. Sarason, & I. G. Sarason (Eds.), *Handbook of social support and the family* (219–248). New York: Plenum.

Rosow, I. (1967). *Social integration of the aged.* New York: Free Press.

Ross, H. K. (1983). The neighborhood family: Community mental health for the older people. *The Gerontologist, 23,* 243–247.

Sampson, R. (1988). Local friendship ties and community attachment in mass society. *American Sociological Review, 53,* 766–779.

Schorr, J. (1991). *The overworked American: The unexpected decline of leisure.* New York: Basic.

Sieber, S. (1974). Toward a theory of role accumulation. *American Sociological Review, 39,* 567–578.

Stack, C. (1974). *All our kin: Strategies for survival in the Black community.* New York: Harper and Row.

Takahashi, K. (1990). Affective relationships and their lifelong development. In P. B. Baltes, D. L. Featherman, & R. M. Lerner (Eds.), *Life-span development and behavior, Vol. 10* (1–29). Hillsdale, NJ: Erlbaum.

Umberson, D. (1987). Family status and health behaviors. *Journal of Health and Social Behavior, 28,* 306–319.

Van Willigen, J. (1989). *Gettin' some age on me.* Lexington: University of Kentucky.

Veroff, J., Douvan, E., & Kulka, R. (1981). *The inner American.* New York: Basic.

Wentowski, M. (1981). Reciprocity and the coping strategies of older people: Cultural dimensions of network building. *The Gerontologist, 21,* 600–609.

Wethington, E., & Kessler, R. C. (1986). Perceived support, received support, and adjustment to stressful life events. *Journal of Health and Social Behavior, 27,* 78–89.

CHAPTER EIGHT

Social Integration and the Move to a Continuing Care Retirement Community

Mary Ann Erickson, Donna Dempster-McClain,
Carol Whitlow, and Phyllis Moen

Although most older Americans wish to "age in place," many individuals in the second half of life will face at least one residential relocation. For an increasing number of older Americans, this move may be to age-segregated, congregate housing, such as a retirement community. Early studies (Bultena, 1974; Lawton, 1970; Rosow, 1967) suggested that older adults in age-segregated settings actually experience higher rates of social interaction and higher levels of social integration and morale compared to residents of age-integrated housing. But the experiences of older adults in the 1960s may or may not be relevant as contemporary cohorts make the decision to move into continuing care retirement communities, an increasingly popular alternative in residential housing. Leaving one's neighborhood to move into a continuing care community is, clearly, a major life transition in later adulthood. What is not clear is whether such a move affects individuals' social integration. In this study we document levels of social integration before and after a move in order to better understand the social consequences of relocation.

The life-course perspective (Giele & Elder, 1998; Moen, 1997) points out the importance of transitions at all ages. Residential relocation is a key life-course transition, often associated with other life-course transitions. For example, adult migration is connected to employment and career opportunities, marital events, and growth in the size of family (Marini, 1996; Speare & Goldscheider, 1987). Triggering events for relocation in later life may include widowhood (Chevan, 1995), divorce (Booth & Amato, 1990), the desire for more amenities or a more suitable home, health problems, and the need for assistance from others (Loomis et al., 1989; Wiseman, 1980).

The life-course focus on timing and context suggests that the effects of relocation may vary according to circumstances surrounding the event and the social and structural characteristics of those involved. For children, the effects of relocation are associated with family structure and characteristics (Eckenrode et al., 1995; Tucker et al., 1998) and parental involvement (Hagan, 1996). For older women, the experience of moving differs by social class. Interviews with forty women who had recently moved to congregate housing revealed that middle-class women viewed their new housing as a "step down" in relation to their previous homes, while working and lower-class women appreciated the security and services of congregate housing (Redfoot, 1987).

Moves in later life are often prompted by increasing illness or disability. Chapter 6 outlines the developmental model of later life migration proposed by Litwak and Longino (1987). According to this model, changes in health status are key triggering factors for later life relocation. Other research confirms that many older persons make no changes in their housing arrangements until health considerations render their current independent housing no longer feasible (Golant, 1992). In a study of movers and nonmovers, using data from the Longitudinal Study on Aging (LSOA) (1984–86), Sommers and Rowell (1992) found no significant effects of health status on relocation. Respondents who owned their own homes and who had lived in one place the longest were less likely to relocate, while those elders with greater numbers of adult children were more likely to move. Decisions to move, where to move, and when to move will continue to be important in the lives of older adults as well as on the public agenda as the baby-boomer cohort begins to consider alternative housing arrangements as they age (Groves & Wilson, 1992; VanderHart, 1995).

A small but increasing number of Americans are relocating in *anticipation* of future health care needs, rather than in reaction to increasing illness or disability (Krout et al., 1998). For those wishing to anticipate future housing and health care needs, one option is relocation to a continuing care retirement community (CCRC). For a substantial entry fee and continuing monthly fees, these facilities offer independent living with a variety of health services and nursing facilities available on site when needed (Sherwood et al., 1997). As CCRCs age, more attention has been focused on the needs of residents who are becoming older and frailer (Bowers, 1989). Sheehan and Karasik's (1995) survey of 184 CCRC residents and 246 waiting list respondents found the most common reasons for moving to a CCRC were guaranteed health care, freedom from home maintenance, and supportive services.

Although relocation is generally classified as a stressful life event (Holmes & Rahe, 1967), most research shows that moves have minimal impacts on well-being. For example, relocation has little effect on the well-being of early adolescents (Brown & Orthner, 1990). Relocation in later adulthood could be more disturbing. However, research on 22,579 Swedish individuals aged 65 and over in 1988–90 shows that residential relocation, except for forced, permanent relocation due to urban renewal, is not associated with increased mortality or morbidity (Danermark et al., 1996). However, data from the Longitudinal Study on Aging (1984–90) on 4,060 adults aged 70 and over show that moving late in life contributes to health deterioration to a small but significant degree (Choi, 1996).

Although there are a number of empirical studies of relocation, little theory is available to guide this research. Much of the research on congregate housing facilities is guided by person-environment models, such as that of Lawton (1982). These models suggest that residents' adaptations to housing depend both on personal and environmental factors, and especially on the fit between the two. However, these models have not been extended to consider changes in social integration across the transition into congregate housing. Golant has proposed a framework for studying change in older people's housing, but his model speaks specifically to individuals' evaluations of their situation rather than their social connectedness (Golant, 1998).

However, two other theories may help us make predictions about relocation and social integration. The social ecological approach of Moos and Lemke (Moos, 1976; Moos & Lemke, 1994; Scheidt, 1998) suggests that physical and social environments affect each other and are inextricably related. Their model links adaptation to group residences for older adults to the social climate of the residence as well as to personal factors, the objective characteristics of the program, and residents' coping responses. Applying these concepts to the study of relocation in later life suggests that changes in both physical and social characteristics of the environment may affect individual outcomes, including social integration.

Atchley has proposed that individuals strive to maintain continuity in psychological and social patterns even in the face of changes in their physical and social environments (Atchley, 1989). In the present context, this would suggest that individuals will be likely to maintain previous levels of social contact, social role participation, and social integration after moving to a different residential arrangement.

As the market for alternative housing arrangements grows, more older Americans will consider relocating to a CCRC. Yet we know little about the way in which social contact, social roles, and social integration are affected by a move to a CCRC. We consider the move to a CCRC to be a "best case scenario"—people moving to a CCRC are generally healthy and have the financial, social, and psychological resources to plan for future health and housing needs. We develop hypotheses about the effects of relocation to a CCRC on social contact, social role participation, and perceived social integration and test them on a sample of older adults before and after their move to a CCRC.

We ground our hypotheses in the social ecological perspective and in continuity theory, coupled with the overarching life-course theme. Specifically, we argue that social structures shape accessibility and availability of opportunities for social integration. Changes in social structure and the constraints associated with a residential move produce corresponding shifts in social contacts, social role participation, and the subjective assessment of social integration. However, individuals will strive to maintain previous levels of these factors.

Availability of Social Contact

A key component of social integration is contact with family, friends, and neighbors. Contact with children can be especially important for older adults, as parents often turn to children for help. Adults moving to a CCRC are usually "downsizing," or moving from a larger home to a smaller one. Typically, individuals have lived in a single family home for many years, often the same one in which their children grew up. The process of "downsizing" may have consequences for visits with children, since the parents' home will no longer have the space to host large family gatherings. However, continuity theory suggests that parents will strive to maintain ties with children despite this change in the physical environment, implying that:

Hypothesis 1: Visits with children will decline after the move to the CCRC. In contrast, we expect no changes in phone or mail contact with children following the move to the CCRC.

The changes in social climate associated with moving to a CCRC may increase the availability of social contact with non-family members. Living in single family homes surrounded by neighbors busy with jobs and families may limit the social integration of older adults. A CCRC, in contrast, may offer more opportunities to make and visit with friends. Living in an age-segregated environment may facilitate friendship formation within the community, as similar others are in more frequent contact. Ethnographic observations and interviews with twenty female residents in a new CCRC identified various stages of friendship development and aspects of the context (large pool of potential friends, abundance of public spaces, communal meals, structured activities) that facilitated the formation of friendship (Perkinson, 1996).

Besides increased opportunities to meet other residents, the time available to spend with other people may increase after moving to a CCRC. In addition to the provision of health care, a popular reason for moving to a CCRC is to avoid worries about the upkeep and maintenance of the previous residence. Residents of a CCRC have fewer domestic responsibilities; their new living arrangements require less upkeep and maintenance, as well as less cooking and cleaning, thus leaving more time for social activities.

Other factors unique to the CCRC we studied may lead to increased contact with friends. All of the participants in the study were moving into a new CCRC. Indeed, some of the study respondents helped bring the CCRC into the community. Many have long-term ties to the area, to nearby universities, and to each other. In these respects, this particular community at this point in time is more like an intentional community than most other congregate facilities for older adults. Thus, several factors lead us to expect that:

Hypothesis 2: Contact with friends and neighbors will increase after moving to the CCRC.

Social Role Participation

Another key indicator of social integration is participation in a variety of roles. Thoits (1983, 1986) found that involvement in multiple roles was associated with increased meaning in life and improved well-being. Moen et al. (1989, 1992) documented the importance of multiple role involvement over the life course, especially social participation in the community: people with more roles benefited in terms of health, well-being, and longevity (see also Chapter 2, this volume). Young and Glasgow (1998) have shown that participation in volunteer work and other forms of instrumental participation is linked to perceived health of the elderly living in nonmetropolitan areas.

Opportunities for employment decrease as one ages. Some people choose to exit the workforce completely in their sixties, while others continue to work as long as possible. None of the physical or social changes associated with moving to a CCRC are likely to influence the employment status of residents. Similarly, church attendance is not likely to be affected by the move to the CCRC, especially for those moving within the local area. However, we do expect changes in volunteer and organizational activities.

As mentioned above, CCRCs are age-segregated environments as well as planned communities. Outsiders are not likely to enter the community without a reason. As Robison and Moen discuss in Chapter 6, age segregation can lead to social isolation from the broader community, suggesting that a move to a CCRC may lead to a decline in volunteering and organizational membership outside the CCRC. However, continuity theory suggests that residents will try to preserve social role participation across the transition to the CCRC. There are many opportunities to be active with volunteering and clubs within the CCRC itself. Indeed, the CCRC organization has an explicit philosophy of leaving activities and events in the hands of residents. These factors shaping the accessibility and availability of volunteer opportunities and organizations lead us to hypothesize a change in the location of these activities rather than in the amount of involvement.

Hypothesis 3: Volunteering and organizational membership will shift from involvement with the outside community to activities within the CCRC.

Perceived Social Integration

It is important to examine not only objective continuity or change in social connectedness but also to examine residents' own evaluations of their social integration. Even if objective levels of social contact and social role participation stay about the same, new residents of a CCRC may feel less socially integrated if the friends they see now are new friends rather than old friends, or if they are on the fringe of a new committee rather than a long-standing member of one. A feeling of "dislocation" may be especially strong for those who have moved to the CCRC from outside the local area. Friends, volunteer opportunities, and clubs from one's previous residence may be too far away to see or engage in regularly. This suggests that:

Hypothesis 4: The perceived social integration of distance movers will decrease more after a residential relocation than the social integration of local movers.

METHODS

Sample

We analyze data collected in the 1995 and 1997 waves of the *Pathways to Life Quality* project (Henderson & Oggins 1999). The respondents in the 1995 wave were 101 individuals from the group that founded a continuing care retirement community in upstate New York, many recruited from a letter sent by the director of the facility. This baseline pre-move sample includes 50 percent of the 204 individuals who were expecting to move into the CCRC during the winter of 1995–96. Of the 101 who participated in the first wave, 4 decided not to move to the CCRC, and 5 died before the summer of 1997. We interviewed all of the remaining 92 individuals in the summer of 1997, about two years after their move into the CCRC.

The average age of respondents at the initial interview was 76.5, with a range in age from 64 to 94. About two thirds of the sample are female (66%), and about two thirds were married at the initial interview (62%). All respondents are white, and median annual income is approximately $75,000. More than half (60%) have a graduate degree. For the 88 percent of respondents with children, the average number of children is 3.5.

Variables

Respondents reported on contact with each child in both years, as well as overall contact with friends and neighbors. For indicators of social roles, we asked respondents if they were currently working, volunteering, or belonged to a club or organization, charting continuity and change from before and after their residential relocation. We also used indicators of the frequency of church attendance and the frequency of participating in religious organizations, to capture potential changes following the move.

A key variable of interest is perceived social integration. In both 1995 and 1997, respondents completed several subscales of the Cutrona Social Provisions Scale, including the four-item Social Integration subscale (Russell et al., 1980). Respondents indicate their agreement with the following items on a four-point scale: "I feel part of a group of people who share my attitudes and beliefs"; "There are people who enjoy the same social activities I do"; "There is no one who shares my interest and concerns"; and "There is no one who likes to do the things I do." Alpha reliabilities for the scales before and after the move are .89 and .79, respectively.

We divide the sample into two groups by marital status: those who are married, and those who are divorced, widowed, or never married in 1995 (before moving). We used two levels of income: above and below the median income of the whole sample. The measure of perceived health asks respondents to rate how their health has been lately on a scale of 0 to 10, with 0 being the very worst and 10 being the very best. We also asked respondents at both interviews about whether they had any problems with a set of eleven daily activities (such as walking six blocks, climbing stairs, doing household tasks, and getting to doctor's appointments). In the analyses, we use the sum of the number of functional limitations reported.

RESULTS

Social Contact

Respondents reported on visits and phone contact with each child both before and after moving to the CCRC. On average, parents in the sample visited at least one child a few times a year and spoke to at least one of their children on the telephone once a week before moving to the CCRC. Contrary to our hypothesis, both visits and phone contact with children stayed about the same for the majority of respondents. About half of the parents (51.9%) in the sample had frequent visits (at least several times a year) with at least one of their children both before and after moving to the CCRC, while more than a quarter (27.8%) had infrequent visits from all of their children at both times. Only a few (2.5%) of the parents reported frequent visits before the move and infrequent visits afterward, while almost one in five (17.7%) reported infrequent visits before the move and frequent visits afterward. However, a high percentage of the parents have at least one child whom they see less than a few times a year (80% before the move, 73% after the move). Telephone contact remained similar despite the residential relocation, with 86.3 percent of parents having frequent phone contact (at least once a week) with at least one of their children and 10.0 percent having infrequent phone contact both before and after the move. Only 1.5 percent of parents had frequent phone contact with at least one child before the move and infrequent contact with all children after the move, while 2.5 percent of parents had infrequent phone contact with all children before the move and frequent phone contact with at least one child after the move.

Visits with children may have changed in ways other than in simple frequency of contact. If our hypothesis that downsizing affects the feasibility of family gatherings is correct, the location of visits may have shifted from the parents' home to the children's homes. Perhaps parents are seeing each child about the same number of times, but this is accomplished by the parents visiting each child in turn rather than children congregating at their parents' home.

Whether the residents see and talk to their children frequently or infrequently is not related to whether the children live nearby or far away. Similarly, change in contact is not related to change in proximity to children. More than half of the respondents did not live near children before or after moving to the CCRC (58%), while 28 percent had children in the local area both before and after moving.

The participants in our study were not asked about the frequency of contact with other family members in both surveys, but after the move we asked them if there had been a change in the amount of contact with other family members. More than half (57.0%) said the amount of contact was the same, about one in ten (10.3%) said they had less contact, and almost one in five (17.8%) said they had more.

Although change in the frequency of contact with friends was not statistically significant after the move to the CCRC, the change is in the hypothesized direction: a higher percentage of respondents report seeing or talking to friends "almost every day" after the move (34.1% to 48.2%). This is not surprising, considering that most respondents in 1995 (73.5%) reported that at least one friend was also moving to the CCRC. Those with friends moving to the CCRC reported that, on average, ten friends also moved to the CCRC. However, change in contact with friends is not significantly related to the number of friends moving to the CCRC. Even if people who were friends before the move now live much closer to each other, they may continue to meet with the same frequency, perhaps for the same kinds of events; they may continue to meet once a month for dinner, have lunch every Friday, or have coffee every morning.

Contact with neighbors changed significantly across the transition to the CCRC, supporting Hypothesis 3. While fewer than one in ten (8.9%) of the people in our study reported visiting with neighbors "almost every day" before moving to the CCRC, fully one in four (25.0%) reported visiting almost daily with neighbors after moving to the CCRC. About two out of five (43.6%) visited with neighbors once a week or more before moving to the CCRC. After the move, 53.3 of the residents in our study visited with neighbors at least once a week.

Social Role Participation

Employment levels remain steady before and after the move to the CCRC, with about 15 percent of respondents employed, while the proportions of residents volunteering and belonging to organizations are higher following the move to the CCRC. This increase is due mostly to opportunities at the CCRC, as levels of volunteering outside the CCRC and membership in clubs or organizations based in the community decrease only slightly (see Figure 8.1). There are no significant differences in the rates of being an employee, a volunteer, or a member of a club or organization by age cohort or marital status. Men are more likely than women to be working for pay at both waves, and are somewhat more likely than women to be volunteering after the move to the CCRC (both within the CCRC and in the community). Social role participation is similar for both local and distance movers with one exception: volunteering outside of the CCRC. Local movers are more likely than distance movers to volunteer in the larger community (63%

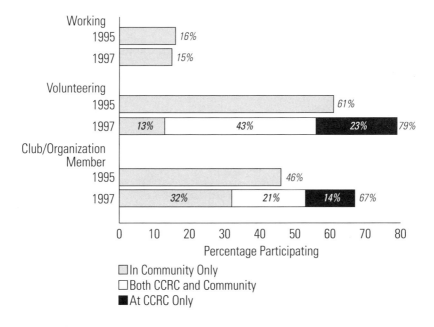

Figure 8.1   Social Role Participation in 1995 and 1997.
Source: Pathways to Life Quality Study, CCRC Sample, N = 92.

vs. 32%; p<.05). Frequency of participating in service organizations, senior center activities, civic groups, and religious groups did not change from before to after the transition to the CCRC. Similarly, frequency of church or synagogue attendance did not change significantly.

We hypothesized that respondents would shift their volunteering and club membership from the larger community to the CCRC. Instead, it appears that volunteering and membership at the CCRC are *added* on to prior commitments. This is also shown by the number of hours respondents spend volunteering. Four out of five (79%) volunteer after the move, with three out of five (61%) volunteering prior to the move. Men who volunteered gave an average of 17.1 hours before moving and 39.9 hours after moving. Women who volunteered did so an average of 15.8 hours before moving and 22.4 hours afterward. Especially for men, volunteer activities at the CCRC have not replaced volunteer activities within the community. Similarly, less than half (46%) of the respondents were members of clubs before they moved; two thirds (67%) were club members after the move.

The availability and accessibility of volunteer opportunities at the

CCRC attracted new volunteers as well as those who had previously volunteered. Although 21 percent of the people in our study did not volunteer either before or after moving to the CCRC, 58 percent continued volunteer activity across the transition and 21 percent started volunteering after moving to the CCRC. Only 3 percent of the respondents stopped volunteering after moving to the CCRC. Those who did not ever volunteer and those who stopped volunteering tend to be somewhat older and have more functional limitations. Those who started volunteering are especially likely to spend their volunteer hours within the CCRC. Those who continued volunteering tend to maintain the hours they volunteered in the community while adding significant hours of volunteer work within the CCRC.

The high rate of volunteering in this sample certainly is partly a function of our highly educated, healthy sample, but the nature of the CCRC does seem to foster volunteering. Only two residents were unwilling to volunteer after the move to the CCRC, and both of these felt that their physical limitations prevented them from volunteering. Although there are a few residents in the sample who feel as if they have done enough in the past, residents are more likely to report that they volunteer at the CCRC to build the community. One reported that the CCRC was a "budding democracy" and wanted to help get it started.

Perceived Social Integration

The findings discussed thus far show that the people in the *Pathways to Life Quality* study tended to maintain their social contacts and social role participation after moving to the CCRC. This suggests that social integration in terms of objective social connectedness was maintained or increased after the move to the CCRC. We now turn to an assessment of *perceived* social integration, as gauged by the Cutrona Social Provisions Scale.

On average, perceived social integration was high before the move to the CCRC (13.5 on a scale of 4 to 16) and did not change significantly after the move to the CCRC. Before relocation, the perceived social integration of married individuals was higher than that of unmarried individuals (13.8 vs. 13.0; p < .05). After the move to the CCRC, however, the perceived social integration of married individuals is slightly lower than that of unmarried individuals (13.7 vs. 13.1; p > .05). Change in perceived social integration is significantly different by marital status (unmarried individuals gain an average of .68 points, while married individuals lose .67 points; p < .01).

Age and gender are not significantly related to perceived social integration before the move to the CCRC, but both are significantly related to perceived social integration after the move. After the move, older individuals and women have significantly *higher* perceived social integration. We find no significant differences in perceived social integration by income, education, or parent status.

Of course, age and gender are significantly related to marital status. The unmarried individuals in the sample are almost all women, and married residents are significantly younger than those who are not married. Leaving out the two unmarried males, we can divide the sample into three groups: thirty-six unmarried women, thirty-three married women, and thirty-two married men. Change in perceived social integration is significantly different for the three groups; the perceived social integration of unmarried women increased (.81) while the perceived social integration of married women and men decreased (−.69 and −.64, p < .05).

Moving to an age-segregated community may put unmarried, older women in touch with more peers than before. Their increase in perceived social integration may be due to finding more close friends at the CCRC. In 1997, we asked respondents if they had close friends at the CCRC. Though not statistically significant (probably due to our small sample), unmarried women are somewhat more likely to have close friends at the CCRC (88.9%), compared to married women (77.4%) and married men (80.6%). In terms of close friends at the CCRC, unmarried women actually report fewer close friends at the CCRC (5.1) than married women (8.5) or married men (7.0), although again the difference is not statistically significant.

To compare the strength of the relationships of these variables with perceived social integration, we estimated regression models. Our models include indicators of demographic factors; physical health; contact with family, friends and neighbors; and social roles. We found that being older, having an annual income of $75,000 or more, being in better health, being married, and attending church often are significantly associated with higher perceived social integration before moving to the CCRC, in 1995. We should note that many things are *not* associated with social integration before the move, including contact with children, friends, and neighbors, as well as volunteering, working, and belonging to a club.

The most important predictor of perceived social integration in 1997 (after the move) is prior perceived social integration (before the move). Thus, the factors that are significant predict *changes* in perceived social integration from before to after the move. Older individuals, those with more contact with neighbors, and those who regularly attend religious services are more apt to see themselves as more socially integrated *after* moving to a CCRC.

We estimated a model for social integration after the move (1997), controlling for social integration before the move (1995) and using indicators of change in health, social contact, and social role participation. Interestingly, a negative change in perceived health is associated with a positive change in perceived social integration. Again, more support may be available in the CCRC environment for those with health problems. Church attendance and volunteering are associated with higher perceived social integration following relocation to a CCRC, while stopping volunteering and employment are associated with declines in social integration. Thus, continuity of roles across the transition may be most important. This also points to the importance of objective social role participation for perceived social integration.

We find no evidence that moving to the CCRC from outside the local area is associated with any deficits in social contact, social roles, or perceived social integration. Distance movers are less likely to volunteer outside the CCRC, but overall rates of volunteering are similar. In addition, we found no evidence that having a child in the local area is related to perceived social integration.

CONCLUSION

In sum, we can say unequivocally that moving to a continuing care retirement community does *not* reduce social integration. In fact, it appears to enhance both objective connectedness and perceptions of being integrated. New residents both visit more with neighbors and volunteer more than they did prior to their relocation. They also feel more integrated, especially those most at risk of isolation (residents who are older, in poor health, or a single female). Taking charge of one's last major residential move by relocating to a continuing care retirement community provides more than guaranteed health care. It also offers availability and accessibility to important ways to remain connected as one ages.

REFERENCES

Atchley, R. C. (1989). A continuity theory of normal aging. *The Gerontologist, 29*, 183–190.

Booth, A., & Amato, P. (1990). Divorce, residential change and stress. *Journal of Divorce and Remarriage, 18*, 205–213.

Bowers, B. J. (1989). Continuing care retirement communities' response to residents aging in place: The reluctantly accommodating model. *Journal of Housing for the Elderly, 5*, 65–81.

Brown, A. C., & Orthner, D. K. (1990). Relocation and personal well-being among early adolescents. *Journal of Early Adolescence, 10*, 366–381.

Bultena, G. (1974). Structural effects on the morale of the aged: A comparison of age-segregated and age-integrated communities. In J. Gubrium (Ed.), *Late life communities and environmental policy* (18–31). Springfield, IL: Charles C. Thomas.

Chevan, A. (1995). Holding on and letting go: Residential mobility during widowhood. *Research on Aging, 17*, 278–302.

Choi, N. G. (1996). Older persons who move: Reasons and health consequences. *Journal of Applied Gerontology, 15*, 325–344.

Danermark, B. D., Ekstrom, M. E., & Bodin, L. L. (1996). Effects of residential relocation on mortality and morbidity among elderly people. *European Journal of Public Health, 6*, 212–217.

Eckenrode, J., Rowe, E., Laird, M., & Brathwaite, J. (1995). Mobility as a mediator of the effects of child maltreatment on academic performance. *Child Development, 66*, 1130–1142.

Erickson, M. A., Robison, J. T., & Moen, P. (1999). *Moving plan and expectations in later life: Differences between community and senior housing residents.* Paper presented to the American Sociological Association Annual Meeting, Chicago.

Giele, J. Z., & Elder, G. H., Jr. (1998). *Methods of life course research: Qualitative and quantitative approaches.* Thousand Oaks, CA: Sage.

Golant, S. M. (1992). *Housing America's elderly: Many possibilities/few choices.* Newbury Park, CA: Sage.

Golant, S. M. (1998). Changing an older person's shelter and care setting: A model to explain personal and environmental outcomes. In R. J. Scheidt (Ed.), *Environment and aging theory: A focus on housing* (33–60). Westport, CT: Greenwood Press.

Groves, M. A., & Wilson, V. F. (1992). To move or not to move? Factors influencing the housing choice of elderly persons. *Journal of Housing for the Elderly, 10*, 33–47.

Hagan, J. M. (1996). New kid in town: Social capital and the life course effects of family migration on children. *American Sociological Review, 61*, 368–385.

Henderson, C. & Oggins, J. (1999). Pathways research and sampling design. *Pathways Working Paper No. 7*. Ithaca: Bronfenbrenner Life Course Center, Cornell University.

Holmes, T. H., & Rahe, R. H. (1967). The social readjustment rating scale. *Journal of Psychosomatic Research, 11*, 213–218.

Krout, J. A., Moen, P., Oggins, J., & Bowen, N. (1998). Reasons for relocation to a continuing care retirement community. *Pathways Working Paper No. 2*. Ithaca: Bronfenbrenner Life Course Center, Cornell University.

Lawton, M. P. (1970). Assessment, integration and environments for older people. *The Gerontologist, 10*, 38–46.

Lawton, M. P. (1982). Competence, environmental press, and the adaptation of older people. In M. P. Lawton, P. G. Windley, & T. O. Byerts (Eds.), *Aging and the environment: Theoretical approaches* (33–59). New York: Springer.

Litwak, E., & Longino, C. F., Jr. (1987). Migration patterns among the elderly: A developmental perspective. *The Gerontologist, 27*, 266–272.

Loomis, L. M., Sorce, P., & Tyler, P. R. (1989). A lifestyle analysis of healthy retirees and their interest in moving to a retirement community. *Journal of Housing for the Elderly, 5*, 19–35.

Marini, M. M. (1996). Adolescent expectations and adult outcomes: Insights from the study of migration. *Research in Sociology of Education and Socialization, 11*, 299–339.

Moen, P. (1997). Women's roles and resilience: Trajectories of advantage or turning points? In I. H. Gottlieb & B. Wheaton (Eds.), *Stress and adversity over the life course: Trajectories and turning points* (133–156). New York: Cambridge University Press.

Moen, P., Dempster-McClain, D., & Williams, R. M., Jr. (1989). Social integration and longevity: An event history analysis of women's roles and resilience. *American Sociological Review, 54*, 635–647.

Moen, P., Dempster-McClain, D., & Williams, R. M., Jr. (1992). Successful aging: A life course perspective on women's multiple roles and health. *American Journal of Sociology, 97*, 1612–1638.

Moos, R. H. (1976). Conceptualizations of human environments. In R. Moos (Ed.), *The human context: Environmental determinants of behavior* (3–35). New York: John Wiley & Sons.

Moos, R. H., & Lemke, S. (1994). *Groups residences for older adults: Physical features, policies, and social climate*. New York: Oxford University Press.

Perkinson, M. A., & Rockerman, D. (1996). Older women living in a continuing care retirement community: Marital status and friendship formation. *Journal of Women and Aging, 8,* 159–177.

Redfoot, D. L. (1987). "On the separatin' place": Social class and relocation among older women. *Social Forces, 66,* 486–500.

Rosow, I. (1967). *Social integration of the aged.* New York: Free Press.

Russell, D., Peplau, L. A., & Cutrona, C. E. (1980). The revised UCLA Loneliness Scale: Concurrent and discriminant validity evidence. *Journal of Personality and Social Psychology, 39,* 471–480.

Scheidt, R. J. (1998). The social ecological approach of Rudolf Moos. In R. J. Scheidt & P. G. Windley (Eds.), *Environment and aging theory: A focus on housing* (111–139). Westport, CT: Greenwood Press.

Sheehan, N. W., & Karasik, R. J. (1995). The decision to move to a continuing care retirement community. *Journal of Housing for the Elderly, 11,* 107–122.

Sherwood, S., Ruchlin, H. S., Sherwood, C. C., & Morris, S. A. (1997). *Continuing care retirement communities.* Baltimore: Johns Hopkins University Press.

Sommers, D. G., & Rowell, K. R. (1992). Factors differentiating elderly residential movers and nonmovers: A longitudinal analysis. *Population Research and Policy Review, 11,* 249–262.

Speare, A., Jr., & Goldscheider, F. K. (1987). Effects of marital status change on residential mobility. *Journal of Marriage and the Family, 49,* 455–464.

Thoits, P. A. (1983). Multiple identities and psychological well-being: A reformulation and test of the social isolation hypothesis. *American Sociological Review, 48,* 174–187.

Thoits, P. A. (1986). Multiple identities: Examining gender and marital status differences in distress. *American Sociological Review, 51,* 259–272.

Tucker, C. J., Marx, J., & Long, L. (1998). "Moving on": Residential mobility and children's school lives. *Sociology of Education, 71,* 111–129.

VanderHart, P. G. (1995). The socioeconomic determinants of the housing decisions of elderly homeowners. *Journal of Housing for the Elderly, 11,* 5–35.

Wiseman, R. F. (1980). Why older people move: Theoretical issues. *Research on Aging, 2,* 141–154.

Young, F. W., & Glasgow, N. (1998). Voluntary social participation and health. *Research on Aging, 20,* 339–362.

PART THREE

Interventions to Promote Social Integration in Later Life

CHAPTER NINE

An Intervention to Improve
Transportation Arrangements

Nina Glasgow

Transportation mobility is critically important to nonmetropolitan older people's social, physical, and psychological well-being.
As is detailed in Chapter 4, transportation is one link that connects
individuals to their social networks and activities. Poor access to
transportation contributes to social isolation, constrains the use of
needed medical care, and limits access to goods and services. In an
effort to improve the transportation arrangements of rural older persons and, hence, their social integration, the *Cornell Transportation
and Social Integration of Nonmetropolitan Older Persons Study* investigated how older persons with differing personal characteristics and household circumstances organize their access to and use of
transportation.

To briefly recapitulate the study design, a two-wave panel survey
was conducted to examine how the use of transportation changes over
time as older individuals experience life-course transitions, and as aspects of their communities may change. A survey of a representative
sample of 737 individuals aged 65 or older from two upstate New York
nonmetropolitan counties was conducted in 1995, and in 1997 the
Wave 2 survey of the panel study was conducted. (Through approximately 50 deaths, severe illnesses of 30 respondents, 10 migrations
out of the study area, an inability to contact 80 individuals, and a refusal rate of approximately 10 percent, the 1997 survey had an N of
476 cases.)

An Educational Intervention

One component of the study was an educational intervention planned and implemented in 1996 for respondents from the Wave 1 survey of the panel study who self-reported being "unable to go places as often as they desired." Their inability to go places as often as they wanted is thought to be a result of the interplay between older individuals' personal or household characteristics and attributes of their communities. The educational intervention was designed to encourage "transportation disadvantaged" survey respondents to modify the organization of their transportation toward arrangements that will be durable over time and that will enhance their social integration. The educational intervention consisted of a workshop series held in each of the two study counties, the purpose of which was to facilitate changes in the way older individuals understand the importance of participating in social activities and to improve effective management of their transportation arrangements. The objectives of the workshops were to enhance older people's sense of control over their personal mobility by increasing their knowledge of available public and volunteer transportation services and to improve their skills in organizing transportation from informal sources. Each three-session workshop series was designed to emphasize transportation within the context of social participation.

In this chapter I discuss the content and methods employed in conducting the educational intervention, evaluate the effectiveness of the workshops, and make recommendations on the content of and uses of future educational interventions. While social interventions have been employed in a number of social contexts (e.g., retirement planning), interventions to educate older people about their transportation options are relatively uncharted territory. Thus, the intervention conducted in conjunction with this study must be considered exploratory.

Background

Literature bridging the areas of transportation and social integration of rural older people is underdeveloped. Previous studies have examined the relationship between the personal characteristics of rural older persons and transportation issues (e.g., Cutler, 1979; Iutcovich & Iutcovich, 1988; Patton, 1975), but few have addressed methods to facilitate change in behavior. Relevant guidance for the intervention design was obtained from the social and community psychology literature on developing social networks and implementing social interventions, as well as research on personal control and independence.

The intervention methodology most frequently cited in the community and social psychology literature embraces social norms related to self-reliance, collective action, and empowerment (Gottlieb, 1988). Gottlieb (1992) outlines a typology of support interventions that includes individual, group, social system, and community levels. Each type of intervention uses mutual aid or self-help strategies to optimize "psychosocial resources" that people exchange with members of their social network. Intervention participants accomplish this by bringing about change within their network or in their personal behavior to improve the quality or quantity of desired support. Commonly used with targeted groups such as widows, widowers, and caregivers, the intervention process helps individuals work through issues related to self-care, social behavior, or perceived control (Baltes & Baltes, 1990; Biegel et al., 1984). The process demands an environment conducive to the sharing of experiences and the expression of support. The length of the intervention process varies depending on specific content.

Older people, as well as people in other age groups, strive to maintain control and independence over their lives. To sustain control over mobility and remain independent, most rural older persons rely on the personal automobile and their ability to drive (see Chapter 4). A disproportionate share of nonmetropolitan compared to metropolitan older people own and rely on personal automobiles for their transportation (Glasgow & Beale, 1985), a situation related to the limited availability of public transportation in rural areas (Talbot, 1985). As their ability to drive diminishes, rural older persons living in areas where public transit does not exist or is limited may have to seek alternative transportation from informal sources.

Developing such alternatives involves determining what one can and cannot do and setting priorities accordingly. Coping with changing circumstances may involve a willingness to accept help from other people to retain some degree of control and independence (Baltes & Baltes, 1990). Older people may employ different methods to maintain control and independence in their lives, despite the inability to personally perform certain activities. Two methods—mutual aid relationships and informal networks—focus on developing reciprocal relationships with others that can provide social interaction, or assist with daily tasks, or provide transportation and other informal services. Helping relationships work best when characterized by balanced reciprocity and equal power (Collins, 1991). Balanced reciprocity and equal power, however, may derive from past helping behavior of an older person who, in a current situation, is the receiver of assistance. It was against this background that we developed the process and content of the educational workshops.

Methods and Procedures

This section provides a discussion of the methods used to identify, select, and recruit participants for the workshop series. It also describes the workshop design and specific activities used to achieve workshop objectives. A discussion of the study counties, or the context of the educational workshops, concludes the section.

Selection Criteria

Initial selection of participants for the educational workshop series was based on respondents' answer to one question from Wave 1 of the panel survey. When asked whether they were able to go places as often as they wanted, 20 percent, or 147 of 737 cases, reported that they were "unable to go places as often as they desired." Compared to persons who were "able to go places as often as they desired," those 147 cases were found to be less socially active, desired to see friends more often, reported poorer health, were less likely to drive under certain driving conditions, and were more likely to have reduced their driving. (Data not shown.) They were not, however, more likely to have stopped driving. Based on this profile, these 147 cases were considered appropriate candidates for participation in a workshop series. We also thought that individuals who indicated they were not getting out as often as they wanted would be motivated to change their situation and would make good candidates for a social intervention.

Two subgroups were identified within the "unable to go" group based on whether they used an aid such as a wheelchair, walker, or cane to get around. Subgroup 1 included those who reported having to use an aid to get around and thus probably had a serious physical mobility limitation. We believed the intervention design could not address the more extensive needs of individuals with substantial physical mobility limitations. Subgroup 2 included those who did not use an aid to get around, and thus they were presumed not to have serious physical disabilities that would limit their mobility. Exclusion of the "unable to go, use an aid" cases narrowed to ninety-one the number of potential participants in the educational intervention. Those ninety-one individuals were assumed to have both the motivation to get out more often and relatively minor, if any, physical mobility limitations. The ninety-one potential participants were further narrowed to eighty-seven when we eliminated one respondent, whose survey interview had been done by a proxy (indicating a serious health problem, if not specifically a physical disability), and three individuals who said at the end of the Wave 1 survey they wished not to participate in the follow-up survey or other components of the study.

Subgroup 2 was further divided for purposes of comparison into (1) a transportation-disadvantaged "intervention group" and (2) a "control group" of those who were transportation disadvantaged and did not receive the intervention. The intervention and control groups were randomly selected from subgroup 2. The "unable to go, no aid," or subgroup 2 respondents, resided approximately equally in Cortland or Seneca Counties. Figure 9.1 outlines the selection process.

Participant Recruitment

Once selected for the intervention group, respondents received an invitation letter and a follow-up telephone call to determine their interest in attending the workshop series.[1] To encourage participation, three incentives were offered to the participants: (1) a monetary payment of $10 for each of the three sessions attended; (2) food and

---

[1] The invitation letter reminded respondents of their participation in the 1995 survey, provided a project overview, and stated the purpose and objectives of the workshop series. They were told their participation would help in developing programs to increase other older people's mobility and their own participation in social activities. The letter concluded with information on the time and location of the workshops, as well as incentives for participation. One week after sending the letter, each person selected for the intervention group received a follow-up telephone call to determine whether they would participate in the workshops. Callers were instructed to use gentle persuasion techniques among those who showed little interest in participation.

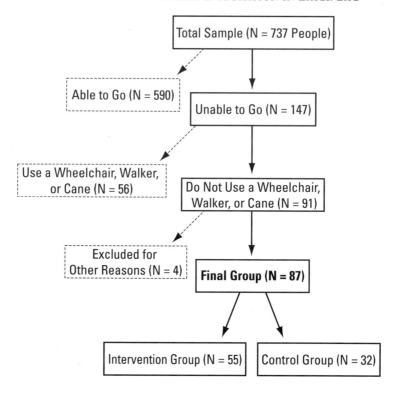

Figure 9.1   Selection Process for Educational Intervention.

beverages during each session; and (3) transportation to and from the workshop sessions. The incentives were included to make it psychologically easier for respondents to participate in the workshop series but modest enough to ensure that participation was not motivated by extrinsic rewards (Gottlieb, 1989).

During the recruitment process, 19 individuals agreed to participate in the workshop series (10 from Cortland County and 9 from Seneca County). In the intervention "refusal" group of 36 respondents, 10 individuals were outright refusals, but the remainder could be considered "ineligible" for participation in the intervention. We felt that individuals could be considered ineligible if they could not participate because of a temporary or permanent health setback. For example, one individual was to enter the hospital for prostate cancer surgery during the scheduled dates of the workshops, and another had recently had a stroke. Other ineligibles had work or other scheduling conflicts, full-time caregiving responsibilities, or we were unable to contact them (e.g., their telephone had been disconnected). The difficulty of recruiting older individuals for a set of group activities will be commented on in the section on recommendations.

Site Selection and Logistics

Churches were selected as the sites for the two workshop series because of their community emphasis, central location to the majority of the participants' homes, and availability. Each site provided small, intimate rooms for the workshops. Church administrators helped with logistics, such as providing access to the church. The workshops spanned four weeks and, to the extent possible, were held on the same day of the week across the three sessions of each workshop series. The first two workshops were held approximately one week apart in each county, and a two-week interval was allowed to elapse between the second and third workshops in the series. Each workshop series consisted of three, two-hour sessions. Each session was held between 10:00 A.M. and noon, and the sessions were broken into one-hour blocks, with a morning break and lunch served immediately after each session.

Workshop Design and Content

Based on Gottlieb's typology (1992), our efforts modeled a group-level approach by bringing together individuals who self-reported the desire to get out more often. The group process approach was used to facilitate dialogue, activities, and panel discussions concerning the development of more effective transportation arrangements and increased social participation. A facilitator and the project's principal investigator (PI) guided the participants through the process using didactic, participatory, and reflective methods. Participants' comments were recorded on a flip chart to create a group memory of the workshop content and process. Information was presented to participants in multiple formats, including verbal, paper, poster, and overhead transparency formats.

The facilitator's primary roles included keeping the group focused, recording participants' comments, and asking probing questions. The PI presented the didactic material included in the workshops. Local public and volunteer transportation providers and representatives from nonprofit organizations introduced participants to available services in the area via interactive panel discussions. The professionals involved in the process made an effort to create an environment for strengthening participants' capacities to cope with changing circumstances by fostering the sharing of mutual experiences, providing new information, and promoting goal-oriented, problem-solving behavior.

The workshop content was divided into three primary areas: participants' experiences, information dissemination, and informal network development. The workshop series was pilot-tested in Tompkins County, also an upstate New York nonmetropolitan county, and minor revisions to content were then made before the two series were conducted in Cortland and Seneca Counties. Session I of each workshop series introduced participants to the goals of the workshops, gathered information on participants' experiences, and highlighted the link between social participation, health, and longevity. Session II focused on informal network development and information dissemination from local public and nonprofit agencies. Session III focused on dissemination of information on available transportation services (a directory prepared on each county's public and volunteer services was distributed, and the contents were explained) and participants' planning of their alternative transportation futures.

Context

Cortland and Seneca Counties in upstate New York are nonmetropolitan counties with open-country rural territory, small villages, and small cities. The City of Cortland is the largest community in the two counties, with a 1990 census population of 19,801. Seneca Falls, New York, the largest place in Seneca County, had a 1990 census population of 9,384.

The degree of urbanization of an area is an important determinant of the array of formally provided transportation and other services for older people (Taietz & Milton, 1979), a situation that holds for Cortland and Seneca Counties. Cortland has a fixed-route public bus system that primarily serves the City of Cortland's inner core, but it also extends one service route into surrounding rural areas a few days each week. As part of the system, limited and costly "dial-a-ride" services are available for Cortland County residents. Cortland County has approximately half a dozen taxi companies, and a few long-distance bus companies serve the area. Seneca County, in contrast, has no public bus system, no long-distance bus company serving the county, and only one taxi company. Seneca County offers senior citizens' van transportation for senior center activities, doctor's appointments, or grocery shopping. The limited availability of public transportation in these two counties is not atypical for nonmetropolitan counties (Talbot, 1985) and constituted a primary reason we emphasized both formal and informal networks of ride providers to the participants in our educational workshops.

EVALUATION OF THE EDUCATIONAL INTERVENTION

The test of whether a social intervention was successful depends on how highly participants rate the experience and whether there is evidence of a change in attitudes or behavior. Thus, the focus of this section is on whether the workshop series made a difference to the older participants. In 1996 the intervention group anonymously evaluated each workshop series immediately following the final session. Those questions were repeated to intervention group respondents only in a supplement to the 1997 Wave 2 survey. This information shows participants' short-term evaluations of the workshop series and their longer-term evaluations. An important question is how well the effects of the workshops held up over time. A second type of analysis focuses on whether particular attitudes and behaviors of the intervention group differ from those of the control group and the "refusal" group. This second type of analysis draws from answers to questions that were asked of all respondents in the 1997 panel survey.

Table 9.1 displays findings on increased knowledge of public and volunteer transportation; whether participants felt better prepared to get around by means other than a car subsequent to attending the workshop series; and perceived usefulness of the information presented in the workshops. A large majority of participants perceived an increase in their knowledge of public and volunteer transportation options as a consequence of having attended the workshop series. Very little erosion occurred over time in the proportion reporting that as their experience (83.3% percent in 1996 and 82.3% in 1997). Immediately following the workshops in 1996, 83.3 percent of the participants felt they were better prepared to get around by means other than a car as a result of having attended the workshops. By 1997, still a large majority felt better prepared to get around by means other than a car (76.5%), but some erosion had occurred.

Table 9.1. Intervention Group's Workshop Series Evaluation (in %)

Evaluation Questions	1996 Post-Workshop Evaluation	1997 Follow-up Evaluation
Increased knowledge of public and volunteer transportation? "Yes"	83.3	82.3
Better prepared to get around by means other than a car? "Yes"	83.3	76.5
How useful was the information presented in the workshop series?		
Very useful	50.0	35.3
Useful	50.0	52.9
Not very useful	0.0	11.8
Not at all useful	0.0	0.0

Participants' evaluation of the usefulness of the workshops is also shown in Table 9.1. In the 1996 post-workshop evaluation, 50 percent of participants rated the workshops as "very useful," and 50 percent as "useful." By 1997, just over 35 percent felt the workshops had been "very useful," nearly 53 percent "useful," and approximately 12 percent "not very useful." In summary, participants' evaluations of the workshops were largely positive, and the positive evaluations held up reasonably well over the nine to ten months of elapsed time between the workshop series and the follow-up survey.

The remaining analyses compare responses to various questions answered by the intervention group, control group, and "refusal" group respondents. Some attrition had occurred in each group by 1997, when the Wave 2 survey was conducted. Seventeen of the nineteen in the intervention group, or workshop series participants, were interviewed in the 1997 survey. The size of the control group diminished from thirty-two to twenty-four by 1997, and the "refusal" group declined from thirty-six to twenty-two individuals. (The 1997 Ns of the three comparison groups are shown in Table 9.2.)

The "refusal" group showed greatest attrition between the two survey waves, the control group was second, and the intervention group had the least attrition. During our efforts to recruit individuals to participate in the educational workshops, we formed impressions about the characteristics and situations of the "refusal" group. The "refusal" group seemed to comprise both the most active and the

Table 9.2. How often are you able to go places you would like to? Is it as often as you'd like, or not as often as you'd like? (in %)

Group Type	As often as I'd like	
	1995 Survey	1997 Survey
Intervention group (N = 17)	0.0	76.5
Control group (N = 24)	0.0	41.7
"Refusal" group (N = 22)	0.0	66.7

least active of those who were originally randomly assigned to the intervention group. Their refusal to participate in the educational workshops was probably partly due to a tendency to refuse participation in research studies. Their overall health status may also have been poorer. Thus, it does not seem surprising that attrition was greater among the "refusal" group compared to the intervention and control groups.

Table 9.2 shows the proportions in each group who reported being "able to get out as often as they want" in 1995 and in 1997. By definition, all of the respondents included in the intervention, control, or "refusal" groups reported in the 1995 survey that they were not getting out as often as they wanted. All three groups, whether or not they received the educational intervention, improved by 1997 in the proportions reporting that they got out as often as they wanted. During the course of conducting the workshops, it became clear that older individuals rapidly experience life-course transitions. For example, a few workshop participants were primary caregivers at the time of the Wave 1 survey in 1995 but were not caregivers by 1996, when the intervention workshops were conducted. Our contacts with the intervention group and the "refusal" group also taught us that older individuals' health setbacks are often only temporary. Full-time caregiving responsibilities and temporary health setbacks are just two examples of situations that can affect the ability to get out as often as one wants. Given that life-course events and transitions may be only temporary, it is not too surprising that older respondents' assessments of whether they were getting out enough changed over time, regardless of whether they participated in the intervention.

Further, older individuals' attitudes may shift frequently regarding whether they are getting out as often as they want, depending on general mood at a particular time. The improvement in the different groups' ability to get out "as often as they wanted" may have been influenced by our having contacted both the intervention and "refusal" groups for participation in the workshops, and the control group for participation in the two waves of the panel survey. We solicited the intervention and "refusal" groups' participation in the educational workshops, stating that it is important for older individuals to have effective transportation mobility and to participate in social activities. All of the comparison groups thus may have been influenced by their participation in the study.

Despite this general trend, the intervention group showed the greatest improvement (76.5%), the "refusal" group the second most improvement (66.7%), and the control group the least improvement (41.7%) in getting out as often as they wanted. The findings presented in Table 9.2 suggest the intervention had the desired effect of helping older people improve the management of their transportation arrangements.

Table 9.3 addresses other questions posed to the intervention, control, and "refusal" groups in 1997 when the Wave 2 survey was conducted. Most in the intervention group reported getting out "almost every day" (82.5%), and others in the intervention group were getting out "once or twice a week." By contrast, only 50 percent of the control group and 63.3 percent of the "refusal" group were getting out "almost every day." Both the control and the "refusal" groups thus reported a lower frequency of trips out of their homes than did the intervention group. Both respondents' subjective assessments of whether they were getting out enough (see Table 9.2) and this measure of frequency of getting out indicate the educational intervention had a positive outcome for the participants.

During the workshop series, information was disseminated to intervention group participants on the availability of older driver retraining courses in their local area. Table 9.3 indicates that including such information in the workshop series may have stimulated the intervention participants to take such a course. Fifty percent of the intervention group, 11.1 percent of the control group, and 31.3 percent of the "refusal" group reported in 1997 that they had taken such a course.

As noted earlier, the workshops stressed the importance of developing effective transportation arrangements and active social participation. That strategy appears to have had an effect, given that 52.9 percent of intervention group compared to 41.7 percent of control group

Table 9.3. Intervention, Control, and "Refusal" Groups' Mobility-Related Activities (in %)

Activity	1997 Survey		
	Intervention Group	Control Group	"Refusal" Group
How often do you get out and away from your house?			
Almost every day	82.5	50.0	63.3
Once or twice a week	17.6	41.7	27.3
Once to a few times a month	0.0	4.2	9.0
Less than once a month but at least yearly	0.0	0.0	0.0
Almost never or never	0.0	4.2	0.0
The American Association of Retired Persons offers an older driver retraining course through local agencies called 55 Alive, and the American Automobile Association offers a similar course in some local areas. Have you taken a driver retraining course?			
Yes	50.0	11.1	31.3
Did you do volunteer work during the past year for any type of organization?			
Yes	52.9	41.7	22.7

and only 22.7 percent of the "refusal" group reported in 1997 that they had done volunteer work during the past twelve months (Table 9.3). The "refusal" group may be especially reluctant to get involved in community activities, as evidenced by their "refusal" to participate in the intervention.

CONCLUSION AND RECOMMENDATIONS

One should keep in mind that the numbers of individuals in each of these three groups is not large. Therefore, this evaluation of the effectiveness of the educational intervention cannot be considered definitive. The evaluation, however, suggests that participants in the educational intervention did undergo changes in attitudes and behavior.

The findings indicate that the educational intervention workshops were successful in increasing the knowledge of available transportation resources among older individuals living in two nonmetropolitan counties of upstate New York. Apparently, the intervention contributed to behaviors conducive to older persons' getting out of their houses frequently and to engaging in community activities. Thus, it is recommended that similar workshops be replicated in other locations. Additional recommendations are as follows:

— The group process methodology provided a supportive environment where older people could freely express their concerns about transportation issues. Although the number of older individuals we were able to recruit for the workshops was disappointingly small, those of us who conducted the workshops observed that the small-group dynamics worked well with regard to older people's willingness to brainstorm solutions to their transportation problems.

— Given the scheduling conflicts that are inevitable when planning a set of group activities, it may be worthwhile to hold ongoing workshops in local areas so that individuals may attend sessions as their schedules permit.

— An ongoing educational and informational group methodology could be used to develop ride-sharing networks among older individuals. We considered development of such networks in the context of our intervention workshops. Given the relatively short duration of our workshops and the lack of a local person to coordinate such an activity, however, we felt a ride-share network could not be developed and sustained within the time frame of our intervention.

— Many older individuals who have full-time caregiving responsibilities, health problems, or other situations that make it difficult for them to attend group activities may benefit from being teleconferenced into group meetings.

— County offices for the aging, other government agencies, or nonprofit organizations, in conjunction with local transportation providers, could develop hotlines to provide information on local public and volunteer transportation options to older people.

— Local aging-oriented organizations could also develop transportation directories of public and volunteer transportation, similar to the directories we developed, to distribute to older individuals in local areas.

— Sterns and colleagues (1997) recommended public marketing campaigns to encourage responsible use of transportation options and to inform older individuals of public transportation availability. Indeed, advertising the resources available in local areas (whether a hotline or actual transportation services) is an important activity in helping older people more effectively manage their arrangements for transportation.

The ability to drive, or the convenient and effective use of other types of transportation, influence the social integration and quality of life of older people, especially those living in rural areas. Thus, educational programs that increase older people's knowledge of transportation options, including perhaps being retrained for safer driving, should continue to be designed and evaluated.

REFERENCES

Baltes, P., & Baltes, M. (1990). *Successful aging: Perspectives from the behavioral sciences.* New York: Cambridge University Press.

Biegel, D. E., Shore, B. K., & Gordon, E. (1984). *Building support networks for the elderly.* Beverly Hills, CA: Sage.

Collins, J. (1991). Power and local community activity. *Journal of Aging Studies, 5,* 209–218.

Cutler, S. J. (1979). The availability of personal transportation, residential location, and life satisfaction among the aged. *Journal of Gerontology, 27,* 383–389.

Glasgow, N., & Beale, C. L. (1985). Rural elderly in demographic perspective. *Rural Development Perspectives, 2,* 22–26.

Gottlieb, B. H. (1988). Support interventions: A typology and agenda for research. In S. W. Duck (Ed.), *Handbook of personal relationships* (519–541). New York: Wiley.

Gottlieb, B. H. (1992). Quandaries in translating support concepts to intervention. In H. O. F. Veiel & U. Baumann (Eds.), *The Meaning and Measurement of Social Support* (293–309). New York: Hemisphere.

Gottlieb, B. H. (Ed.). (1989). *Marshalling social support: Formats, processes and effects.* Newbury Park, CA: Sage.

Iutcovich, J. M., & Iutcovich, M. (1988). Assessment of the transportation needs of Pennsylvania's elderly population. *Journal of Gerontology, 7,* 515–529.

Patton, C. V. (1975). Age groupings and travel in rural areas. *Rural Sociology, 40,* 55–63.

Sterns, H. L., Sterns, R., Aizenberg, R., & Anapolle, J. (1997). *Family and friends concerned about an older driver.* Final Report. Akron, OH: U.S. Department of Transportation, National Highway Traffic Safety Administration.

Taietz, P., & Milton, S. (1979). Rural-urban differences in the structure of services for the elderly in upstate New York. *Journal of Gerontology, 34,* 429–437.

Talbot, D. M. (1985). Assessing the needs of the rural elderly. *Journal of Gerontological Nursing, 11,* 39–43.

CHAPTER TEN

Fostering Integration

A Case Study of the Cornell Retirees Volunteering in Service (CRVIS) Program

Phyllis Moen, Vivian Fields, Rhoda Meador, and Helene Rosenblatt

In this chapter we draw on qualitative data describing a unique arrangement to foster the volunteer participation of retirees, supplementing this case example with survey data from the *Cornell Retirement and Well-Being Study* to document factors that shape the circumstances, motivation, and volunteer participation of a sample of retirees. Following our case example, we offer implications for policy, research, and practice, concluding with the potential that this untapped portion of the population—retirees—offers for themselves, their communities, and society.

Clearly, retirees conceive of retirement not simply as a time of leisure but also as a time of continued productive engagement. Harnessing the full productive potential of these younger, better educated, and healthier retirees will require new social institutions that can take advantage of their talents and energies. A number of scholars (e.g., Freedman, 1994; Herzog & Morgan, 1993a, 1993b; Moen, 1998; Moen & Fields, 2000; Musick et al., 1999) are investigating social integration in the form of productive engagement beyond retirement, including volunteer community service. Increasingly, employers and their retirees are recognizing and exploring ways to tap retiree talents in service to their communities. Corporate Retiree Volunteer Programs (Anderson, 1993), offering strategies for workers from particular organizations to move from paid work for their company to volunteer service as they retire, are an excellent example of this. We present a case study of a retiree volunteer group organized on such a "corporate" model. We begin by examining the research literature on retirement, aging, and volunteering, relating it to the benefits of a volunteer model that helps workers retain their bond with the workplace.

RETIREES: AVAILABLE AND READY

Many discussions of the "aging of America" conclude with dire predictions about its consequences. However, as Marc Freedman (1994: 1) points out, "This transformation presents both challenges and opportunities." Other scholars also advocate viewing retirees as a *resource* rather than a *problem* (Herzog & Morgan 1993a, 1993b; Caro & Bass, 1995; Moen, 1994; Riley & Riley, 1994). Current cohorts of retirees represent the healthiest and best educated in history. These retirees, and those to follow from the baby-boom generation, will be creating new models that challenge existing ideas about midlife, aging, older workers, retirees, and volunteer work (Moen, 1998). A recent national survey of baby boomers found that almost four out of five expect to volunteer after they retire.

Americans are now retiring earlier than ever before. In the *Cornell Retirement and Well-Being Study* (described in Chapter 3) we asked respondents about when their fathers retired. Three in ten of their fathers never retired, frequently dying before age 65. Most other fathers retired either on or after age 65. By contrast, almost two thirds of those in our survey retired (or expect to do so) *before* age 62! A national survey found that three out of four retirees did in fact retire before age 65 (Hunt, 1999).

Although contemporary retirees welcome the flexibility afforded by freedom from a fixed work schedule, many wish to continue with productive activities after leaving their primary "career" jobs. A 1991 study of Americans aged 60 and older found that 41 percent did some volunteer work. Thirty-eight percent of those not volunteering indicated that they might be willing to volunteer if asked to do so and if the conditions were "right" (ICR Survey Research Group, 1991). In addition, 25.6 percent of *current* volunteers in this age group report that they "would have preferred to volunteer more."

In the *Cornell Retirement and Well-Being Study* we asked all respondents what they consider to be important elements in "the *ideal* retirement lifestyle." While respondents chose "life of leisure" more

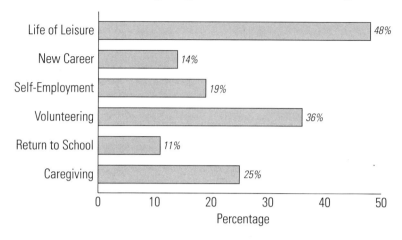

Figure 10.1   Elements of an Ideal Retirement. *Source: Cornell Retirement and Well-Being Study,* Wave 1 (1994–95), N~450.

than any other category (see Figure 10.1), fully 66 percent *also* chose some form of formal productive activity (in terms of a new career, self-employment, or volunteer service). Volunteering was the activity most often chosen.

Research has shown the importance of volunteer service and social participation more generally for health, psychological well-being, and general life quality (see discussions in Chapters 2 and 3). The challenge we face is to design more effective social opportunities and roles for older people in our society. Since Americans now spend almost a third of their lives beyond retirement, the question of productive roles in these years becomes especially critical as a matter of both public and private policy.

ONE SOLUTION: PUTTING RETIREES TO "WORK"

Employers and retirees are recognizing and exploring ways to bridge the social transition between paid work and post-retirement productivity. Both groups are forming partnerships to create new models to facilitate this shift, building on the pre-existing social support provided by the workplace community. Donna Anderson, founder and president of the National Retirees Volunteer Coalition (NRVC) was one of the pioneers of the corporate model in which retirees, with support from their former employers, serve community agencies. The model involves (1) the identification and recruitment of leadership among retirees of a particular firm, (2) the launching of an informational program, and (3) the creation of a framework to encourage retirees' volunteer efforts. The NRVC has helped to develop more than sixty-six corporate retiree volunteer programs in twenty-six states.

Many good ideas for volunteer programs have failed because of what has been called "fervor without infrastructure" (Freedman, 1993). The enduring structure created by the corporate retiree model is advantageous to the sponsoring company, the retirees, and the community agencies being served. First, it recognizes the need for continued support by and participation of the corporation, hospital, or university from which the retirees have retired. The (former) employer benefits in terms of improved public relations with the community and through enhancing the environment in which their retirees and current employees live. The community benefits from an infusion of stable and long-lasting service. The retirees themselves also profit from the social network of ongoing relationships and continued productive engagement.

Social theory provides some insight into the mechanisms by which such a model helps to smooth the transition into retirement. Loss of the role of employee deprives people of ready access to colleagues and friends. For example, fully 73 percent of the retired men and women in the *Cornell Retirement and Well-Being Study* report that "missing co-workers" is a disadvantage of retirement.

Corporate retiree volunteer programs provide a way for retirees to sustain important ties with co-workers, as well as their identity as a member of the corporate community. The value of this model is that it both builds on and extends workers' existing occupational identity and provides formal organizational support for volunteer work. This becomes a vehicle for bridging the transition from paid work to retirement, an adaptive strategy that provides continuity rather than discontinuity in identity and productivity (see Atchley, 1989).

As part of our ongoing study of ways to promote productive engagement, we have systematically observed, using participant observation and other ethnographic techniques, the creation and development of an organization fashioned along the NRVC model, one that brings together corporate (in this case, university) retirees. The Cornell Retirees Volunteering in Service (CRVIS—pronounced "service") provides an important case study of the corporate model.

CRVIS: EVOLUTION OF A MODEL FOR RETIREE INVOLVEMENT

In 1994, Cornell University and a coterie of its retirees began a volunteer initiative under the guidance of representatives from the NRVC. The initial step in the development of CRVIS was the identification of a group of retirees who had played leadership roles in the workplace prior to retirement. This group of leaders met regularly to consider the potential for and value of establishing a formal retiree volunteer program in association with Cornell University. The retiree group participated in a variety of activities that led to setting up an organizational structure and an explicit statement of shared group values. (NRVC representatives played a minor role in facilitating these monthly meetings.) The group explored alternative ways of serving the broader community, inviting representatives from several community organizations to assess the "fit" between the interests and capabilities of the Cornell retirees and community needs.

After a number of meetings, the focus of the group narrowed and the decision was made to serve youth aged 5–12 through the elementary schools. The group devised a name (CRVIS) and a mission statement (see Figure 10.2). They invited principals from the area to talk about the possibilities of service to their schools. After interviewing a number of principals, they selected one school, Cayuga Heights Elementary School, in which to begin a pilot program. The group has been explicit about the desire to be involved in activities that offer a significant "value-added" benefit to the educational environment and not simply a reduction of teachers' workload. CRVIS consciously chooses to work in schools where volunteers are viewed as "full collaborative partners." (Most retirees don't want to simply "push a cart" or stamp incoming mail. Rather, they want to be engaged in activities that both challenge them and use their talents.) What is unique about the Cornell program is that it is a *group* effort, with retirees working together with a common purpose and the conscious goal of making the experience "fun."

WHY CRVIS WORKS

Four main points from the research literature on volunteerism are relevant in analyzing the success of CRVIS. First, perennial non-

Vision of the Cornell Retirees Volunteering in Service

Cornell retirees can and will contribute significantly to community betterment by joining others in addressing common needs. By doing so, we will add value to the community while enjoying the satisfaction of volunteering. Our combined energy and enthusiasm can a make a difference to important local projects and increase the effectiveness of other groups working in a variety of community initiatives. We especially relish the chance to interact helpfully with younger people. Our desire to build positive relationships with younger people, and other community members, springs from a strong feeling of responsibility. We have gained much from our community over the years and feel the need to give something in return. We confidently expect to utilize the talents of the people with whom we address common challenges and benefit from their experiences. We seek to increase mutual respect and trust among all members of our community as we work to enhance the quality of Cornell s relations with its employees and retirees, and between Cornell and the larger community.

CRVIS Mission
To enhance the quality of life and relationships in Tompkins and surrounding counties through volunteer leadership and service by retired members of the Cornell community.

CRVIS Goals
■ To enrich educational experiences for children aged 5-12 years.
■ To develop and maintain an effective retiree organization/collaboration that will ensure continuing leadership.
■ To build an organization that can be replicated in other areas.

Figure 10.2   CRVIS' Statement of Mission and Group Values.
Source: CRVIS Volunteer Handbook, 1997–98.

volunteers are likely to be more difficult to recruit compared with those who have volunteered (Fischer & Schaffer, 1993). However, Caro and Bass (1997) point out that the timing of recruitment can be crucial. In their study, retired non-volunteers who are approached within the first two years after retirement were almost twice as likely to be receptive to volunteering as other non-volunteering retirees. The

"corporate" model affords the opportunity to make specific information about volunteering part of the pre-retirement process. Part of the
difficulty in recruiting and retaining older volunteers is that most
people do not visualize the kind of social life they might desire following retirement. Our society typically prepares individuals for moving
into new roles, whether it is kindergarten or employment, but we do
not prepare individuals for role disengagement, such as that involved
in leaving the world of work (Ebaugh, 1988; Kahn, 1994).

In the case of CRVIS, board members receive lists of recent retirees from the university and target recruitment efforts to them. Information about CRVIS is also included in pre-retirement literature. Qualitative data from focus groups and in-depth interviews in the *Cornell
Retirement and Well-Being Study* suggest that many retirees want to
travel and spend time with family before settling into a schedule that
includes volunteering. CRVIS is in a position to approach retirees early
while recognizing that they may not be ready to begin to volunteer
until they have had a chance to experience fully the freedom that
retirement may offer. When asked when people are most receptive to
requests to participate, one member of the CRVIS steering board told
us that, in his experience, "When they first retire they want to have
fun, but you have to catch them before they turn into couch potatoes."

Second, there appears to be little targeted recruitment aimed at
the older population. Moreover, existing programs indicate some ambivalence about the range of activities appropriate for the retirement
age population (Freedman, 1993, 1994; Caro & Bass, 1995). Barfield
and Morgan (1968) found that more men expected to increase their
volunteer activity following retirement than actually did so. There
appear to be significant numbers of potential volunteers who would
be willing to volunteer if someone asked them, but retirees are sel-
dom asked (Herzog & Morgan, 1993a).

Third, personal contact has been found to be an important recruitment mechanism (Fischer & Schaffer, 1993; Gallup, 1991). When CRVIS
members identify potential volunteers, they approach them with personal phone calls. As often as possible, friends or acquaintances do the
actual recruiting. Data from the *Cornell Retirement and Well-Being
Study* provide support for the efficacy of this method. More than two
fifths (44%) of the volunteers in our sample indicate that they started
their current volunteer job because an organization had approached
them (see Figure 10.3).

And fourth, some degree in choice in type of volunteering and the

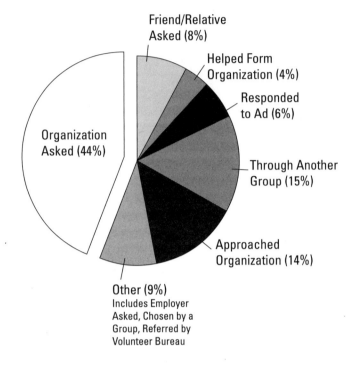

Figure 10.3   How Did Volunteers Start at Current Job? *Source: Cornell Retirement and Well-Being Study*, Wave 1 (1994–95).

matching of skills and interests of the volunteer with the volunteer work may be important for recruitment and retention (Francies, 1983; Morrow-Howell & Mui, 1989). Consideration of the needs and interests of potential volunteers is also an important factor in the number of hours people are willing to devote to volunteer work (ICR Survey Research Group, 1991; Smith, 1981). The CRVIS Steering Committee provides a formal structure through which the school administration can address requests and through which the retirees can propose activities to the school. When retirees choose and develop their own programs, not only is the likelihood of making full use of their talents and know-how enhanced but the volunteers are also most likely to find the activities rewarding.

Although many programs find that volunteers are better at "signing up than showing up" (Freedman, 1993; 79), CRVIS has been extremely successful in retaining committed volunteers. We interviewed members of the CRVIS Steering Committee, who stressed that CRVIS "works in partnership with" the schools and went "to them with the things we were interested in doing. It was collaborative." There is a great effort made to match individual interests with the needs of the school. One board member explained "There is a questionnaire that lists the hobbies. We use this to make placements." Individual retirees carve out tasks for themselves after establishing contact with an individual teacher, forming a collaboration. Another committee member described an example of an activity developed by the volunteers themselves: "We find out what the person is interested in doing. We fit the task with the personality. One couple loves bird walks and they are well received and appreciated by the children."

When we asked how the organization deals with "no-shows," the chair of the Steering Committee emphasized, "We have had very little of that. There is a sense of commitment." Another board member concurs that "the meetings are well attended. We have been lucky with attendance in schools." "It [absenteeism] hasn't been too much of a problem." CRVIS' success with volunteer retention and commitment supports the findings of the research literature, which indicates the relationship between commitment and working on personally meaningful tasks.

IMPLICATIONS FOR PRACTICE, POLICY, AND RESEARCH

Recruitment and Retention

Little is known about volunteer recruitment in terms of differences across the life course, couple (or family) volunteering, and gender differences. We reviewed what research has found, including data from the *Cornell Retirement and Well-Being Study.*

Life-course considerations. Theoretical and empirical work on factors affecting the likelihood of volunteering suggests that personal gain, not *merely* altruism, is frequently an important motivator. Some scholars have suggested that occupational development or social status concerns may be important in the decision to volunteer (Mueller, 1975). However, in the *Cornell Retirement and Well-Being Study,* we found that helping others and wanting to do something useful for a good cause are principal reasons volunteers give for volunteering (see also

Gallup, 1981). One would expect motivations to volunteer to change over the life course. According to a 1995 national survey of American youth (Prudential Youth Survey on Community Involvement, 1995), the most important reasons students volunteer are (1) to list activity on college applications (87%), and (2) to learn new skills (81%). By contrast, those in their fifties, sixties, and seventies in the *Cornell Retirement and Well-Being Study* mention helping others, accomplishing something, and believing in the cause as key motivators (see Figure 10.4). These results suggest that recruitment issues (and strategies) may vary over the life course.

Family considerations. Although recruitment and retention are approached from the perspective of individuals, volunteer service may well be a family project. A poll of 1,002 family households conducted by the Gallup International Institute in cooperation with the Family Matters Program of the Points of Light Foundation found that in more than 36 percent of American households, family volunteering is a part of family life. This is equally true in young families (adults aged 18–34), in the middle years (aged 35–49), and in older families (aged 50 or older). The top reason agencies say families give for volunteering together is "to teach values of service and community involvement" (Search Institute, 1994). The most common partnership in families volunteering is, however, between husband and wife—60 percent (Gallup International Institute, 1997).

Many of the married respondents participating in the *Cornell Retirement and Well-Being Study* tell us that spending time together as a couple is one of the most satisfying aspects of retirement. The sentiments expressed by a large number of the participants in the study are typified by remarks like:

We do things together to help each other and be together more often.

We're more of a partnership.

We can do things together we were not able to do before.

CRVIS encourages couples to volunteer together. One steering committee member told us that volunteering with her husband is part of her motivation for her involvement with CRVIS: "My husband came along when I became involved. We saw the pleasure in the children

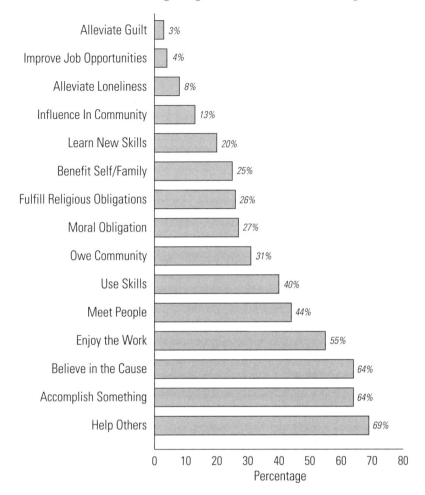

Figure 10.4 Why Older Workers and Retirees Volunteer: Percent Citing Reason as Very Important. *Source: Cornell Retirement and Well-Being Study,* Wave 1 (1994–95), N~340 (current volunteers).

and found pleasure in volunteering. We worked hard to put CRVIS together."

To date, there has been no systematic research addressing the issue of whether volunteer recruitment efforts are enhanced by directing them toward couples (or families). Neither is much known about the recruitment of people who are single, widowed, or divorced. Organizations may well need different strategies for their recruitment. Since a fairly large proportion of older people are widowed or divorced, it is important that they not be forgotten in thinking about how different people can be recruited.

Gender considerations. We know little about how recruitment and retention vary by gender. But a look at participation rates by gender in three other volunteer programs designed for older Americans reveals that different activities attract varying proportions of men and women. Whereas only 11 percent of Foster Grandparents and 15 percent of Senior Companions are men, men comprise 34 percent of those involved in the Community Service Employment Program (Freedman, 1994: 5). In 1997, fully 48 percent of CRVIS' active volunteers were men. We might predict that volunteer groups offering a greater range of individual choice would result in higher participation rates of both men and women.

"Structured" Flexibility

Lifestyle. The founders of CRVIS recognized that retirees, while wanting to remain productive, also find it important to have the freedom to pursue activities they were unable to pursue while working. Qualitative data from the *Cornell Retirement and Well-Being Study* document the importance to retirees of retaining flexibility and freedom. We asked retirees what they found most satisfying about retirement. Typical responses included:

I'm pleased with my life and the new-found freedom.

I have freedom—tremendous amounts of freedom—and am very happy.

One wife related her husband's satisfaction with his retirement to his ability to "do what he wants to do, when and how he wants to do it."

For many retirees, the ability to travel and spend extended time with family is a very important part of their retirement plans. CRVIS' literature explicitly states that the volunteer commitment should not encroach upon these activities. Important mechanisms facilitating this flexibility are built into the CRVIS organizational structure. First, "multiple coverage" ensures that when one volunteer is away or ill, another volunteer is available to fulfill the commitment. Second, the volunteer responsibilities are set up so that "each volunteer position has a beginning and an end"; "We have schedules and everyone works together. Each person decides how many hours they want to volunteer." The volunteer program includes some short-term projects and long-term activities that are divided up among volunteers according to individual vacation and travel schedules. Thus, potential volunteers who are reluctant to become involved because they are out of town for long stretches of time are assured that they can still make a contribution to the volunteer effort. Positions are made to fit the individual's schedule in terms of "times, days, and months" of the year. This built-in flexibility is likely to be another important factor in CRVIS' success in recruitment and its high retention rate.

But this very desire for flexibility might be seen by organizations as a liability rather than an asset. Some community organizations may not seek out retirees as volunteers precisely because they are seen as "unreliable." One solution is for organizations to create modules of volunteer work. Individuals (of all ages) might be particularly receptive to volunteering for a fixed project or a fixed time period—a year, six months, two months, two weeks, or even a day. Provisions could be made that would facilitate signing on for yet another module of fixed duration.

Formal participation. We know that many retirees identify with the place where they worked and often miss the collegiality of the workplace and the respect that paid work is accorded in our society. The corporate model of retiree volunteering takes advantage of a valuable community asset while providing a means for retirees to be productive under conditions where the value of their contribution is recognized both formally and informally. To be sure, retirees, our "seasoned citizens," can volunteer as individuals, performing needed work in hospitals, schools, and other institutions, but most of us are used to being productive in jobs that involve working with co-workers. As one CRVIS member tells us, "CRVIS provides a level of response that is similar to what they had at work. I'm still needed. For me it is trying to give something back. I want to participate with other people. It doesn't fit for me to sit at home."

The efforts of volunteers are formally acknowledged at awards presentations and through publicity in the local media. Both CRVIS members and Cornell University staff ensure that the organization remains in the public eye through articles in the local paper and spots on the radio. Perhaps more important, however, the volunteers' work is informally acknowledged as volunteers validate one another's efforts.

It is both touching and striking to hear how often volunteers point with pride to the achievements of other group members and relay stories of one another's successes.

Community links. CRVIS is careful to filter out requests from schools that are not willing to consider them full and valuable partners, ensuring that they are valued as unpaid workers. As the group expands, they interview and at times reject requests for help when, in the opinion of the steering committee, the particular school administration or staff is not enthusiastic about their participation. A recent poll of Philadelphians by the Pew Research Foundation found that respondents who believed that they could "make a difference" were especially likely to volunteer (Galston & Levine, 1997). By careful selection of schools the organization is able to control the volunteer experience so that the individuals feel they do have an impact. As the chair of the CRVIS Steering Committee commented, "[CRVIS volunteers] realize they are doing something that matters."

The Corporate Model and the Agency Being Served

The principal of the school involved in the CRVIS pilot project describes how her initial guarded and somewhat skeptical attitude toward the initiative turned into delight as she discovered the advantages of CRVIS' organizational structure. One of the reservations many agencies have about placing volunteers in key positions is a concern about dependability. The CRVIS organization helps to enhance the effectiveness of the volunteer effort in several ways. First, the framework ensures reliability by providing for substitute coverage. Second, the leaders of the organization serve as a conduit through which both the school and volunteers can channel problems and concerns. One steering committee member told us: "We keep in contact with the volunteers and find out what problems they may have had." By serving as an intermediary, the organization deals with potential problems before they become serious.

Moreover, CRVIS also helps individual volunteers limit their commitments by acting as a filter, that is, a conduit through which requests for aid can be processed. The CRVIS chairman pointed out, "We set limits to be most effective." He describes the learning process the group went through as they first "spread out a little too much in the Cayuga Heights School and so we set more bounds when we expanded to the Enfield School." This observation is in line with research findings on limit setting. For example, Wuthnow (1993) reports on the conflict in American society between individualism and self-interest on the one hand and compassion and caring on the other hand. He cites various studies pointing to the deleterious health consequences to Americans who fail to "place boundaries around their caring" (Wuthnow, 1991: 193).

Analysis of data from the *Cornell Retirement and Well-Being Study* provides empirical evidence for Wuthnow's hypothesis. We find that formal volunteering (in the context of membership in an organization) is particularly beneficial to psychological well-being of retirees (Moen & Fields, 2000). Those who do community volunteer work report higher levels of self-efficacy, self-esteem, general life satisfaction, and overall energy than retirees who are neither organization members nor volunteers; those who volunteer informally do not score significantly higher than non-volunteers on these measures of well-being.

CONCLUSIONS

America is a work-oriented society in which most people derive a large part of their identity and sense of self-worth from their employment. The role of worker is the way we become integrated and acknowledged as adult members of the larger community. Employment is not only a central role in American society, it is virtually isomorphic with contemporary notions of productivity and achievement. The changes our society is undergoing call forcefully for a thoughtful re-examination of existing—and increasingly inappropriate—life patterns. Occupational careers are what Pearlin (1988) describes as "durable arrangements" that serve to "organize experience over time." In turn, it is precisely this organized experience that "is the basis for how we see the world around us, how we think about it and act toward it." We need similar such durable arrangements for the post-career years. Americans equate productivity with paid work, yet an increasingly larger portion of the life course is being spent in the "post-employment" period. Mature adulthood is vital involvement in generative activities, active participation in meaningful roles (e.g., Erikson et al., 1986), regardless of whether that meaningful work is paid or unpaid. As more people make the (earlier) transition to retirement, it is vital that new institutional arrangements encourage people to remain productive and active (Morris, 1993).

Retirees—now younger, healthier, more capable than ever in history—are constructing a new life stage (see Bronfenbrenner et al., 1996). As such, they constitute an important untapped reserve of human capital that can be put to work in community service. Doing so is not only advantageous to society, but it also promotes the social integration of this (growing) segment of the population. How can our nation give to volunteer work the same sense of purposive activity, collegiality, and salience it accords to paid work? One answer is through new organizations, such as employer-sponsored retiree programs like CRVIS.

REFERENCES

Anderson, D. (1993). *Building community: National Retiree Volunteer Coalition, 1993 annual report.* Minneapolis: National Retiree Volunteer Coalition.

Atchley, R. C. (1989). A continuity theory of normal aging. *Journal of Personality and Social Psychology, 29,* 183–190.

Barfield, R., & Morgan, J. N. (1968). *Early retirement: The decision and the experiences.* Ann Arbor, MI: Institute for Social Research.

Bronfenbrenner, U., McClelland, P., Wethington, E., Moen, P., & Ceci, S. J. (1996). *The state of Americans: This generation and the next.* New York: Free Press.

Caro, F. G., & Bass, S. A. (1995). Increasing volunteering among older people. In S. A. Bass (Ed.), *Older and active: How Americans over 55 are contributing to society* (71–96). New Haven: Yale University Press.

Caro, F. G., & Bass, S. A. (1997). Receptivity to volunteering in the immediate postretirement period. *Journal of Applied Gerontology, 16,* 427–444.

Ebaugh, H. R. F. (1988). *Becoming an ex: The process of role exit.* Chicago: University of Chicago Press.

Erikson, E. H., Erikson, J. M., & Kivnick, H. Q. (1986). *Vital involvement in old age.* New York: Norton.

Fischer, L. R., & Schaffer, K. B. (1993). *Older volunteers: A guide to research and practice.* Newbury Park, CA: Sage.

Francies, G. R. (1983). The volunteer needs profile: A tool for reducing turnover. *Journal of Volunteer Administration, 2,* 17–23.

Freedman, M. (1993). *The kindness of strangers: Adult mentors, urban youth, and the new voluntarism.* San Francisco: Jossey-Bass.

Freedman, M. (1994). *Seniors in national and community service.* Report prepared for the Commonwealth Fund's Americans over 55 at Work program. Philadelphia: Public/Private Ventures.

Gallup International Institute. (1997). *Family volunteering.* Conducted in cooperation with the Family Matters program of the Points of Light Foundation. http://vp.libertynet.org/resources/volstat.htm.

Gallup Organization. (1981). *Americans volunteer 1981.* Princeton: Gallup Organization.

Gallup Organization. (1991). *Americans volunteer 1991.* Princeton: Gallup Organization.

Galston, W. A., & Levine, P. (1997). America's civic condition: A glance at the evidence. *Brookings Review, 15,* 23–26.

Herzog, A. R., & Morgan, J. N. (1993a). Formal volunteer work among older Americans. In S. A. Bass, F. G. Caro, & Y.-P. Chen (Eds.), *Achieving a productive aging society* (119–142). Westport, CT: Auburn House.

Herzog, A. R., & Morgan, J. N. (1993b). Age and gender differences in the value of productive activities: Four different approaches. *Research on Aging, 14,* 169–198.

Hunt, A. R. (1999). Fundamental shift in what it means to be a senior: "Third age" elderly begin to give a new definition to "retirement." *Wall Street Journal,* March 11, 1999.

ICR Survey Research Group. (1991). Marriott's Seniors Volunteerism Study. Washington, DC: Marriott Senior Living Services.

Kahn, R. L. (1994). Opportunities, aspirations, and goodness of fit. In M. W. Riley, R. L. Kahn & A. Foner (Eds.), *Age and structural lag: The mismatch between people's lives and opportunities in work, family, and leisure* (37–53). New York: Wiley.

Moen, P. (1994). Women, work and family: A sociological perspective on changing roles. In M. W. Riley, R. L. Kahn, & A. Foner (Eds.), *Age and structural lag: The mismatch between people's lives and opportunities in work, family, and leisure* (151–70). New York: Wiley.

Moen, P. (1998). Recasting careers: Changing reference groups, risks, and realities. *Generations, 22,* 40–45.

Moen, P., & Fields, V. (2000). Retirement and well-being: Does community participation replace paid work? Unpublished manuscript.

Morris, R. (1993). Defining the place of the elderly in the twenty-first century. In S. A. Bass, F. G. Caro, & Y.-P. Chen (Eds.), *Achieving a productive aging society* (287–293). Westport, CT: Auburn House.

Morrow-Howell, N., & Mui, A. (1989). Elderly volunteers: Reasons for initiating and terminating service. *Journal of Gerontological Social Work, 13,* 21–34.

Mueller, M. W. (1975). Economic determinants of volunteer work by women. *Signs, 1,* 325–338.

Musick, M. A., Herzog, A. R., & House, J. S. (1999). Volunteering and mortality among older adults: Findings from a national sample. *Journal of Gerontology: Social Sciences, 54B*, S173–S180.

Pearlin, L. (1988). Social structure and social values: The regulation of structural effects. In H. J. O'Gorman (Ed.), *Surveying social life* (252–264). Middletown, CT: Wesleyan University.

Prudential Youth Survey on Community Involvement. (1995).

Riley, M. W., & Riley, J. W. Jr. (1994). Structural lag: Past and future. In M. W. Riley, R. L. Kahn, & A. Foner (Eds.), *Age and structural lag: The mismatch between people's lives and opportunities in work, family, and leisure* (15–36). New York: Wiley.

Search Institute. (1994). Involving families in service. http://www. searchinstitute.org/archives/ifis.htm.

Smith, D. H. (1981). Altruism, volunteers and volunteerism. *Journal of Voluntary Action Research, 10*, 21–36.

Wuthnow, R. (1991). *Acts of compassion: Caring for others and helping ourselves.* Princeton: Princeton University Press.

Wuthnow, R. (1993). Altruism and sociological theory. *Social Service Review, 67*, 344–357.

CHAPTER ELEVEN

Peer Support for Alzheimer's Caregivers

Lessons from an Intervention Study

Karl Pillemer, J. Jill Suitor, L. Todd Landreneau,
Charles R. Henderson, Jr., and Sharon Brangman

ALZHEIMER'S CAREGIVING: THE NEED FOR SUPPORT INTERVENTIONS

Over the past two decades, interest in supporting caregivers of frail elderly family members has increased. Partly fueling the attention to family caregiving is a demographic imperative: the dramatic growth in the elderly population will create unprecedented demands on formal health and welfare systems, as well as on families who provide the bulk of care. This concern is also an outgrowth of extensive research indicating that family caregivers are at elevated risk for such negative outcomes as psychological distress, physical illness, and economic strain, all of which may disrupt social relationships (for reviews, see Chapter 5, this volume; Pillemer & Suitor, 1996; Schulz & Williamson, 1994).

Nowhere are these problems so great as among family caregivers for persons with Alzheimer's disease (AD) and other related types of dementia. The consequences of AD for victims are devastating: irreversible memory loss is usually accompanied by profound declines in intellectual skills, judgment, and language (Morris, 1996). The prevalence of dementia supports attention to this subgroup, with 2–3 percent of the population affected at age 65 and 30 percent or more of persons aged 85 and over (Barker, 1992).

Research (reviewed in Chapter 5, this volume) has also demonstrated the burden and stress experienced by family caregivers to AD patients. As the disease progresses, demands for assistance increase, typically involving dependency for personal care, as well as for activities such as shopping, household maintenance, and financial management. Equally or more distressing for family caregivers are the behaviors that frequently accompany the disease, for example, agitation, wandering, sleeplessness, delusions, obsessive behavior, and verbal and physical aggression (Buckwalter, 1996). Further, the family experiences the loss of the loved one as a companion or confidant, as their role is reduced to that of care provider (Fiore et al., 1986).

Most relevant to the present chapter is that caregiving responsibility negatively affects social relationships. As was demonstrated in Chapter 5, three characteristics of AD caregiving point to the need for a support intervention that focuses on social relationships. First, AD caregivers experience decreased social contact and support. Second, the degree of perceived support from others has a beneficial impact on caregivers' well-being. And third, negative interactions with network members cause distress for care providers. AD caregivers thus face a paradoxical situation: although social integration is of great importance to them, their network of social support and relationships are threatened by their adoption of this role, and social ties can become strained as a result.

Interventions that support caregivers have been seen as a primary response to preventing, postponing, or reversing the negative sequelae of caregiving. Most of the programs designed for caregivers feature professionally led support groups (Gottlieb, 1998; Lakey & Lutz, 1996; Rogers, 1999). Empirical findings regarding the effectiveness of such groups have been mixed, however. Research on support interventions for caregivers shows a general pattern: participants often report high levels of satisfaction with support groups but fail to improve significantly on various outcome measures (Kane & Penrod, 1995; Pillemer, 1996). Studies have typically failed to find significant differences between participants and controls on outcome variables such as the burden on caregivers and psychological well-being (Demers & Lavoie, 1996; Haley et al., 1987; Whitlach et al., 1991; Zarit et al., 1989).

We suggest that there are several conceptual and methodological reasons for the equivocal findings. First, most caregiver support interventions have not been theoretically grounded but rather have typically constructed program models based on social work practice or clinical impressions. Below, we argue that sociological and psychological research on the role of similar others in the lives of persons undergoing life-course transitions provides a sound basis for designing a caregiver support project. The intervention program detailed in this article was developed specifically according to these theoretical guidelines.

Second, caregiver support programs usually include a variety of intervention components. Most programs involve a mixture of advice from a professional (such as a social worker), educational sessions, information and referral regarding community services, and peer support, among other components. As is discussed further below, it is important to begin to isolate these various aspects of support, so that we can ascertain which components are effective and which are not.

Third, studies have typically not addressed the issue of who benefits most from social support interventions (Bass et al., 1998). That is, we do not know if different sub-groups of caregivers are more likely to benefit from support programs. In the study analyzed here, we examine the degree to which factors such as gender and the strength of the pre-existing social network affect outcomes.

In sum, the goal of the intervention study discussed in this chapter was to fill conceptual and methodological gaps by designing and evaluating a program for caregivers that is grounded in theory and research relating to life-course transitions and their impact on interpersonal relationships. Below we review the theoretical framework we have developed for studying the effects of caregiving and discuss how that framework was used to design a support intervention for Alzheimer's caregivers.

THEORETICAL BACKGROUND: TRANSITIONS, SOCIAL SUPPORT, AND PSYCHOLOGICAL WELL-BEING

Considerable research has demonstrated that social support serves as a buffer against stressful life events and chronic stressful conditions (Cohen & Wills, 1985; Eckenrode & Gore, 1990; Kaplan, 1996). Comparable findings exist regarding family caregiving (see Chapter 5). However, understanding the conditions under which support is most effective is a key to designing successful interventions. As discussed in Chapter 5, one factor that is likely to enhance the value of social support is similarity between the support provider and the recipient. Indeed, several researchers have suggested that similarity may be relevant for support interventions (cf. Lakey & Lutz, 1996; Thoits, 1986).

However, there is little experience with programs based exclusively on the benefits of similar others. As Lakey and Lutz note, "Although similarity appears to be a powerful determinant of perceived support judgements, much more needs to be understood about this effect before we can use it optimally in intervention" (1996: 460).

To briefly restate our argument in Chapter 5, we proposed that both sociological theory and empirical research encourage attention to the role of similar others as effective supporters. Support from similar associates may be especially important when an individual has recently experienced a life-course transition, such as becoming a family caregiver. Particularly critical is similarity of *experience*. Our studies of AD caregivers (Suitor & Pillemer, 1993, 1996, in press; Suitor et al., 1995) demonstrated that network members who had caregiving experience were more likely to be sources of emotional support, and they were less likely to be sources of interpersonal stress. We also examined whether the presence of experientially similar others affected psychological distress. The study found that a larger number of fellow caregivers in the respondents' social networks was associated with lower levels of depression (Pillemer & Suitor, 1996), especially among individuals in more stressful caregiving situations. In light of this evidence, it is plausible to hypothesize that increasing the number of network members who share the caregiving status would have a positive effect on social and psychological well-being among AD caregivers.

Although few interventions have specifically examined the effects of similarity, several reports suggest that contact with similar others is the major benefit of organized support programs. For example, Glosser and Wexler (1985) reported that "getting a chance to meet people with similar problems" (233) was one of the two most frequent reasons the members found group participation helpful. Two surveys by Wright et al. (1987) and Gonyea (1989) had similar findings: among the aspects of AD support groups cited as being most helpful were seeing how others dealt with their problems, feeling less isolated in performing caregiving, and talking with others who understood their experiences. However, the design of these studies precluded the possibility of systematically examining the effects of such participation. Isolating the impact of support from experientially similar others appears to be a worthy intervention goal.

Intervention Design

Conceptual Approach

To examine the benefits of introducing similar others into caregivers' networks, we designed a model program called the Peer Support Project (PSP). The PSP differed from previous caregiver support interventions in four major ways. First, unlike most previous programs, the PSP did not involve professional intervention of any kind. Instead, it emphasized "indigenous social support," that is, behaviors which persons in the same life situation can provide to one another without professional intervention (Heller et al., 1991).

Second, most caregiver support interventions have focused on what Gottlieb (1988) termed *directed* support. These programs provide considerable guidance about the precise form of support and how it should be delivered. In the case of family caregiving, the modal intervention has been groups with a psychoeducational focus, emphasizing training in caregiving skills and the use of community resources. The PSP took a different approach by providing *diffuse* support (Gottlieb, 1988). This type of intervention involves grafting on a social tie to reduce isolation. As Gottlieb (1988) notes, such interventions provide units of companionship that encourage the formation of friendships. The PSP's focus on increasing numbers of status-similar social ties is in contrast to the traditional emphasis on highly specific components of didactic information or social support to improve their coping ability. Gottlieb describes the distinction between the two types of interventions: "In effect, directed support interventions marshal the partner's specialized social supportive resources while diffuse interventions compensate for a generally impoverished social field" (526). The impoverishment in the context of the project described here is a lack of status-similar others in the network. Therefore, the primary component of the PSP intervention was making available regular contact with another person who shared the status of caregiver.

Third, the study was part of a much-needed effort to isolate the various features of caregiver support programs (peer support, education, professional counseling, etc.), to ascertain which components are effective and which are not. This issue is of special importance in light of what may be termed "dosage-response" issues in support interventions. That is, it is critical to ascertain more precisely the amount of support needed to bring about positive outcomes. If, as our theoretical framework suggested, the most effective aspect of support groups is increasing interaction with others who are similar, then complex group interventions with didactic content may be unnecessary. Instead, more simple mutual aid and "friendly visiting" approaches could be equally effective at lower cost. Conceivably, there is a "minimum threshold" of support, with only marginal improvements for amounts of support that exceed the threshold (Schiaffino, 1991). Our goal in this study was to test the specific benefits of support from similar others, in the absence of other program components.

Finally, we designed the program as a dyadic rather than a group intervention, for two reasons. First, persons who, because of temperament or past experience, are less inclined toward group participation may tend to avoid group interventions. It is nevertheless possible that they could benefit substantially from a supportive relationship with someone with similar problems. Second, support groups can increase the possibility that a participant will experience miscarried support, such as unwanted advice. For example, group members are usually in very different stages of the caregiving process; it can be distressing when a person whose relative is experiencing mild memory loss must participate in discussions of nursing home placement or autopsy (Wasow, 1986). We hypothesized that a dyadic intervention might avoid some of these difficulties.

Specific Intervention Components

The design of the program was based on the experience of friendly visiting programs for the elderly and disabled (cf. Biegel et al., 1984; Korte & Gupta, 1991; Thornton, 1991). The PSP used community volunteers who had themselves been caregivers to a relative with AD. Volunteers were recruited to the program by the Alzheimer's Association of Central New York and were provided with training in communication and listening skills. After training, the volunteers were matched with family caregivers to persons who had been diagnosed with AD at the State University of New York Health Science Center (SUNY-HSC), a major medical center with a large dementia screening program in Syracuse, New York. Recruiting subjects through SUNY-HSC also allowed us to avoid a problem evident in some research efforts on dementia caregivers: lack of firm diagnostic criteria (Zarit, 1989). A comprehensive neuropsychiatric examination is conducted on all patients at SUNY-HSC in accordance with strict research diagnosis criteria. This rigor in establishing diagnosis ensured to the greatest extent possible that our sample was not contaminated with non-dementia cases.

It was expected that the volunteer and the caregiver would meet for eight weekly sessions lasting between one and two hours each. Specific components of the intervention were designed to correspond as closely as possible to the theoretical framework we outlined above. To this end, the project had a number of special features that attempted to maximize the benefits of similarity between the volunteer and the caregiver. These were as follows.

Training of volunteers. Volunteers received 5–7 hours of training (depending on the size of the training group). The volunteer training focused on enhancing positive aspects of similarity. First, the conceptual underpinnings of the PSP were reviewed; in this discussion, the importance of experiential similarity was stressed. Selected research findings were presented demonstrating the importance of similar others in promoting caregivers' well-being. The volunteers were characterized as "true experts" on handling the stress of caregiving and were encouraged to draw on their own experiences when interacting with their partners. Our intent was to make volunteers consciously aware of the benefits of similar experience and to suggest that they emphasize this fact to the caregivers.

The second major portion of the training program was devoted to clarifying and understanding the volunteers' own experiences as caregivers. A family therapist with expertise in aging designed several exercises for use in this phase of training. The exercises included having each trainee tell his or her "caregiving story" and reflect on how similar others had influenced his or her caregiving experience. These activities helped volunteers identify which aspects of their own experiences were particularly sensitive or emotionally charged and to examine their own levels of comfort in disclosing information about themselves.

A third feature of the training was to create awareness of stages in the caregiving experience. Because many volunteers were caring for persons in very advanced stages of the disease (and in some cases, their care recipients had died), it was important to stress the need for approaching newer caregivers "at their own stage." Volunteers were trained not to anticipate future stages for the caregiver but rather to focus on aspects of experience that corresponded to the current stage of their partner.

Finally, the volunteer training included activities designed to improve communication and active listening skills. Volunteers engaged in role-playing exercises that simulated discussions they might have with their partner. These exercises emphasized the need to avoid giving advice or trying to solve the caregivers' problems for them. Instead, following each role-playing session, the trainer discussed the need for empathic listening and reassurance regarding the caregiver's strengths and coping abilities. Further, the role plays allowed the volunteers to identify appropriate boundaries of contact between them and the caregivers.

Matching. Both the volunteers and the recipients shared the characteristic of having been a caregiver to a person with AD. However, to maximize similarity between the volunteer and the caregiver, they also were matched on gender and on relationship to the care recipient (spouse or adult child). In addition, volunteers and caregivers were matched according to county of residence. This led, in effect, to a regional match, with caregivers and volunteers from similar areas matched with one another.

Content. Because the goal of the intervention was to encourage the exchange of social support and the formation of friendships, it was decided that the meetings of the pairs would primarily involve unstructured time that allowed for sharing of experiences and the development of relationships. The only exception to this emphasis on unscripted interaction was the first meeting between the partners. A protocol was developed for the initial visit, in which the volunteer encouraged the caregiver to discuss his or her reaction to the diagnosis and did a preliminary exploration of social network resources. The goal of this session was to increase the partner's comfort and to reduce awkwardness.

In the event that the volunteer desired additional assistance in planning the visit, we created a manual with additional exercises that could be conducted with the caregiver. The exercises included an exploration of social network problems and a guided discussion about future plans that could be used by volunteers any time after the first session at their discretion. Very few volunteers chose to use any of these exercises, preferring instead to engage in open-ended dialogue with their partners.

During the initial session, the volunteers discussed how the caregiver would prefer to spend the time, and attempted to follow these suggestions as much as possible. Although it was suggested to the volunteers that they focus a part of each meeting on a discussion of caregiving concerns, purely social visits were also permitted. In the majority of visits, the volunteer met the caregiver either at the caregiver's home or in a restaurant, with conversation typically focused on caregiving issues. However, a minority of pairs engaged in other activities. In some cases, this was a mutually satisfying leisure pursuit. (For example, two women met early in the morning for a power walk, and another pair met for lunch during the workday.) In other cases, the volunteer accompanied the caregiver on visits to a nursing home, adult day center, or other possible service providers for the patient.

An important decision in the design was the duration of the intervention. On the one hand, it was important to include a sufficient number of meetings to produce effects. On the other hand, too extensive a program might be perceived as burdensome by both volunteers and caregivers, and would therefore be more difficult to replicate. Based on the existing literature and the experience of practitioners, we established eight sessions as the target number of visits. However, we recognized that some matches might continue for fewer visits, depending on the needs and commitments of the caregivers.

Monitoring and tracking. Based on the experiences of other visitation programs, we believed it was important to keep in close contact with the volunteer visitors. We anticipated that volunteers who were placed in a more difficult or initially awkward match might be inclined to skip visits or end their involvement entirely. Therefore, a check-in program was instituted in which research assistants called each volunteer on a weekly basis during the period that the match was taking place. This procedure allowed for trouble-shooting (for example, in the case of transportation problems or difficulty contacting the caregiver), as well as affording an opportunity to learn about the content of visits. The research assistant recorded the volunteers' answers to a set of questions regarding the issues discussed in the visit, any problems encountered, and how enjoyable the volunteer felt the visit had been. We considered conducting a similar weekly contact with the caregivers, but it became clear that such an effort would be perceived as overly invasive and time-consuming.

Methods

Design

After a patient received a diagnosis of AD at the SUNY-HSC, the patient's caregiver was contacted by the program social worker, who provided him or her with literature about the project. If the caregiver refused to participate, refusal conversion was attempted by a member of the research staff. Caregivers who agreed to participate were randomly assigned to either the treatment group or the control group. The outcome evaluation was based on a pre-intervention interview (T1) and a post-intervention interview (T2). After completing the T1 interview, the treatment group member was matched with a volunteer, and the visits began. Post-test interviews took place approximately six months later (3–4 months after the final visit).

Sample

To be included in the study, a subject had to be the primary caregiver to a diagnosed AD patient who did not reside in a nursing home at T1. There were no other eligibility restrictions, such as residing with the care recipient or being in a particular relationship (spouse or child, for example). A total of 147 caregivers agreed to participate in the study, representing a response rate of approximately 50 percent. Although a higher acceptance rate would have been desirable, the refusal rate in this study was comparable to a number of other similar efforts.

A unique feature of the present study was the ability to conduct a detailed analysis of refusals (Pillemer et al., 1996b). The SUNY-HSC maintains fairly extensive data on all patients and their primary caregivers. Using this data base, we found that refusals did not significantly differ from participants on basic demographic variables. However, the two groups did vary on one important dimension. Contrary to the view that support programs attract persons whose needs are less acute, caregivers in more stressful caregiving situations (as measured by the severity of the patient's behavioral symptoms) were more likely to agree to participate, as were caregivers whose relatives had experienced a sudden deterioration in memory. Further, participants were somewhat more likely to report that they were the only person providing care to the relative. Thus, to the extent that any self-selection bias existed, it led to participation of persons whose need for support appears to have been greater.

A total of 115 persons completed both the pre-test and post-test interviews (54 in the treatment group and 61 in the control group); it is on these respondents that our data analyses were based. Attrition between T1 and T2 was 28 percent, which is comparable to or better than most caregiver intervention projects (Demers & Lavoie, 1996). Similar to Zarit et al. (1989), we found no differences between participants who completed both interviews and those who did not on any of the outcome indicators used in this study or on any other variable of interest.

Of the 115 respondents, 71 percent were female and 29 percent male. Respondents ranged in age from 35 to 87, with a mean of 58 years. Most of the respondents (84%) were married. Only 5 percent of respondents had less than a high school education, while 64 percent had completed high school, and 30 percent had completed college. Forty percent of respondents were caring for their spouse, and 60 percent for their parent. In 61 percent of cases, the caregiver and care recipient lived together. The age of care recipients ranged from 59 to 90, with a mean of 77. Sixty-one percent of the care recipients were female; 39 percent were male.

In terms of equivalency at Time 1, no significant differences in any of the outcome variables were found between the treatment and control groups on the pretest. The groups were also very similar on demographic variables and on variables related to the caregiving experience (for example, level of impairment of the care recipient, number of hours spent daily providing care, and severity of behavioral symptoms). However, caregivers in the intervention group were disproportionately likely to be spousal caregivers; the control group had a greater concentration of adult-child caregivers. Analyses were conducted dividing the sample to control for this difference.

Measures

Outcome variables. The evaluation focused on three major outcome variables. Two measures of caregiver psychological well-being were employed: the Center for Epidemiologic Studies Depression (CES-D) scale (Radloff, 1977), and the Rosenberg Self-Esteem Scale (Rosenberg, 1986). Based on previous research, including our own studies, we expected that these measures should be sensitive to increases in the supportiveness of the network.

Data on satisfaction with social support were also collected as a more proximal outcome than psychological well-being. We used a three-item scale that measured the caregivers' satisfaction with support from their social networks. The items composing the scale were (1) How satisfied are you with the overall emotional support you have in caring for [RELATIVE]?; (2) How satisfied are you with the overall support you have for talking about problems involving [RELATIVE]?; and (3) How satisfied are you with the overall support you have for dealing with personal or day-to-day problems? Answer categories for these four variables were: 4 = very satisfied, 3 = fairly satisfied, 2 = a little satisfied, and 1 = not satisfied at all. Reliability of this scale was high (Chronbach's alpha > .78).

One goal of the study was to examine differences in the effectiveness of the intervention for various subgroups. Most substantively important, we examined subgroup differences in the degree of stress in the caregiving situation. Research shows that the best indicator of demands on the caregiver is the extent of the relative's disruptive behaviors (cf. Deimling & Bass, 1986; Pillemer & Suitor, 1992; Rabins, 1989; Stephens et al., 1991). Further, in a previous study, we found that in situations where disruptive behaviors were low, the presence of other caregivers in the network had only limited positive effects on the caregivers' well-being. When disruptive behaviors were high, persons with larger concentrations of caregivers in their networks experienced substantially lower levels of distress (Pillemer & Suitor, 1996). We therefore anticipated that the PSP intervention might have greater effects among caregivers in more stressful situations.

A shortened version of George's index of disruptive behaviors was used in the present study (George & Gwyther, 1986). The scale consists of eight items that ask how often problematic behaviors occur (1 = never; 2 = rarely; 3 = occasionally; 4 = frequently). The behaviors include the following: wanders or gets lost, is agitated or fidgety, does not recognize family or friends, has problems expressing thoughts, is depressed, does not like to be left alone with strangers, hears voices or sees things that aren't there, and cannot control bladder or bowels. The scale ranged from a score of 10 to 31 ($M = 20.3$; $SD = 4.3$).

Satisfaction with PSP. Two global satisfaction items were asked of respondents: whether they would recommend the PSP to another caregiver, and whether participation in the PSP had made them feel less alone in their situation. They were also asked a set of items that measured the caregiver's perceptions of the volunteer's sensitivity and responsiveness. Respondents were asked: "I am going to read you a list of ways in which your volunteer might have felt or behaved during your visits together. For each item, please tell me whether this occurred very often, fairly often, sometimes, rarely, or never." "Showed an interest," "shared similar experiences," and "expressed support" were the positive items. "Got impatient," "got embarrassed," and "got frustrated" were the negative items.

Finally, caregivers were asked a number of open-ended items regarding their views of the project, including what they liked most and least about participation, and why they would or would not recommend the PSP to another caregiver.

Implementation Evaluation

An evaluation of the process of implementation was carried out to ensure that the intervention was conducted in the way it was intended. Extensive data were therefore collected on the operation of the program. As noted earlier, volunteers reported on each visit with the caregivers, usually in short weekly telephone interviews (or occasionally on a prepared response card). Following completion of the intervention, meetings were held with volunteers to discuss their experiences in a focus group format; these meetings were videotaped and analyzed. In addition, the post-test interviews with caregivers contained a number of open-ended questions regarding the activities carried out with the volunteer, satisfaction with the program, and suggestions for improvement.

In general, the intervention appears to have been conducted according to plan. Volunteers were matched with the caregivers, and in most cases, the relationship continued for multiple sessions. The mean number of visits was 6.7, and 80 percent of the pairs met four or more times. Three reasons account for why matches did not complete the suggested eight visits. First, the matches sometimes ended for practical reasons, including (a) the caregiver's schedule was so hectic that it was impossible to continue weekly meetings; (b) a change in the care recipient's status led the caregiver to feel that the meetings were no longer necessary (usually when the patient was institutionalized or died); or (c) changes in the situation of the caregiver occurred (health problems or moving out of the area). A second reason was that the caregiver felt that he or she had benefited from the visits that had already taken place and that no more benefit could be achieved. In these situations, the volunteer tried to encourage additional visits and, when unsuccessful, typically followed up with one or more telephone calls. A third reason was cited in six of the fifty-four matches: incompatibility between volunteer and caregiver. It should be noted that only in one case did this incompatibility lead to the termination of the match after just one visit. Even in the remaining five cases, the match continued for two or more visits, and all of these caregivers reported at least a somewhat positive experience in the project.

The content of the weekly visits, as reported by the volunteers, followed our expectations in designing the project. Although there were differences in the quality and duration of individual matches, the content of interactions was quite uniform across the matches. Topics of discussion fell generally into three categories: (1) the relative's condition and stresses resulting from it; (2) relationships with other members of the social network, both positive and negative; and (3) practical issues, such as finding needed services, financial planning, seeking medical opinions, etc. In about one quarter of the matches, the volunteer and caregiver engaged at least once in some kind of activity together. For example, one pair went together to pick up a window for the caregiver's house. Another volunteer suggested to his isolated caregiver that he consider attending a nearby senior center, and both men went together to visit.

In terms of quality of the interactions, the volunteers were asked to rate each visit in terms of how enjoyable they felt the visit was for them and their partners. In addition, they reported whether there were any "difficulties and problems" with the visit. In the 301 visits on which we have data, 82 percent were reported by the volunteer as having been very enjoyable, and only 1 percent were reported as not enjoyable. Further, difficulties and problems were reported less than 7 percent of the time. (The problems most often cited were scheduling difficulties and the disruptive presence of the care recipient.)

RESULTS

Intervention Effects

The goal of the statistical analysis was to evaluate effects of the intervention on the three primary outcome variables: caregiver depression, caregiver's satisfaction with support, and caregiver's self-esteem.

These variables were measured at both baseline prior to entry into the Peer Support Project and approximately 3–4 months after its completion. Using a multivariate analysis (primarily a 2×2 repeated measures design for time by treatment), we found no treatment main effects for the three major outcome variables. Statistically significant improvements did not occur on either the CES-D scale or the Rosenberg Self-Esteem Scale for either the treatment or the control group. Further, although the perceived social support scale showed borderline improvement between the pre-test and the post-test for the treatment group, an almost identical improvement occurred in the control group.

However, trends were identified at the level of interactions, suggesting that the Peer Support Project benefited members of particular subgroups. Most interesting was the finding that program participation appeared to mediate the effect of stress (as measured by disruptive behaviors) on depression. At Time 1, there was a strong and significant relationship between the frequency of disruptive behaviors and depression in both the treatment and the control groups. At Time 2, disruptive behaviors still strongly predicted depression for control group members. However, in the treatment group, this relationship disappeared. Thus, it appears that participation in the project buffered the impact of stress in the caregiving situation on depression. Interestingly, this finding mirrors that of Bass and colleagues (1998), who found that communication support through a computer network had a similar buffering effect when caregivers were in more stressful situations.

Further, in several subgroups, a trend toward improvement in self-esteem was found over the control group when the caregiver was the child of the care recipient, when the care recipient was female, and when the caregiver was male. It is important to interpret these findings cautiously, however, because the difference in changes in self-esteem between the two groups was generally small and of borderline statistical significance. They do, however, show a pattern of positive program effects on self-esteem. No consistent effect from participation in the program was found for satisfaction with support.

Satisfaction with the PSP

Despite the mixed effects of treatment on our outcome measures, it is important to note the high degree of satisfaction reported by participants. We asked whether they would recommend the program to others, what changes they would suggest, and whether the patterns of interaction with the volunteers were positive or negative. On all dimensions, the large majority of the treatment group was highly satisfied with the intervention. For example, 96 percent of the caregivers reported that they would recommend the project to another caregiver, and more than 93 percent identified specific dimensions of the intervention that they found to be positive. Further, more than 90 percent of the treatment participants reported that the volunteer showed an interest in them and expressed support; less than 5 percent reported that the volunteer got impatient or embarrassed.

The qualitative data confirmed our prediction that caregivers would highlight similarity with the volunteer as a key component of their experience in the project. When asked to describe the most positive features of the project, many caregivers expressly mentioned experiential similarity. Some illustrative quotes range from the simple to the elaborate on this issue:

> What I did like most about the project was talking to somebody who, you know, had the same problems that I have.

> It was good, just to sit there and talk to somebody else who was going through it.

> I guess the opportunity to have someone listen to me with some degree of sympathy, yes, because she had been through it and knows how a person who has Alzheimer's is. Because you get the impression from other family members and from personal friends that sometimes they don't really believe what you're going through.

> The fact that you find that there's other people out there that have gone through the same things that you're going through and can kind of help you through some of the rough spots.

> I guess the main thing was we had something in common, and I was able to relate to her, and to find out that she herself has gone through what I'm going through now. . . . If I tell her that some of my relatives weren't too supportive, not so much on my side, but on my husband's, she would say that she herself had gone through the same thing, and the best thing to do was just ignore it.

It is interesting to note that although men and women were equally likely to evaluate the intervention positively and to recognize the salience of similarity of caregiving experience, they explained the importance of that experience somewhat differently. Women typically emphasized the effects of similarity on the volunteer's emotional supportiveness and their ability to "know just how I feel," as illustrated in the quotations above. In contrast, men emphasized the effects of similarity on their ability to talk about meeting the patients' needs (see Chapter 5, this volume).

In sum, both men and women appear to have recognized and acknowledged the major mechanism of the intervention. Further, a parallel analysis of the experience of the volunteers echoes this finding. The volunteers reported that they considered the sharing of similar experiences to be the key feature of the project (Landreneau, 1996; Pillemer et al., 1996a).

DISCUSSION

The PSP used a rigorous research design to test the effects of providing an experientially similar associate to AD caregivers. Overall, the findings on the ability of the intervention to improve psychological well-being or satisfaction with social support were limited, at least in terms of main effects. However, participant assessment of the benefits of the program were very high. We suggest two possible explanations for this pattern: our measures were not sufficiently sensitive to change; or the intervention should have been stronger.

It is possible that more sensitive measures would have been successful in uncovering treatment effects of the PSP. For example, the intervention might have had an impact on loneliness or on anxiety about the future progress of the caregiving situation (Cicirelli, 1988). Further, our measure of perceived social support was relatively simple; a multidimensional assessment that examined various components of social support might have revealed the program's impact more successfully.

Further, Heller et alia's (1991) suggestion that this type of intervention may result in subtle mood changes or changes in satisfaction with support that have short-term positive effects is persuasive. The qualitative responses from the caregivers indicate that this may have been the case. When asked about benefits of the project, they typically mentioned positive feelings about talking to someone who "really understands." However, they almost never noted that major changes occurred in the caregiving situation or in the stress it created in their lives, which might in turn produce enduring changes in psychological well-being. Thus, effects on mood may have occurred immediately following the visit but then dissipated over time. A daily diary might reveal such changes (see Chapter 2), although we doubt that many family caregivers could be persuaded to add daily recordkeeping to their already hectic schedules.

The explanation that the intervention was too weak is also possible. As noted earlier, the persons who agreed to participate tended to be in more difficult caregiving situations and to have less social support in caring for their relatives. It may be that the psychological distress brought on by the caregiving situation was too overwhelming to be ameliorated by a time-limited interaction with a friendly visitor. Indeed, several caregivers mentioned this fact when asked for their feelings about the PSP. They noted that although the visits had been helpful, the objective characteristics of their stressful situations had remained the same. To benefit over the long-term from the social support offered by the PSP, more concrete support (in the form of financial assistance or services) may first be necessary to make caregiving more manageable.

In conclusion, despite the mixed findings of the present study, we suggest that further attempts be made to study the effects of increasing social integration for caregivers. Two directions in particular may be fruitful for additional intervention research. First, given the basic research findings showing the importance of similar others to caregivers, we continue to view enhancement of this dimension of social relationships as promising. However, similarity may be beneficial primarily among members of the already existing social network. An intervention could assist caregivers in activating support from such persons. Second, studies that experimentally compare support enhancement with other caregiver support services (such as education or material assistance) would shed light on the specific role social integration plays in the lives of caregivers.

REFERENCES

Barker, W. H. (1992). Prevention of disability in older persons. In J. M. Last & R. B. Wallace (Eds.), *Public health and preventive medicine*, 13th ed. (973–981). Norwalk, CT: Appleton and Lange.

Bass, D. M., McClendon, M. J., Brennan, P. F., & McCarthy, C. (1998). The buffering effect of a computer support network on caregiver strain. *Journal of Aging and Health, 10,* 20–43.

Bell, R. (1981). *Worlds of friendship.* Beverly Hills: Sage.

Biegel, D. E., Shore, B. K., & Gordon, E. (1984). *Building support networks for the elderly: Theory and applications.* Newbury Park, CA: Sage.

Buckwalter, K. C. (1996). An overview of psychological factors contributing to stress of family caregivers. In Z. S. Khachaturian & T. S. Radebaugh (Eds.), *Alzheimer's disease: Cause(s), diagnosis, treatment, and care* (305–312). Boca Raton, FL: CRC Press.

Cicirelli, V. G. (1988). A measure of filial anxiety regarding anticipated care of elderly parents. *The Gerontologist, 28,* 478–482.

Clipp, E. C., & George, L. K. (1993). Dementia and cancer: A comparison of spousal caregivers. *The Gerontologist, 33,* 534–541.

Cohen, S. & Wills, T. A. (1985). Stress, social support, and the buffering hypothesis. *Psychological Bulletin 98,* 310–357.

Deimling, G. T., & Bass, D. M. (1986). Symptoms of mental impairment among elderly adults and their effects on family caregivers. *Journal of Gerontology, 41,* 778–784.

Demers, A., & Lavoie, J. (1996). The effect of support groups on family caregivers to the frail elderly. *Canadian Journal on Aging, 15,* 129–144.

Eckenrode, J., & Gore, S. (1990). *Stress between work and family.* New York: Plenum.

Fiore, J., Coppel, D. B., Becker, J., & Cox, G. B. (1986). Social support as a multifaceted concept: Examination of important dimensions for adjustment. *American Journal of Community Psychology 14,* 93–111.

George, L. K., & Gwyther, L. P. (1986). Caregiver well-being: A multidimensional examination of family caregivers of demented adults. *The Gerontologist, 26,* 253–259.

Glosser, G., & Wexler, D. (1985). Participants' evaluation of educational support groups for families of patients with Alzheimer's disease and other dementias. *The Gerontologist, 25,* 232–236.

Gonyea, J. G. (1989). Alzheimer's disease support groups: An analysis of their structure, format and perceived benefits. *Social Work in Health Care, 14,* 61–72.

Gottlieb, B. H. (1988). Support interventions: A typology and agenda for research. In S. W. Duck (Ed.), *Handbook of personal relationships* (519–541).

Gottlieb, B. H. (1998). Support groups. *Encyclopedia of mental health. Volume 3.* New York: Academic Press.

Gottlieb, B. H., & Pancer, S. M. (1988). Social networks and the transition to parenthood. In G. Y. Michaels & W. A. Goldberg (Eds.), *The transition to parenthood: Current theory and research.* New York: Cambridge University Press.

Haley, W. E., Brown, S. L., & Levine, E. G. (1987). Experimental evaluation of the effectiveness of group intervention for dementia caregivers. *The Gerontologist 27,* 376–382.

Heller, K., Thompson, M. G., Trueba, P. E., Hogg, J. R., & Vlachos-Weber, I. (1991). Peer support telephone dyads for elderly women: Was this the wrong intervention. *American Journal of Community Psychology 19,* 53–74.

Kane, R. A., & Penrod, J. D. (1995). *Family caregiving in an aging society.* Thousand Oaks, CA: Sage.

Kaplan, H. B. (Ed.) (1996). *Psychosocial stress: Perspectives on structure, theory, lifecourse, and methods.* San Diego: Academic Press.

Korte, C., & Gupta, V. (1991). A program of friendly visitors as network builders. *The Gerontologist 33,* 404–407.

Lakey, B., & Lutz, C. J. (1996). Social support and preventive and therapeutic interventions. In G. R. Pierce, B. R. Sarason, & I. G. Sarason (Eds.), *Handbook of social support and the family* (435–465). Plenum series on stress and coping. New York: Plenum.

Landreneau, L. T. (1996). *Volunteer participants in the peer support project: An evaluation of their experiences.* Unpublished doctoral dissertation, Cornell University.

Morris, J. C. (1996). A diagnosis of Alzheimer's disease. In Z. S. Khachaturian & T. S. Radebaugh (Eds.), *Alzheimer's disease: Cause(s), diagnosis, treatment, and care* (75–84). Boca Raton, FL: CRC Press.

Pillemer, K. (1996). Family caregiving: What would a Martian say? *The Gerontologist, 36,* 269–271.

Pillemer, K., Landreneau, L. T., & Suitor, J. J. (1996a). Volunteers in a peer support project for family caregivers: What motivates them? *American Journal of Alzheimer's Disease, 11,* 13–19.

Pillemer, K., Landreneau, L. T., & Suitor, J. J. (1996b). *Why do caregivers refuse support interventions?* Paper presented to the Gerontological Society of America Annual Meeting, Washington, DC, November 1996.

Pillemer, K. A., & Suitor, J. J. (1992). Violence and violent feelings: What causes them among family caregivers? *Journal of Gerontology: Social Sciences, 47,* S165–S172.

Pillemer, K., & Suitor, J. J. (1996). It takes one to help one: Status similarity and well-being of family caregivers to relatives with dementia. *Journal of Gerontology: Social Sciences, 51,* S250–257.

Rabins, P. V. (1989). Behavioral problems in the demented. In E. Light & B. Lebowitz (Eds.), *Alzheimer's disease treatment and family stress: Directions for research.* Washington, DC: National Institute of Mental Health.

Radloff, Lenore S. (1977). The CES-D Scale: A self-report depression scale for research in the general population. *Applied Psychological Measurement, 11,* 385–401.

Rogers, Nancy. (1999). Caring for those who care: Achieving family caregiver wellness through social support programs. *Activities, Adaptation, and Aging, 24,* 1–12.

Rosenberg, M. (1986). *Conceiving the self.* Melbourne, FL: Academic Press.

Schiaffino, K. M. (1991). Fine-tuning theory to the needs of the world: Responding to Heller et al., *American Journal of Community Psychology, 19,* 99–102.

Schulz, R., & Williamson, G. (1994). Health effects of caregiving: Prevalence of mental and physical illness in Alzheimer's caregivers. In E. Light, G. Niederehe, & B. D. Lebowitz (Eds.), *Stress effects on family caregivers of Alzheimer's patients* (38–63). New York: Springer.

Stephens, M. A. P., Kinney, J. M., & Ogrocki, P. K. (1991). Stressors and well-being among caregivers to older adults with dementia: The in-home versus nursing home experience. *The Gerontologist, 31,* 217–223.

Suitor, J. J., & Pillemer, K. (1993). Support and interpersonal stress in the social networks of married daughters caring for parents with dementia. *Journal of Gerontology: Social Sciences, 48,* S1–S8.

Suitor, J. J., & Pillemer, K. (1996). Sources of support and interpersonal stress in the networks of married caregiving daughters: Findings from a 2-year longitudinal study. *Journal of Gerontology: Social Sciences, 52,* S297–306.

Suitor, J. J., & Pillemer, K. (in Press). Gender, social support, and experiential similarity during chronic stress: The case of family caregivers. In B. Pescosolido & J. Levey (Eds.), *Advances in medical sociology: Social networks.* New York: JAI Press.

Suitor, J. J., Pillemer, K., & Keeton, S. A. (1995). When experience counts: The effects of experiential and structural similarity on patterns of support and interpersonal stress. *Social Forces, 73,* 1573–1588.

Thoits, P. A. (1986). Social support as coping assistance. *Journal of Consulting and Clinical Psychology, 54,* 416–423.

Thornton, P. (1991). Subject to contract?: Volunteers as providers of community care for elderly people and their supporters. *Journal of Aging Studies, 5,* 181–194.

Wasow, M. (1986). Support groups for family caregivers of patients with Alzheimer's disease. *Social Work, 31,* 93–97.

Whitlach, C. J., Zarit, S. H., & von Eye, A. (1991). Efficacy of interventions with caregivers: A reanalysis. *The Gerontologist, 31,* 9–14.

Wright, S. D., Lund, D. A., Pett, M. A., & Caserta, M. S. (1987). The assessment of support group experiences by caregivers of dementia patients. *Clinical Gerontologist, 6,* 5–59.

Zarit, S. H. (1989). Issues and directions in family intervention research. In E. Light & B. D. Lebowitz (Eds.), *Alzheimer's disease treatment and family stress: Directions for research* (458–486). Washington, DC: U.S. Department of Health and Human Services, National Institute of Mental Health.

Zarit, S. H., Anthony, C. R., & Boutselis, B. (1989). Interventions with care givers of dementia patients: Comparison of two approaches. *Psychology and Aging, 2,* 225–232

CHAPTER TWELVE

Closing Thoughts and Future Directions

Phyllis Moen, Karl Pillemer, Elaine Wethington,
Nina Glasgow, and Galyn Vesey

Human beings have long pondered the question, What makes people happy and healthy in later life? Two thousand years ago, the Roman statesman Cicero (1971) in the essay "De Senectute" ("On Old Age") declared his intention to examine "on what principles we may most support the weight of increasing years" (15). He raised the issue of whether a felicitous old age was in fact only possible because of "resources, means, and social position, and that these are advantages which cannot fall to the many" (17). In the United States in the twenty-first century we continue to debate, investigate, and legislate conditions aimed at improving the prospects of those in the second half of life.

This volume focused on one crucial piece of the successful aging puzzle: *social integration.* In the previous chapters we examined factors that promote or inhibit the social connectedness of older Americans, as well as the implications of this integration for their well-being. Chapter authors have approached the issue in a variety of ways, from examining specific dimensions of social integration to considering ways (interventions) to promote it. The book's life-course theme provides important insight into both the causes and consequences of social integration in the later years.

Our life-course perspective highlights the historical, cultural, and social contexts in which older people have become the focus of public and political concern. This perspective recognizes the dynamic nature of roles and circumstances as individuals move through their life course, and the interdependence of lives and life choices among family members. The life-course perspective also focuses attention on situational imperatives confronting families, the possibility for substantial change during crisis and transition, and the accumulation of advantage or disadvantage in individuals' life experiences.

This life-course theme highlights the notion of a "career" of social integration, consisting of shifts in roles, relationships, and responsibilities over time, with concomitant shifts in family needs, resources, and vulnerabilities. Even normative role exits, such as workers moving into retirement, can generate strains and challenges to their integration into society. Unexpected events—one's own illness or that of a family member, widowhood, the inability to continue to drive—are even more apt to place older adults in crisis. Individuals' and families' response to such challenges and their subsequent adaptation influence their integration and life quality in both direct and indirect ways.

In this closing chapter, we highlight several common themes that run throughout the book, suggesting implications for research, intervention, practice, and policy. We also point out gaps in our treatment of the issues, which can be addressed in future work.

Major Themes

1. Rapid social change challenges older people's social integration

Some middle-aged and older individuals have richly rewarding social networks and social roles, and they remain socially integrated well into old age. Many others, however, are socially isolated or are at risk of social isolation. It is not an oversimplification to state that social integration in later life is uniquely challenging. Moreover, it is not a "golden-age" fantasy to argue that older people in past times were typically embedded in family, work, and community life until (or almost until) the close of their own life spans. Indeed, given the much shorter life expectancy, the end of work and family responsibilities typically coincided with the end of life itself (Kertzer & Laslett, 1995). And although very old persons were sometimes neglected or abandoned (Pillemer & Wolf, 1986), the aged typically lived in small communities or ethnic enclaves rich in kin and social exchange ties. During this century, we have seen unprecedented gains in average life expectancy and improvements in health status, but opportunities for older people to participate in meaningful social roles have not kept pace with the positive changes in their health and longevity. Structural lags in older individuals' opportunities to occupy productive social roles while still capable of doing so jeopardize their social integration (Riley & Riley, 1994; Moen, 1998).

This century has seen dramatic changes, touched on throughout this volume, that present unique challenges to staying socially integrated during the second half of life. Early retirement, increased propensity to live alone after divorce or widowhood, geographic mobility of offspring, and—in the baby-boom generation who are now growing old—smaller family sizes, create a large group of older persons for whom social integration is a *task to be accomplished,* rather than a given. Tillie Olsen's story "Tell Me a Riddle," with which we began this volume provides a classic example. In the Old World, relationships may have been good or bad, satisfying or conflictual, but they were at least *there.* In late life, the couple featured in the story must *work* to remain socially integrated, whether by nomadically shuttling among distant children, chasing down old acquaintances, or moving into a retirement community. Complacency and failure to actively reach out lead to isolation.

To point out this difference does not necessarily mean comparing our social situation negatively to that of earlier times. But it does mean that contemporary Americans face historically novel challenges in the second half of life. Finding and sustaining meaningful roles and relationships is a challenge for many, perhaps most, older individuals in contemporary society.

Some might argue that the changes over the past century that threaten social integration are relieved or mitigated by technological advances that allow improved communication over distance. It is beyond the scope of this volume to speculate on the impact of advances in computer and telecommunications technology (e.g., internet, fax) that are now available to older people. We would comment, however, that there is no convincing evidence that such long-distance communication modalities effectively substitute for sustained face-to-face interaction. We are reminded of Sigmund Freud's insight when he posed this hypothetical question seventy years ago:

One would like to ask: is there, then, no positive gain in pleasure, no unequivocal increase in my feeling of happiness, if I can, as often as I please, hear the voice of a child of mine who is living hundreds of miles away, or if I can learn in the shortest possible time after a friend has reached his destination that he has come through the long and difficult voyage unharmed? (Freud [1929], 1961: 35)

Freud responded:

If there had been no railway to conquer distances, my child would never have left his native town, and I should need no telephone to hear his voice; if travelling across the ocean by ship had not been introduced, my friend would not have embarked on his sea-voyage and I should not need a cable to relieve my anxiety about him. (35)

Thus, technology can be a double-edged sword. To be sure, communication technologies allow older persons and their intimates to "keep in touch." But contemporary society has created a fluidity of social relations and an atmosphere of continual changes that make social integration in later life an effort and an achievement.

2. Older persons, as a group, risk social isolation

In earlier chapters, we asked the question, Are older people at greater risk of social isolation than younger age groups? While acknowledging large individual differences, we would answer this question in the affirmative. Age has its impact in at least two ways. Age is a marker of biological and, to some degree, psychological functioning that forms the context for social behavior. Thus, to the extent that increasing age is associated with declines (or perceived declines) in physical or mental health, it limits possibilities for social integration. Throughout this volume, increasing age (especially into the "oldest-old" group of persons, aged 85 and older) is associated with diminished social embeddedness, as networks shrink and the ability to create new ties is diminished by health limitations.

Second, age helps determine social roles, over and above the capacities of individual persons. The loss of work and family roles decreases the number of social ties and can pose a threat to a sense of meaning and self-esteem. For some, retirement also often brings a drop in income that in turn may constrain social activities. Further, American culture and institutions continue to systematically discount older adults. Social scientists have documented both the absence of meaningful integration of older people into productive activities valued by the broader society and its corollary—social isolation and its consequences.

3. Sustaining social integration is problematic for certain subgroups of the older population

The chapters in this volume make it clear that vulnerability to social isolation is not evenly distributed. Some subgroups of older adults are more at risk of social isolation than are others. To be sure, it is difficult to generalize, because certain subgroups have *both* strengths and weaknesses (for example, retirees may lose the work role but gain freedom from demanding or boring jobs, as well as time for volunteer activity, returning to school, active grandparenting, or travel with elder hostels). However, our findings, reviewed below, underscore the heterogeneity of the older segment of the population, with its correspondingly unequal social integration.

Gender matters. Older women are more likely to be without a spouse, to be living alone, and to be unable to drive. They are also less likely to have a continuous work history, with both the social relationships and economic support this implies. Women are more likely to assume family caregiving responsibilities, which we have shown tends to reduce social contacts. However, consistent with their lifetime roles as kinkeepers, women may be able to compensate more successfully for network losses, primarily by maintaining close emotional ties with family members.

Health matters. Perhaps no characteristic is so important a determinant of social integration as health. Physical and psychological impairment, this volume shows, lead to poorer transportation mobility, the inability to stay in one's home, difficulty maintaining friend and neighboring relationships, and difficulty participating in work or volunteer roles. Although these consequences may appear obvious, we are aware of few social integration-enhancement programs that particularly target ill and impaired older persons. Poor health also has a ripple effect on family members, many of whom are also in late middle and old age. People in poor health appear to benefit from social participation, suggesting the importance of interventions for the less healthy segment of the older population.

Geographical context matters. Rural older persons appear to encounter special challenges in their quest to remain socially integrated. Mobility, for example, is more problematic for those living in rural areas—especially in those places that have weak infrastructures of community services. The risk of social isolation in nonmetropolitan areas is greater than in more urban environments, given the low population density and widely scattered settlement patterns. In addition, out-migration of the young in nonmetropolitan communities reduces the availability of close-at-hand, supportive family relationships, particularly between adult children and their older parents. Although rural residents are currently at greater risk of social isolation, older people aging in their individual suburban homes may well face a similar risk for social isolation in the future, especially those who are childless or whose few children live in other parts of the country.

4. Supportive contexts can foster social integration

In this book, we have pointed to how the contexts and environments in which people grow old affect their social integration. For example, safer and more stable neighborhoods have higher rates of neighboring activity. Church and voluntary group memberships facilitate meaningful social participation. The physical and social characteristics of the environment of retirement communities can promote social integration. Community-based services, such as high quality transportation services, facilitate social engagement. And employers can contribute to the social integration of their retirees through the promotion of systemic programs of community service as well as opportunities for post-retirement employment.

The importance of certain ecologies as supportive of social integration, whether in living environments, neighborhoods, or organizations, is a promising and hopeful sign. Interventions that alter these ecologies are a promising way to both enhance the lives of older people and to exploit the talents and energies of this neglected segment of the population.

5. Lives typically reflect cumulative advantage or disadvantage

Individuals who are advantaged in one area of their lives tend to be advantaged in other social roles and relationships. For example, individuals who have (or had) rewarding careers tend also to have better incomes, larger networks of friends and social acquaintances, and greater resources to age successfully. Conversely, disadvantages in employment status, health, income, and even driving status tend to cumulate and compound one another.

The persistence, indeed the widening, of social inequality across the general population of the United States that characterized the last third of the twentieth century has promoted inequality in the lives of older people as well. Reflections of lifetimes of advantage or disadvantage will also color the futures of adults soon moving into their later adult years. Take, for example, the coming development of congregate housing for seniors. Although the burgeoning of new independent living, assisted care, and life care options for older people can be expected to continue, such housing and care options are only available for those who can afford to pay for them. Non-profit and subsidized care for older people with lower incomes must rely upon community largesse, strong volunteer support, and the involvement of family members to produce comparable benefits. Housing and care institutions for the less advantaged are physically separated and segregated from high income and luxury care. To be sure, some institutions and organizations succeed in offering outstanding services to older people in low resource environments. The aging of the baby-boom generation will challenge current housing arrangements and may accentuate the accumulation of disadvantage in the life quality of those already economically disadvantaged.

6. Heterogeneity in the processes of growing old and in the composition of the older population is increasing, with concomitant challenges to social integration

Pathways to and through the later years of adulthood are no longer standardized or routinized. Rather, older Americans are customizing the second halves of their life course, retiring early or never retiring, returning to school, starting second careers, or starting a new career of community participation. One-size-fits-all institutions, policies, and practices are already obsolete. For example, the increase in women's participation in the paid labor force means that retirement can no longer be treated as a one-time, one-way male exit (Han & Moen, 1999). Non-married women must chart their paths through retirement, and two-career couples must coordinate two retirements. Continuous employment during the working years and subsequent retirement from career jobs are relatively new phenomena among women, and we do not yet fully understand what effects these changes will have on their subsequent social integration. The joint retirement decisions of dual-earner couples are frequently problematic, given that spouses may not agree as to the timing of their retirements or the nature of their lives after retirement.

Heterogeneity in the pathways through later adulthood is underscored by the growing ethnic and cultural diversity of the United States as a whole that is mirrored in its aging population. The increasing numbers and proportions of minority older people will lead to greater diversity in life styles, resources, and options of older people. Members of minority groups often enter later adulthood with lower incomes, higher poverty rates, and other accumulated disadvantages. Those living in ethnic enclaves benefit from the social and financial support available in such communities. But members of ethnic or cultural minorities may be at special risk of social isolation, compared to non-Hispanic whites (especially males).

IMPLICATIONS FOR INTERVENTIONS AND SOCIAL INVENTIONS

The findings presented in this volume have a number of implications for intervention. Although social isolation and loneliness constitute significant social problems among older persons, there are no systematic strategies for addressing them. Instead, a number of programs funded by public and private sources have had varying degrees of impact on social isolation. Although practitioners have attempted social support interventions aimed at particular segments of the older population, such efforts (and the technologies to carry them out and evaluate them) are not yet well developed. Developing and assessing efforts to promote social support and meaningful roles among older adults makes sense, given the weight of the evidence that social integration leads to positive outcomes for health and well-being.

To some extent, federal and state governments have responded to the challenge of social isolation among older people. Funding through the Older Americans Act (OAA) for senior centers is perhaps the most notable example (Krout, 1989). These centers have the goal of providing opportunities for social relationships and activity. The congregate meals program funded through the OAA, in addition to nutritional goals, also offers opportunities for socializing. Another federally funded program, the Retired Senior Volunteer Program, provides opportunities for volunteerism on a wide scale. Some communities have implemented specialized transportation services for older people, which link older individuals to social activities, volunteer opportunities, and other services.

At the community level, a range of institutional innovations as well as small-scale voluntary efforts aim at increasing the social integration of older people. Experience Corps, fostered by the non-profit organization Civic Ventures, engages older adults in community services, including tutoring and helping out in neighborhood schools. Some corporations are responding to the needs for continued productive involvement of their retirees, both through rehiring them on a part-time or temporary basis, and by developing special programs that encourage and facilitate volunteering. The National Retiree Volunteer Coalition promotes in-house volunteer programs in corporations for retirees.

Other community-level social support programs include friendly visiting and telephone reassurance projects, as well as support groups targeted toward persons suffering from a particular problem or disease. The past decade has also witnessed growth in intergenerational programs that link older Americans with young people to engage in activities and share experiences.

Our evidence suggests the value of such programs, as well as the need to institutionalize such programs so that they become more widely available. Also needed is systematic evaluation of their effectiveness. What is required are new social inventions aimed at integrating older people into the social fabric of American society. Indeed, the intervention possibilities are as large as the creativity of those who wish to develop them. The three interventions reported on in this volume all point to some possible future directions and ways in which programs can lead to enhanced social integration.

Figure 2.1 in Chapter 2 of this volume suggests an approach for considering priorities for interventions to enhance social integration. Potential goals of social integration interventions are indicated in the middle column: increasing membership in new groups or organizations, expanding networks of friends and supporters, and raising the degree of received functional support (e.g., companionship, information). All of these are measurable outcomes that could be positively influenced by interventions aimed at changing the ecology of later adulthood.

The left column of Figure 2.1 shows where an intervention could have a direct effect on social well-being by increasing support from family and friends and increasing meaningful roles in institutions and organizations. The right column in the figure suggests that interventions can attempt to buffer the effects of threats and disruptions to social well-being. That is, interventions can attempt to reduce the negative impacts of both unpredicted events and predictable life-course transitions.

The intervention programs detailed in Part 3 of this volume describe three different levels of interventions designed to address social integration at three different levels. The educational workshops on transportation (Chapter 9) attempted change at the *individual* level by altering the ways in which individuals conceive of and organize their personal transportation. The Peer Support Project (Chapter 11) focused on change at the level of the *social network*, experimenting with the grafting on of a new social tie to the existing network. The CRVIS project (Chapter 10) investigated change at the *organizational* level by creating a new employer-based organization fostering volunteerism among retirees.

In our view, the key task for future policies and programs is one of *targeting*. We are now at a stage in our knowledge where we must move beyond "scattershot" interventions that seek to promote social integration among persons who are already well integrated to focus on groups with particular needs (such as women living alone, caregivers, persons in poor health or in institutions, isolated rural older persons). Carefully targeted interventions will be the most likely to produce measurable effects.

At the same time, however, systemic, institutionalized structures fostering the connectedness, support, and meaningful engagement of all older Americans should be a national priority. Too often, social integration is viewed as a private trouble, not a public issue. But the ways paid work and retirement are organized, the lack of support for those persons becoming caregivers, the ways volunteers are recruited and volunteer activities are structured, the absence of adequate transportation for older adults in rural and (frequently) urban areas, the lack of housing options for an aging population—all point to the need for social interventions that keep pace with an aging America. We believe that it is important to attempt to match the level of the intervention to the need it addresses. Such social interventions can occur at different levels—national, organizational, community, or household.

Relationships might also be the target of intervention, rather than individuals or social structures. Household members, close kin, and even close friends can be trained to provide regular respite for caregivers in addition to institutionalized, formal respite care, information, and resources for caregivers. Attention to the level of intervention is critical to the invention of new policies and practices and the design of interventions to promote social integration.

RESEARCH IMPLICATIONS

Our life-course focus on social integration points to the need for research focused on the *pathways* by which social relationships enhance or protect health. This refocusing is critical to understanding not only the causes and consequences of social integration in later life but also to informing more targeted and effective interventions.

In Chapter 2 we suggested specific approaches to improve and target research on social integration. Research must begin to develop and use direct, rather than indirect, measures of the mechanisms by which older people remain or become integrated at all levels of society. Although it is abundantly clear that social integration is associated with better health, we believe researchers should target measures of social integration for particular health outcomes (e.g., worsening of degenerative disease versus onset of depression), specific contexts (e.g., urban-suburban-rural), and different subgroups (e.g., men versus women; within as well as across race and ethnicity lines).

The process of social integration unfolds over time, and among older people it is frequently dependent on experiences earlier in the life course (George, 1996; Moen, 1997). Similarly, the course of health in the later adult years is dependent on risks accumulated in youth and middle age. Given the risk that poor health poses to social integration (documented throughout this volume), researchers should conceive of health and integration as dynamically related to one another, with changes in one fostering changes in the other over time. Thus, when estimating models of the impact of social integration on health, researchers should account for the impact of *social selection due to health and life-course factors.*

An important implication is that research designs must account for the possibility of social selection. Researchers can do this in a variety of ways, but the most efficient is the increased use of quasi-experimental designs that can rule out selection factors as an explanation for the findings. At a minimum, researchers should utilize theory and measures sophisticated enough to measure social selection processes.

Changing demographics, economies, and policies render four (related) topics as especially important for future research agendas: caregiving, the aging of the baby-boom population, aging experiences of minority subgroups, and policies aimed at older Americans.

1. Caregiving

The role of kin in caring for family members has been—and remains—an important research topic for scholars of the family and aging. Research that informs the design of interventions to aid family caregivers will require an understanding of family needs across different types of groups, and the level at which different types of intervention should take place.

The problem, however, is that we do not yet fully understand the processes and dynamics of how families assist and care for older family members. We know that many family members choose to care for elderly relatives in their households. But family caregivers and caregiving situations are diverse and in flux. Do adult children commute long or short distances to aid ailing older parents, and is this proportion increasing? Or is it more common for older parents who are alone to move near adult children as their health starts to fail? What are the implications for social integration if older parents move to be closer to their adult children but at the same time lose long-standing social relationships?

Findings in the preceding chapters suggest that family caregiving may follow patterns determined by important life-course factors such as the course of physical decline, the availability of family members in close proximity, the pre-existing closeness of parent-child relationships, place of residence, and the accumulation of advantage or disadvantage.

2. Aging Baby Boomers

Another important gap in research is the knowledge required to make projections about future behavior. Baby boomers are confronting a different world from those who are now retired (Moen 1999).

What is not clear is whether baby boomers will make the same retirement—and life style—choices as their parents. For example, some baby boomers who provide long-distance care for aging parents may make specific plans to remain more physically proximate to relatives, rather than move to a Sunbelt retirement community. Baby boomers who have no or fewer children may have to take active steps to maintain social integration as they age. Those in second marriages or with step-children may follow very different strategies for investing in relationships with children than those who have only their own biological children. Researchers have only begun tracking the impact that sequential, multiple marriages will have on parent-child relationships in the second half of life.

Similarly, even among current retirees, we see workers in younger cohorts expecting to retire earlier than those in later cohorts, and those in their fifties and sixties tend to actually retire earlier than they anticipated (Han & Moen, 1999; Quick & Moen, 1998). Future retirees will be even healthier, better educated, and more vigorous than the currently retired. What do they expect, plan for, and prefer in terms of retirement timing, post-retirement work, housing, and community participation?

3. Minority Groups

A notable gap in the present volume is the lack of specific attention to social integration in minority populations. Our geographical location (in upstate New York) resulted in samples that were almost exclusively white, so we could not generalize the findings to minority group members. Thus, a clear and critically important next step is to examine issues of integration among African American, Hispanic, and other minority groups. For example, the greater likelihood of African American older women to be unmarried, and to have lower incomes over the life course, may place them at higher risk of social isolation in later life (Bronfenbrenner et al., 1996).

Scientific interest in aging in minority communities has grown over the past several decades. Researchers have made significant contributions to our understanding of the experience of minority group members in such areas as health status, family relationships, and service utilization (cf. Jackson, 1980; Markides et al., 1990). Attention has also been devoted to differentials in health status and health care between non-Hispanic whites and minority group members. Much less attention has been paid to conducting research on social integration with minority populations, especially using a life-course perspective. Such efforts should take highest priority in the future.

4. Policies for Older Americans

The issue of social integration in the second half of life is not only prominent among practitioners and researchers, it is also in the political spotlight in the United States at all levels of government. A life-course approach can inform the study of policies related to the later years of adulthood in at least two ways. First, social policies expanding or restricting the older adult's strategies of adaptation can have enduring and possibly unanticipated influences. The timing of government programs and entitlements in the life course may be consequential in fostering the accumulation of advantage or disadvantage over time. Second is the location of individuals and policies in historical context. Policy makers are frequently called upon to respond to the pressure of larger cohorts passing through the social service system, as when the large baby-boom cohorts moved through the educational system and will soon move through the retirement system. Public awareness of increasing longevity is already pointing to the pressures on the retirement system as the baby-boom cohorts move into their later years.

The pervasive intervention of government in so many aspects of contemporary individual and family life is a relatively new phenomenon, concomitant with the rise of the modern welfare state. Federal, state, and local governments touch the lives of those in the second half of life in every aspect of decision making—from educational opportunities, jobs, housing, health care, income security and transfers, to widowhood. This mounting body of public regulation and influence, however, represents in the United States a series of incremental decisions and creates a tacit, often contradictory, rather than explicit set of policies.

Moreover, governments usually provide services and benefits to individuals, not families. Retirement, health care, housing, transportation, and disability, however, are apt to involve families as well as individuals. Thus, it is important for researchers to sort out how policies and programs will affect individuals and their families as both caregivers and receivers of care. Policies and programs that foster a supportive context for individuals and their families are likely to promote the social integration and overall quality of life of people in the second half of life.

Regional, ethnic, and religious differences in values have precluded a consensus on the role of government in the second half of life, much less a common understanding of the "proper" roles of families or of older women and men within society. Similarly, the layered structure of government—city, county, state, federal, as well as executive, legislative, and judicial—encourages a patchwork of often incompatible legislation and regulation in lieu of a national policy addressing the needs and well-being of older Americans. What is required is visionary research and thinking—looking across the life course to anticipate how policies will affect overall well-being and social integration during different stages of the life course.

A FINAL WORD

Taken together, the chapters in this volume suggest several components of a new vision of older people in contemporary America. What is clear is that growing numbers of older Americans and their families are confronting outmoded structures and belief systems regarding aging that are no longer in step with today's—and tomorrow's—realities. The gaps between the social organization and culture of old age and the experiences and preferences of those in later adulthood are becoming increasingly apparent. The question is, What is the role of government in bridging these gaps?

We in the United States, individually and collectively, remain uncertain, if not divided, as to what the role of government should be in supporting older Americans. Attitudes about employment, aging, and the role of adult children are ambivalent and contradictory. This uncertainty is of pivotal importance in seeking to understand the lack of any coherent political or private sector response to the changing age structure in this country. For example, because of the absence of consensus about retirement and employment, or about the role of government in these matters, we are markedly reluctant to adopt social policies and institutional arrangements designed to provide "bridge" jobs, which would ease the transition from full time career work to full time retirement, or options to reduce work hours among those wanting to remain in their career jobs but work less (Quinn, 1999). Clearly, however, policies to promote job opportunities and more flexible job arrangements among older workers would capture the productive capacity of older individuals while also fostering the social integration of older Americans.

The United States does have a policy to promote the welfare and well-being of the older population, as exemplified by Social Security and Medicare (Bronfenbrenner et al., 1996). As a consequence, the poverty rate of older people is much lower in this new millennium than was the case in the middle of the twentieth century. Particular subgroups of the older population, such as women, minorities, oldest-old, rural residents, and individuals who live alone, however, have not shared equally in the overall rising affluence of the older population. A fresh vision of social policy is needed to address the realities of older people who are economically secure and who can make valuable contributions to society in paid work, volunteer, educational, and other productive roles, provided opportunities to do so are available to them. For those older people in contemporary America who are economically insecure, the more immediate concern of policy makers is to promote their economic well-being, but in doing so, the social integration of disadvantaged groups within our society can also be promoted.

How can we, as a nation, provide support for individuals and families in the second half of life without at the same time promoting dependency rather than independence? How can government programs work in partnership with families to promote social integration and well-being without constraining options and opportunities? As we move through the early twenty-first century, these are the kinds of questions facing citizens in and out of government who are concerned with social integration in the second half of life. The dramatic growth in the aging population makes a concerted approach to research, intervention, and policy necessary. We hope that the present volume has provided a starting point for future efforts on these fronts.

REFERENCES

Bronfenbrenner, U., McClelland, P., Wethington, E., Moen, P., & Ceci, S. J. (1996). *The state of Americans: This generation and the next.* New York: Free Press.

Cicero, M. T. (1971). *De senectute, De amicitia, De divinatione.* Trans. W. A. Falconer. Cambridge: Harvard University Press.

Freud, Sigmund. ([1929], 1961). *Civilization and its discontents*. New York: W. W. Norton.

George, L. K. (1996). Social factors and illness. In R. H. Binstock et al. (Eds.), *Handbook of aging and the social sciences*, 4th ed. (229–252). San Diego: Academic Press.

Han, S.-K., & Moen, P. (1999). Clocking out: Temporal patterning of retirement. *American Journal of Sociology, 105*, 191–236.

Hill, R. (1970). *Family development in three generations*. Cambridge, MA: Schenkman Publishing.

Jackson, J. J. (1980). *Minorities and aging*. Belmont, CA: Wadsworth.

Kertzer, D. I., & Laslett, P. (Eds.) (1995). *Aging in the past: Demography, society, and old age*. Berkeley: University of California Press.

Krout, J. A. (1989). *Senior centers in America*. New York: Greenwood Press.

Laslett, Peter. (1991). *A fresh map of life: The emergence of the third age*. Cambridge: Harvard University Press.

Litwak, E. (1985). *Helping the elderly: The complementary roles of informal networks and formal systems*. New York: Guilford.

Litwak, E., & Szelenyi, I. (1969). Primary group structures and functions: Kin, neighbors and friends. *American Sociological Review, 34*, 465–481.

Markides, K. S., Liang, J., & Jackson, J. S. (1990). Race, ethnicity, and aging: Conceptual and methodological issues. In R. H. Binstock & L. K. George (Eds.), *Handbook of aging and the social sciences*, 3rd ed. (112–129). San Diego: Academic Press.

McCubbin, H. I. (1979). Integrating coping behavior in family stress theory. *Journal of Marriage and the Family, 41*, 237–244.

Moen, P. (1997). Women's roles and resilience: Trajectories of advantage or turning points? In I. H. Gotlib & B. Wheaton (Eds.), *Stress and adversity over the life course: Trajectories and turning points* (133–156). New York: Cambridge University Press.

Moen, P. (1998). Recasting careers: Changing reference groups, risks, and realities. *Generations, 22*, 40–45.

Moen, P. (1999). *The Cornell Couples and Careers Study*. Ithaca: Cornell Employment and Family Careers Institute.

Moen, P., Robison, J., & Dempster-McClain, D. (1995). Caregiving and women's well-being: A life course approach. *Journal of Health and Social Behavior, 36*, 259–273.

Moen, P., Robison, J., & Fields, V. (1994). Women's work and caregiving roles: A life course approach. *Journal of Gerontology: Social Sciences, 49*, S176–S186.

Mogey, J. (1990). *Aiding and aging: The coming crisis in support for the elderly by kin and state.* New York: Greenwood.

Pillemer, K., & Wolf, R. (1986). *Elder abuse: Conflict in the family.* Dover, MA: Auburn House.

Quick, H. E., & Moen, P. (1998). Gender, employment, and retirement quality: A life-course approach to the differential experiences of men and women. *Journal of Occupational Health Psychology, 3,* 44–64.

Quinn, Joseph F. (1999). *Retirement patterns and bridge jobs in the 1990s.* Employee Benefit Research Institute Policy Brief No. 206. Washington, DC: EBRI.

Riley, M. W., & Riley, J. W., Jr. (1994). Structural lag: Past and future. In M. W. Riley, R. L. Kahn, & A. Foner (Eds.), *Age and structural lag: Society's failure to provide meaningful opportunities in work, family and leisure* (15–36). New York: Wiley.

Robison, J., Moen, P., and Dempster-McClain, D. (1995). Women's caregiving: Changing profiles and pathways. *Journal of Gerontology: Social Sciences, 50B,* S362–373.

Shanas, E., & Sussman, M. B. (1977). *Family, bureaucracy, and the elderly.* Durham, NC: Duke University Press.

Stack, C. B. (1974). *All our kin: Strategies for survival in a black community.* New York: Harper and Row.

Stone, R., Cafferata, G. L., & Sangl, J. (1987). Caregivers of the frail elderly: A national profile. *The Gerontologist, 17,* 486–491.

U.S. House of Representatives Select Committee on Aging. (1988). Exploding the myths: Caregiving in America Publication. No. 100–665. Washington, DC: U.S. Government Printing Office.

Author Index

Adelman, P. K., 25
Aizenberg, R., 245
Ajzen, I., 166, 182n.2
Akiyama, H., 35
Albright, B., 5
Allen, J., 88
Almeida, D. M., 63
Amato, P., 212
Anapolle, 245
Anderson, D., 247
Anderson, K. H., 89
Angelelli, J. J., 30
Anthony, C. R., 266, 275
Antonucci, T. C., 24, 35, 39, 82, 84, 97, 139
Arbuckle, N. W., 4
Archbold, P. G., 134
Arndt, L., 49, 65
Artis, J. E., 88
Atchley, R. C., 89, 159, 214, 250
Avery, R., 162

Baltes, M. M., 84, 233
Baltes, P. B., 84, 233
Barbee, A. P., 146
Barfield, R., 89, 253
Barker, W. H., 265
Barley, S. R., 79
Barnett, R. C., 98
Barrera, M., Jr., 9
Barrett, A. L., 35
Baruch, G. K., 98
Bass, D. M., 267, 276
Bass, S. A., 248, 252, 253
Beale, C. L., 113, 120, 233
Becker, J., 136, 137, 266

Beckman, J., 166
Bell, R. R., 141
Bellah, R., 20
Belle, D., 193
Belsky, J., 141
Berg, S., 4
Berger, A. M., 108, 110, 114, 121
Berkman, L. F., 24, 26, 56, 96, 123, 134, 137
Biegel, D. E., 233, 270
Bielby, D., 64
Bielby, W. T., 64
Birkel, R. C., 134
Blakely, R., 111–12
Blum, C., 137
Bodin, L. L., 213
Bolger, N., 49, 51, 63
Bongaarts, J., 31
Bookwala, J., 133
Booth, A., 8, 53, 212
Bosworth, H. D., 24
Bound, J., 89
Bourdieu, P., 80
Boutselis, B., 266, 275
Bowen, N., 160, 212
Bowers, B. J., 213
Bowlby, J., 56
Bowling, A., 24
Bradsher, J. E., 161, 162
Brathwaite, J., 212
Brecht, B., 1–2
Breiger, R., 80
Brennan, P. F., 267
Breslow, L., 96
Brinton, M., 81
Brody, E. M., 88, 134

Bronfenbrenner, U., 4, 27, 28, 262, 299, 302
Brown, A. C., 213
Brown, D. L., 7, 110, 122
Brown, G. W., 57, 61, 66
Brown, K. H., 89
Brown, S. L., 266
Bruce, M. L., 24, 49, 66
Buckwalter, K. C., 266
Bull, C. N., 113
Bultena, G. L., 33, 211
Burch, T. K., 33
Burchett, B. M., 81, 89
Burkhardt, J. E., 108, 110, 114, 121
Burkhauser, R. V., 37, 81, 89
Butler, R. N., 101, 192
Bylund, R. A., 114

Campbell, K. E., 35
Cantor, M., 134, 191, 192, 194, 195
Cantor, N., 48
Caro, F. G., 248, 252, 253
Carp, F., 108, 111, 112, 113, 126, 128
Carr, D., 51
Carstensen, L., 198
Caserta, M. S., 268
Casper, L., 192
Cassidy, M. L., 7, 113
Catalano, R., 78
Catternach, L., 135
Ceci, S. J., 4, 27, 28, 262, 299, 302
Chaikin, A., 196, 197
Chambré, S. M., 39, 96
Chatters, L., 193, 195, 196
Chen, M. D., 58
Chenoweth, B., 134
Cherlin, A., 192
Chevan, A., 212
Chirikos, T. N., 81, 89
Choi, N. G., 213
Chriboga, D. A., 137
Cicero, M. T., 287
Cicirelli, V. G., 140, 281
Clark, M. S., 192, 197
Clipp, E. C., 79, 135
Cohen, B., 48, 59
Cohen, C., 137

Cohen, R., 123
Cohen, S., 59, 61, 192, 197, 267
Collins, J., 233
Colsher, P. L., 164
Cooney, L. M., Jr., 110
Coppel, D. B., 136, 137, 266
Cordes, S. M., 112
Coriell, M., 48, 59
Coser, R. L., 25
Coward, R. T., 7, 33, 111, 113
Cox, G. B., 136, 266
Cox, M., 141
Cox, R., 141
Coyne, J. C., 197
Crawford, C. O., 114
Creasey, G. L., 136, 138
Crimmins, E. M., 4, 186
Crystal, S., 140
Cumming, E., 21
Cunningham, M. R., 146
Cutler, S. J., 7, 113, 232
Cutrona, C. E., 48, 59, 218

Danermark, B. D., 213
Davies, R., 37
de Vries, B., 4
Dean, A., 36
Deimling, G. T., 276
DeLongis, A., 51
Demers, A., 275, 266
Dempster-McClain, D., 25, 26, 38, 48, 50, 51, 52, 54, 56, 61, 63, 82, 89, 96, 123, 216
Derlega, V. J., 146, 196, 197
Derogatis, L., 198
DeViney, S., 81
Dewit, D. J., 33
Dooley, D., 78
Douvan, E., 197
Druen, P. B., 146
Dugan, E., 24
Dunkel-Shetter, C., 146
Durkheim, E., 19–20, 40, 50
Dwyer, J. W., 7, 33
Dykstra, P. A., 4

Easterlin, R. A., 4, 31, 32
Ebaugh, H. R. F., 84, 253
Eckenrode, J., 24, 63, 65, 196, 212, 267
Eckert, J. K., 197
Edwards, J. N., 8
Eisenhandler, S. A., 109
Ekerdt, D. J., 82
Ekstrom, M. E., 213
Elder, G. H., Jr., 6, 51, 75, 77, 79, 80, 81, 159, 160, 167, 211
Ellard, J. H., 60
Ellison, C. G., 96
Epperson, M. J., 136, 138
Erikson, E. H., 101, 261
Erikson, J. M., 101, 261
Evans, D. R., 4
Eysenck, H. B., 197, 199
Eysenck, S. B. G., 197, 199

Farquhar, M., 24
Fawzy, N., 49, 65
Fawzy, R. I., 49, 65
Featherman, D. L., 84
Feinleib, M., 53
Fengler, A. P., 126, 134
Fernandez, M. E., 24
Field, D., 36
Fields, V., 50, 60, 78, 88, 96, 97, 139, 247, 261
Filenbaum, G. G., 81, 89
Fiore, J., 136, 137, 266
Fischer, C. S., 36, 192, 193, 199
Fischer, L. R., 96, 252, 253
Fishbein, M., 166, 182n
Fisher, J. D., 197
Fiske, A. P., 193
Fleisher, D., 206
Fleissner, K., 133
Fligstein, N., 81
Foley, D. J., 110
Foner, A., 4, 22, 52, 77, 80, 84
Francies, G. R., 254
Franks, M. M., 138
Freedman, M., 247, 250, 253, 254, 258
Freud, S., 289–90
Fullinwider, R. K., 20

Gall, T. L., 4
Gallagher, S. K., 146
Galliher, G. M., 113
Galston, W. A., 260
Gatz, M., 4
George, L. K., 4, 6, 24, 48, 49, 75, 77, 81, 89, 135, 136, 140, 276, 297
Gerson, K., 64
Gerstel, N., 146
Giele, J., 51, 159, 211
Glaser, R., 133
Glasgow, N., 7, 26, 33, 34, 38, 96, 110, 111, 112, 113, 120, 122, 124, 161, 216, 233
Glass, T., 163
Gleason, H. P., 101
Glosser, G., 268
Gober, P., 160
Golant, S. M., 212, 213
Goldscheider, F. K., 211
Gonyea, J. G., 268
Goode, W., 198
Goodrich, N., 134
Gordon, E., 233, 270
Gore, S., 24, 267
Gotay, C. C., 197
Gottlieb, B. H., 233, 236, 266, 269
Gouldner, H., 141
Gove, W. R., 26
Grafstroem, M., 134
Gray, L. N., 164
Greenberger, E., 51
Groves, M. A., 212
Guacci, N., 35
Gubrium, J. F., 140
Gulley, M. R., 146
Gupta, V., 270
Guralnik, J., 123
Gwyther, L. P., 135, 136, 276

Haas, W. H., III, 161
Hade-Kaplan, B., 206
Hagan, J. M., 212
Hagestad, G. O., 78
Haley, W. E., 133, 134, 266
Han, S.-K., 76, 81, 293, 299
Hareven, T. K., 30

Haring, M. J., 96
Harlow, R. E., 48
Harris, T. O., 57, 61, 66
Harrison, J., 36, 146
Haven, C., 3, 48
Havighurst, R., 3, 22
Haynes, S. G., 53
Hegeman, C., 5
Heller, K., 269, 281
Henderson, C., 5, 217
Henry, W., 21
Herbert, T., 61
Herzog, A. R., 38, 39, 84, 247, 248, 253
Hetherington, E. M., 141
Hochschild, A. R., 22, 192, 195
Hofferth, S. L., 7
Hofmeister, H., 81, 93, 94
Hogg, J. R., 269, 281
Holden, C., 110
Holden, K., 7
Holmes, T. H., 213
Hong, J., 25
Hopkins, K., 58
Horowitz, A., 88
House, J. S., 38, 49, 52, 57, 58, 66, 96, 192, 193, 195, 198, 247
Howard, J., 4
Hull, J. G., 24
Hunt, A. R., 248

Iceland, J., 7
Ingeneri, D. G., 186
Ingersoll-Dayton, B., 192, 199
Ingram, S., 48, 59
Iutcovich, J. M., 110, 111, 232
Iutcovich, M., 110, 111, 232

Jackson, D. J., 161, 162
Jackson, J. J., 299
Jackson, J. S., 39, 84, 193, 195, 196, 299
Janoski, T., 38
Jarrett, W. H., 140
Jarrott, S. E., 140
Jensen, L., 126
Jette, A. M., 4
Jewson, R. H., 84
Johansson, L., 140

Johnson, D. R., 8
Jones, C. J., 134
Jourard, S., 196
Juster, F. T., 169

Kahana, E., 97
Kahn, R. L., 1, 4, 22, 39, 52, 60, 80, 84, 192, 253
Kahneman, D., 164, 165, 167, 182n
Kain, E. L., 80, 81
Kaiser, M. A., 195
Kalish, R. A., 4
Kane, R. A., 266
Kaplan, G. A., 123
Kaplan, H. B., 267
Karasik, R. J., 213
Kasl, S. V., 134, 137, 163
Katz, D., 60
Keeton, S., 30, 141, 149, 268
Keith, V. M., 36, 146
Kertzer, D. I., 30, 288
Kessler, R. B., 4, 24, 48, 51, 57, 58, 61, 62, 63
Kessler, R. C., 51, 57, 62, 197
Kiecolt-Glaser, J. K., 133
Kilty, K. M., 94
Kim, J., 81, 92–93, 94, 95
Kinney, J. M., 276
Kivett, V. R., 24
Kivnick, H. Q., 101, 261
Knight, B. G., 140
Knudsen, L., 123
Kohn, M. L., 63, 79
Korte, C., 270
Krause, N., 35
Krout, J. A., 7, 33, 160, 212, 294
Kuhl, J., 166
Kukulka, G., 113
Kulka, R., 197

Laird, M., 212
Lakey, B., 266, 267, 268
Landis, K. L., 192, 193, 195
Landis, K. R., 49, 52, 57, 58, 66
Landreneau, L. T., 274, 281
Lane, M., 36
Lang, A., 134

Larson, R. D., 63
Laslett, P., 30, 37, 288
Lavoie, J., 275, 266
Lawton, L., 162
Lawton, M. P., 140, 211, 213
Lee, G. R., 7, 8, 33, 84, 113
Lehman, D. R., 60, 197
Lemke, S., 213
Lent, R. W., 166
Lepore, S., 51
Levine, E. G., 266
Levine, P., 260
Levitt, M. J., 35
Liang, J., 123, 299
Lichenstein, P., 4
Lieberman, M., 195, 197
Light, S. C., 141
Lin, N., 141
Link, B. G., 58
Linville, P. W., 59
Litwak, E., 55, 56, 160, 161, 194, 195, 212
Lloyd, K., 81
Logan, J. R., 33, 190
Long, L., 212
Longino, C. F., Jr., 24, 34, 160, 161, 162, 212
Loomis, L. M., 212
Lowe, J. C., 78
Lowenthal, M., 3, 48
Lu, X., 123
Lund, D. A., 268
Lutz, C. J., 266, 267, 268
Lynch, J. A., 35
Lynch, S. A., 146

Macdonald, C., 4
Mace, N., 134
Macunovich, D. J., 4
Madsen, R., 20
Maguire, P., 36, 146
Manton, K. G., 4
Marini, M. M., 211
Marino, F., 36
Markides, K. S., 299
Marottoli, R. A., 110
Marsden, P. V., 35

Marshall, V., 24
Martin Matthews, A., 89
Marx, J., 212
Matt, G. E., 36
Mattlin, J., 199
McAvay, G. J., 24, 49, 66
McCarthy, C., 267
McClearn, G. E., 4
McClelland, P., 4, 27, 28, 262, 299, 302
McClendon, M. J., 267
McGavok, A. T., 110, 121
McGhee, J. L., 126
McHugh, K. E., 160
McLanahan, S. A., 192
McLaughlin, D., 7
McLeod, J. D., 57
Meddaugh, D. L., 135
Menaghan, E. G., 98
Mendes de Leon, C., 163
Menken, J. A., 31
Merril, S. S., 110
Merton, R. K., 84
Messeri, P., 55, 56, 195
Metzner, H. L., 96
Mickelson, K. D., 62
Miller, J. B., 36
Mills, J., 197
Milton, S., 112, 238
Miner, S., 32
Minkler, M., 36
Moen, P., 4, 6, 7, 25, 26, 27, 28, 37, 38, 48, 50, 51, 52, 54, 56, 60, 61, 63, 76, 77, 78, 80, 81, 82, 84, 88, 89, 90, 92, 93, 94, 95, 96, 97, 100, 101, 110, 120, 123, 139, 159, 160, 211, 212, 216, 247, 248, 261, 262, 289, 293, 297, 298, 299, 302
Moore, J. W., 78
Moorman, J. E., 192
Moos, R. H., 213
Morgan, D. L., 34
Morgan, J. N., 39, 84, 89, 247, 248, 253
Moritz, D. J., 134, 137
Morris, J. C., 265
Morris, R., 261
Morris, S. A., 213
Morrow-Howell, N., 254

Mossey, J., 24
Mueller, M. W., 255
Mui, A., 254
Mullan, J. T., 191
Mullins, L. G., 24
Musick, M. A., 38, 247
Mutran, E., 24
Myers, B., 136, 138

Nadler, A., 197
Neilsen, K., 137
Nestel, G., 81, 89
Neugarten, B. L., 78
Newby-Clark, I., 61
Newman, S. J., 161
Nisbet, R. A., 20
Noburn, J. E., 24
Norris-Baker, C., 114
Norton, A. J., 192

O'Brien, A. T., 133
O'Bryant, S. L., 135
O'Conner, P., 36
Oggins, J., 160, 212, 217
Ogrocki, P. K., 276
Okun, M. A., 36, 96, 146
Oliker, S. J., 36
Olsen, Tillie, 2, 289
O'Neil, R., 51
O'Rand, A. M., 81
Orthner, D. K., 213
Ostfeld, A. M., 110
Oxman, T. E., 24

Palmore, E. B., 81, 89
Parkes, C. T., 58
Pasnau, R. O., 49, 65
Patton, C. V., 110, 120, 232
Pavalko, E. K., 79, 88
Pearlin, L. I., 191, 261
Pedersen, N. L., 4
Penrod, J. D., 266
Peplau, L. A., 218
Perkinson, M. A., 215
Perlman, G. D., 110
Peters, G. R., 195
Peterson, J. G., 84

Pett, M. A., 268
Pezzin, L. E., 32
Phelan, J., 58
Pierce, G. R., 48
Pillemer, K., 5, 30, 132, 138, 139, 140,
    141, 142, 143, 147, 149, 151, 265, 266,
    268, 274, 276, 281, 288
Pitceathly, C., 36, 146
Poon, L. W., 61
Putnam, R., 20
Pynoos, J., 206

Quadagno, J., 78
Quick, H., 84, 89, 90, 299
Quinn, J. F., 37, 81, 301
Qureshi, H., 88

Rabins, P. V., 276
Radloff, L. S., 275
Rahal, T. A., 61
Rahe, R. H., 213
Redfoot, D. L., 212
Reid, N., 160
Reitzes, D. C., 24
Reshovsky, J. D., 161
Revis, B. D., 110, 112, 120
Revis, J. A., 110, 112, 120
Richardson, H., 110, 120
Richardson, V., 94
Riggio, R. E., 146
Riley, J. W., Jr., 248, 289
Riley, M. W., 4, 22, 52, 77, 78, 80, 84,
    248, 289
Robbins, C. A., 96
Robison, J., 25, 30, 50, 60, 78, 88, 96, 97,
    139, 160, 163, 216
Rockerman, D., 215
Rogers, A., 162
Rogers, N., 266
Rook, K. S., 56, 59, 78, 137, 194, 195
Rose, A. M., 22
Rosenberg, M., 275
Rosenbloom, S., 112, 118, 121
Rosow, I., 3, 22–24, 75, 84, 163, 191,
    193, 196, 211
Ross, H. K., 191, 197, 206
Ross, M., 61

Rossi, A. S., 33, 146
Rossi, P. H., 33, 146, 160
Rovine, M., 141
Rowe, E., 212
Rowe, J. W., 1
Rowell, K. R., 212
Rowles, G., 7
Rubin, D., 61
Ruchlin, H. S., 213
Ruggles, S., 30
Russell, D., 218
Ryder, N. B., 78

Sampson, R., 193
Sarason, B. A., 48
Sarason, I. G., 48
Schaffer, K. B., 96, 252, 253
Schaie, K. W., 24
Scheidt, R. J., 114, 213
Schiaffino, K. M., 270
Schneider, C. J., 89
Schone, B. S., 32
Schooler, C., 63
Schorr, J., 198
Schudson, M., 20
Schulz, R., 133, 265
Schuster, S., 194, 195
Schuster, T. L., 56
Scott, A., 37
Secombe, K., 84
Seeman, T. E., 24, 49, 66, 123
Selzer, M. M., 25
Semple, S. J., 138, 191
Serow, W. J., 161
Shahtahmasebi, S., 37
Shanahan, M. J., 6, 75, 77
Shaver, P. R., 62
Shaw, L. B., 135
Sheehan, N. W., 213
Sherrod, D., 192, 197
Sherwood, C. C., 213
Sherwood, S., 213
Shore, B. K., 233, 270
Sieber, S., 50, 59, 198
Siegel, J. S., 26, 27, 28, 29, 30, 33, 34, 37
Silverstein, M., 30, 55, 56
Skaff, M. N., 191

Slaten, E., 58
Slater, P., 20
Slocum, W. L., 79
Slokan, L., 146
Smith, D. B., 81
Smith, D. H., 254
Smith, J., 84
Smith, K. J., 162
Smyth, K. A., 136, 137
Sommers, D. G., 212
Sorce, P., 212
Speare, A., Jr., 162, 211
Spencer, R., 134
Spitze, G., 33, 190
Stack, C., 193
Stephens, M. A. P., 4, 138, 276
Sterns, H. L., 245
Sterns, R., 245
Stock, W. A., 96
Strain, L., 36
Strecher, V., 96
Streib, G. F., 89
Strong, M. S., 141
Stuckey, J. C., 136, 137
Sugisawa, H., 123
Suitor, J. J., 30, 132, 138, 139, 140, 141, 142, 143, 147, 149, 151, 265, 268, 274, 276, 281
Sullivan, W. M., 20
Swidler, A., 20, 80
Syme, L., 56
Syme, S. L., 26, 123
Szelenyi, I., 194

Taietz, P., 112, 238
Takahashi, K., 197
Talbot, D. M., 112, 233, 239
Tallman, I., 164
Taylor, J., 136, 138
Taylor, R. J., 193, 195, 196
Tebes, J. K., 135
Teresi, J., 137
Thaler, R. H., 165
Thoits, P. A., 25, 49, 50, 56, 57, 58, 59, 60, 62, 65, 66, 82, 84, 98, 124, 141, 142, 215, 267
Thompson, M. G., 269, 281

Thornton, P., 270
Tipton, S. M., 20
Todd, P. A., 97, 136
Toennies, Ferdinand, 20
Tomaskovic-Devey, D., 81
Townsend, A. L., 138
Trueba, P. E., 269, 281
Tucker, C. J., 212
Tucker, R., 24
Turner, R. J., 36, 81
Tversky, A., 164, 165, 167, 182n
Tyler, P. R., 212

Uhlenberg, P., 31, 32, 33
Umberson, D., 4, 49, 52, 57, 58, 59, 66, 192, 193, 195, 206

Van Arsdol, M. D., Jr., 160
Van Willigen, J., 193
VanderHart, P. G., 212
Verbrugge, L., 52, 53
Veroff, J., 197
Vilhjalmsson, R., 57
Vinick, B. H., 82
Vlachos-Weber, I., 269, 281
von Eye, A., 266

Walker, A., 88
Wallace, R. B., 164
Wallman, L. M., 81, 89
Waring, J., 77
Wasow, M., 270
Watkins, S. C., 31
Weber, R. A., 35
Weiler, P. G., 137
Weinick, R. M., 186
Weiss, R. S., 58
Welch, S., 53
Wenger, C. G., 37

Wentowski, M., 193
Wethington, E., 4, 24, 27, 28, 48, 51, 57, 58, 61, 62, 63, 65, 81, 160, 192, 196, 197, 199, 262, 299, 302
Wexler, D., 268
Wheaton, B., 81, 82
Whitbeck, L. B., 7, 8, 113
Whitlach, C. J., 266
Williams, R. M., 25, 26, 38, 48, 50, 51, 52, 54, 56, 61, 63, 82, 89, 96, 123, 216
Williamson, G., 265
Wills, T. A., 267
Wilson, V. F., 212
Winblad, B., 134
Winstead, B. A., 146
Wiseman, R. F., 212
Wister, A. V., 33, 36
Witchner-Alagna, S., 197
Witter, R. A., 96
Woelfel, M. W., 141
Wolf, D. A., 4
Wolf, R. S., 140, 288
Wolf, W., 81
Wortman, C. B., 4, 60, 197
Wright, S. D., 268
Wuthnow, R., 261

Yankleelov, P. A., 146
Yee, W., 160
Yordy, G. A., 166
Youmans, E. G., 33, 112
Young, F. W., 26, 38, 96, 123, 216
Young, R., 97

Zarit, J. M., 97, 136
Zarit, S. H., 97, 136, 140, 266, 270–71, 275
Zimmerman, J., 146
Zimmerman, R. S., 161, 162

Subject Index

African Americans: home improvement and, 176; housing expectations and, 173–84; marital status and, 28; migration and, 162; neighboring and, 196

age: continuing care retirement community and, 223; driving status and, 119–22; housing expectations and, 172–84; and the life course, 77–78; marriage and, 26–28; neighboring and, 199–200; retirement and, 80–100; social integration and, 290–91; social networks, 35; volunteering and, 39

ageism, 23, 41

Alzheimer's disease, 133–34, 265–66. *See also* caregivers

baby-boom generation: intergenerational relationships and, 31–32; and longevity, 31–32; marriage and, 4, 29–30, 31–32; neighboring and, 191–92; research agenda about, 298–99; social integration and, 4; volunteering and, 248

boredom and retirement, 91–92, 97

caregivers: Alzheimer's, 132–52, 265–82; changes across time, 148–51; and educational attainment, 136; family as, 5, 132–52, 265–82; and gender, 138, 146–48, 281; health of, 133–34, 136–38, 151–52, 268; housing expectations and, 173–82; and income level, 136; interventions for, 266, 269–73; and life-course theory, 139–43; literature review of, 133–38, 267–

68; and marriage, 138; neighboring and, 204–5; research agenda, 298; research examples, 143–52; retirement and, 88, 97; social integration of, 5, 132–52; social networks of, 134–36; social support of, 136–38, 144–52; theories about, 139–43, 267–68; transition to, 140–41; transportation and, 124–26

Caregivers Across Time study, 143–52

children. *See* family

church. *See* religious participation

city. *See* metropolitan areas

club membership: continuing care retirement communities and, 220–22; and gender, 86; neighboring and, 200–201; retirement and, 86, 96, 98–100; transportation and, 124–26

contextual measurement approach, 57–60

continuing care retirement communities, 211–24; and age, 223; and club membership, 220–22; and family, 218–19; and friendships, 220; and gender, 220–21, 223; and health, 224; and loneliness, 216–17, 222–24; and marriage, 222–23; and neighboring, 220, 221, 224; and roles, 215–16, 220–22; and social networks, 214–15; and social support, 215–17; and volunteering, 220–22, 224; and work, 220–22, 224

continuity theory, 214

Cornell Retirees Volunteering in Service program, 247–62

Cornell Retirement and Well-Being Study, 83–100, 164–84, 247–262
Cornell Transportation and Social Integration of Nonmetropolitan Older Persons Study, 115–27, 231
crime, neighboring and, 193, 198, 201–2

data: from the *Caregivers Across Time* study, 143–52; from the *Cornell Retirement and Well-Being Study*, 83–100, 164–84, 247–62; from the *Cornell Transportation and Social Integration of Nonmetropolitan Older Persons Study*, 115–27, 231; from the *General Social Survey*, 34–35; life history, 61; longitudinal, 61–63; from the *Longitudinal Study on Aging*, 161–62, 212–13; from the *National Long-Term Care Survey*, 33; from the *National Survey of Families and Households*, 33; on neighboring, 198–99; from the *New Haven Established Population for Epidemiologic Studies of the Elderly*, 163; from the *Pathways to Life Quality* project, 217–18; from the *Peer Support Project*, 144–52; SUNY-HSC data about Alzheimer's patients, 270–71; from the *Understanding Senior Housing for the 1990s* survey, 169
death, 3–4. *See also* longevity
disengagement theory, 21-22
divorce, 26–28, 32
driving by older persons. *See* transportation of older persons

economic costs of family caregiving, 134
educational attainment: caregivers and, 136; migration and, 161; neighboring and, 199–200; retirement and, 90, 99
empirical strategies. *See* research methods

family: as caregivers, 5, 132–52, 265–82; continuing care retirement communities and, 218–19; finances of, 81;

geographic proximity of children, 3, 33–34; health and, 96–97; housing expectations and, 173–82; living arrangements of, 28–29, 30–31; neighboring and, 194–96; retirement and, 87–88, 90–91, 96; social support and, 35–36, 55–57; transportation and, 111–12, 118, 124–26; volunteering and, 256. *See also* intergenerational relationships
friendships: continuing care retirement communities and, 220; neighboring and, 202–3; social support and, 35–36, 55–57; transportation and, 111–12, 118, 124–26

gender: Alzheimer's caregivers and, 138, 146–48, 281; club participation of retirees and, 86; continuing care retirement communities and, 220–21, 223; driving status and, 119–23, 127; housing expectations and, 172–83; marriage and, 28, 87; neighboring and, 199–200, 203–4; religious participation of retirees and, 86; retirement and, 87–88, 90–100; social integration and, 291; social support and, 36; transportation and, 110–12, 116–18, 126–27; volunteering and, 86, 258; and widowhood, 26–28; work and, 37, 53
General Social Survey, 34–35
geographic proximity of children: literature review of, 33–34; neighboring and, 202; and social networks, 3; trends, 33–34

Habits of the Heart (Robert Bellah et al), 20
health: of caregivers, 133–34, 136–38, 151–52, 268; continuing care retirement communities and, 224; defined, 59; driving status and, 119–20; and family participation, 96–97; housing expectations and, 173–84; housing types and, 162; marriage and, 26–30; migration and, 213; multiple

roles and, 22–25, 48–66, 98–100;
neighboring and, 192–93, 200;
religious participation and, 96;
retirement and, 82–83, 89, 95–100;
social integration and, 3–4, 24–25, 48–
66, 291; social support and, 34, 36,
56–57; transportation and, 126–27;
volunteering and, 38, 261
hobbies, 90–91
home improvement, 172, 176
housing for older persons, 158–86, 211–
24; and health, 162; literature review
of, 160–63; and social networks, 162.
See also continuing care retirement
communities

income level: caregiver support and,
136; driving status and, 119–20;
housing expectations and, 172–83;
migration and, 161; neighboring and,
193, 199–200; in nonmetropolitan
areas, 7; social integration and, 293;
social network participation and, 34–
35; transportation and, 110
insurance for long-term-care, 172–73,
176, 185
intergenerational relationships, 30–32;
and baby-boomers, 31–32; and
divorce, 32; interventions to promote,
295; retirement and, 87–88, 90–91
interventions: agenda for, 294–97; for
caregivers of Alzheimer's patients,
266, 269–73; design of, 234–39, 269–
73; evaluation of, 239–43; for
intergenerational relationships, 295;
as a research method, 65; for
transportation of older persons, 231–
45; for volunteering, 249–50
isolation. *See* social integration

life-course theory: Alzheimer's
caregivers and, 139–43; and context,
78, 111–13, 160; and data collection,
60–65; defined, 6, 51–54; housing
decisions and, 159–60, 211–12; and
process, 76–77, 113–14; retirement
and, 75–80; and roles, 51–54; and

timing, 77–78, 110–11; transportation
transitions and, 109–14; volunteering
and, 255–56
life span trends, 28
literature reviews: on Alzheimer's
caregivers, 133–38, 267–68; on
caregivers, 133–38, 267–68; on
geographic proximity, 33–34; on
health, 59–60; on migration, 160–62,
211–14; on multiple roles, 24–25; on
neighboring, 191–98; on social
integration, 3, 8, 20–41; on social
networks, 34–37; on social support,
24, 58; on transportation of older
persons, 108–14, 232–33; on volunteerism among older persons, 38–39,
248–49, 255–61
living arrangements, 28–29, 30–31
loneliness: continuing care retirement
communities and, 216–17, 222–24;
and retirement, 91–92, 97
longevity: baby-boom generation and,
31–32; marriage and, 26–30; migration and, 213; religious participation
and, 96; retirement and, 89; roles and,
24–25; social support and, 24; volunteering and, 38; work and, 37. *See
also* health
Longitudinal Study on Aging, 161–62,
212–13

marriage: and African Americans, 28;
Alzheimer's caregivers and, 138; and
the baby boom generation, 4, 29–30,
31–32; continuing care retirement
communities and, 222–23; driving
status and, 119–20, 122–23; and
gender, 28, 87; and health, 26–30;
housing expectations and, 173–84;
neighboring and, 201–2; and retirement, 92–94; and social integration,
26–30; volunteering and, 256–57
men. *See* gender
mental health. *See* health
metropolitan areas, 33. *See also*
nonmetropolitan areas

migration: and educational attainment, 161; and health, 213; and income level, 161; of older persons to the Sunbelt, 33–34; theory, 160–62, 164–69, 211–14; of younger persons from the Midwest, 33. *See also* geographic proximity of children

minority groups, 294, 299-300

mobility. *See* transportation of older persons

moving. *See* migration

National Long-Term Care Survey, 33

National Survey of Families and Households, 33

neighboring: and age, 199–200; and the baby boom generation, 191–92; and caregivers, 204–5; and club membership, 200–201; continuing care retirement communities and, 220; and crime, 193, 198, 201–2; data, 198–99; and educational attainment, 199–200; and family, 194–96; and friendships, 202–3; and gender, 199–200, 203–4; and geographic proximity of children, 202; and health, 192–93, 200; housing expectations and, 173–82; and income level, 193, 199–200; literature review of, 191–98; and marriage, 201–2; and personality characteristics, 196–98, 204; and religious participation, 193, 200–201; retirement and, 92; social integration and, 190–207, 292; and social support, 201–4; transportation and, 118, 124–26; and volunteering, 193, 200–201; and work, 204–5

New Haven Established Population for Epidemiologic Studies of the Elderly, 163

nonmetropolitan areas: driving status and, 119–20; housing expectations and, 172–82; and income level, 7; migration of younger persons from, 33; social integration and, 291–92; transportation in, 112–13

older persons, defined, 6, 9

organizational participation. *See* club membership

Pathways to Life Quality project, 217–18

peer support, for Alzheimer's caregivers, 265–82

Peer Support Project, 144–52, 265–82

personality characteristics for neighboring, 196–98, 204

policy: and housing of older persons, 184–86; nonmetropolitan areas and, 7; for older Americans, 300–301; retirement and, 37; and structural lag, 22; and transportation of older persons, 244–45; and volunteerism among older persons, 39, 255–61

poverty. *See* income level

prospect theory, 164

psychological health. *See* health

Pursuit of Loneliness, The (Philip Slater), 20

religious participation: continuing care retirement communities and, 221, 224; and gender, 86; and health, 96; housing expectations and, 173–82; neighboring and, 193, 200–201; retirement and, 86, 92, 96, 98; transportation and, 116–17, 124–26

research agenda, 60–65, 152–53, 297–301

research methods: and intervention studies, 65; and life history data, 61; and longitudinal data, 61–63; and natural experiments, 64–65

retirement: and caregivers, 88, 97; and club membership, 86, 96, 98–100; and community involvement, 86, 90–91; and educational attainment, 90, 99; and family finances, 81; and family roles, 87–88, 90–91, 96; and gender, 87–88, 90–100; and health, 82–83, 89, 95–100; housing expectations and, 172–84; and intergenerational relationships, 87–88, 90–91; and life-course theory, 75–80; and marriage, 92–94; and migration, 160–62; and multiple roles, 98–100; and neighboring, 92; policy about, 37; and post-retirement work, 86–87, 92, 95, 98–100; and religious participation, 86, 92, 96, 98; and roles, 81–82, 88, 90–91, 98–100; and social integration, 4, 75–101; and stress, 82–83; theories of, 80–83; trends, 37–38, 248; and volunteering, 85–86, 96, 98–100, 248–49

reverse mortgage, 173

roles: continuing care retirement communities and, 215–16, 220–22; of family caregivers, 140–41, 146; and health, 22–25, 48–66, 98–100; and housing, 216; and life course theory, 52; literature review of, 24–25; retirement and, 81–82, 88, 90–91, 98–100; theory about, 50–54; transportation and, 123–26; work and, 37–38

similar others, 141–43, 268

social-ecological perspective, 213

social integration: of Alzheimer's caregivers, 5, 132–52; of the baby-boom generation, 4; and boredom, 92, 97; defined, 8–9; and gender, 291; and health, 3–4, 24–25, 48–66, 291; and housing, 224; housing expectations and, 173–83; and income level, 293; indicators of, 25–39; and living arrangements, 30–31; and loneliness, 92, 97; and marriage, 26–30; mechanisms of, 58–59; migration and, 214–17; and minorities, 294; negative outcomes of, 50–54, 60; neighboring and, 190–207, 292; and nonmetropolitan areas, 291–92; retirement and, 4, 75–101; and sociological theory, 19–25; summary of problems with, 3–5, 40–41; technology and, 288–90; theory, 19–25, 50–54; transportation of older persons and, 115–27, 292; and volunteering, 38–39, 292; and work, 4, 37–38

Social Integration of the Aged (Irving Rosow), 22–24

social networks: of Alzheimer's caregivers, 134–36; continuing care retirement communities and, 214–15, 218–20; geographic proximity of children and, 3; housing types and, 162; and income level, 34–35; literature review of, 34–37; model of, 55–57; transportation and, 110–14, 118

social security, 302

social support: of Alzheimer's caregivers, 136–38, 144–52; continuing care retirement communities and, 215–17, 220–22; and family, 35–36, 55–57; and friendships, 35–36, 55–57; and gender, 36; and health, 34, 36, 56–57; literature review of, 24; model of, 55–57; neighboring and, 201–4; social network participation and, 35; transportation and, 124–26

socioeconomic status. *See* income level

structural lag, 22, 289

suicide, 19–20

Suicide (Emile Durkheim), 19–20, 40

technology, 288–90

Tell Me a Riddle (Tillie Olsen), 2, 289

transportation of older persons, 108–28, 231–45; and caregivers, 124–26; cessation of driving, 110–11, 114, 126; and club membership, 124–26; and income level, 110, 119–20; interventions to improve, 231–45; and family, 111–12, 118, 124–26; and friendships, 111–12, 118, 124–26; and gender, 110–12, 116–18, 126–27; and health, 126–27; and life-course theory, 109–14; literature review of, 108–14, 232–33; modes, 115–18; and neighboring, 118, 124–26; in nonmetropolitan areas, 112–13; public, 118, 239–40; and religious participation, 116–17, 124–26; and roles, 123–26; and social integration, 115–27, 292; and social

transportation of older persons
(continued)
networks, 110–14, 118; and social
support, 124–26
trends: and the baby boom generation,
31–32; in geographic proximity of
children, 33–34; in living arrangements, 30–31; in marriage, 26–30,
31–32; in migration, 33–34, 160–62,
211–14; policy about, 244–45; in
retirement, 37–38, 248; in social
integration, 19–41, 288–90; in social
network participation, 34–37; in
volunteering, 38–39, 248–49; in work,
37–38

*Understanding Senior Housing for the
1990s* survey, 169
Unseemly Old Lady, The (Bertolt
Brecht), 1–2

volunteering: and the baby-boomer
generation, 248; case study, 247–62;
continuing care retirement communities and, 220–22, 224; corporate
model, 249–50; and family, 256; and
gender, 86, 258; and health, 38, 261;
housing expectations and, 173–82;
interventions to improve, 249–50; and
life-course considerations, 255–56;
literature review of, 38–39, 248–49,
255–61; and marriage, 256–57;
neighboring and, 193, 200–201; policy
about, 39, 255–61; recruitment and
retention strategies, 251–55; retirement and, 85–86, 96, 98–100, 248–49;
social integration and, 38–39, 292;
transportation and, 116–17, 124–26;
trends, 38–39, 248–49

widowhood: and African Americans, 28;
driving status and, 122; gender and,
26–28; housing expectations and, 176;
trends, 26–28
women. *See* gender
work: continuing care retirement
communities and, 220–22, 224; and
gender, 37, 53; housing expectations
and, 172–84; neighboring and, 204–5;
post-retirement, 86–87, 92, 95, 98–
100; and roles, 37–38; social integration and, 4, 37–38; theories of, 79–80;
transportation and, 116–17; trends,
37–38

Library of Congress Cataloging-in-Publication Data

Social integration in the second half of life / edited by Karl Pillemer . . . [et al.].
    p.   cm.
  Includes index.
  ISBN 0-8018-6453-4 (alk. paper) — ISBN 0-8018-6454-2 (pbk. : alk. paper)
  1. Aged—Social conditions. 2. Aged—Family relationships. 3. Aging—Social
aspects. I. Pillemer, Karl A.
HQ1061 .S64817 2000
305.26—dc21   00-042417